NO-NONSENSE
NUTRITION

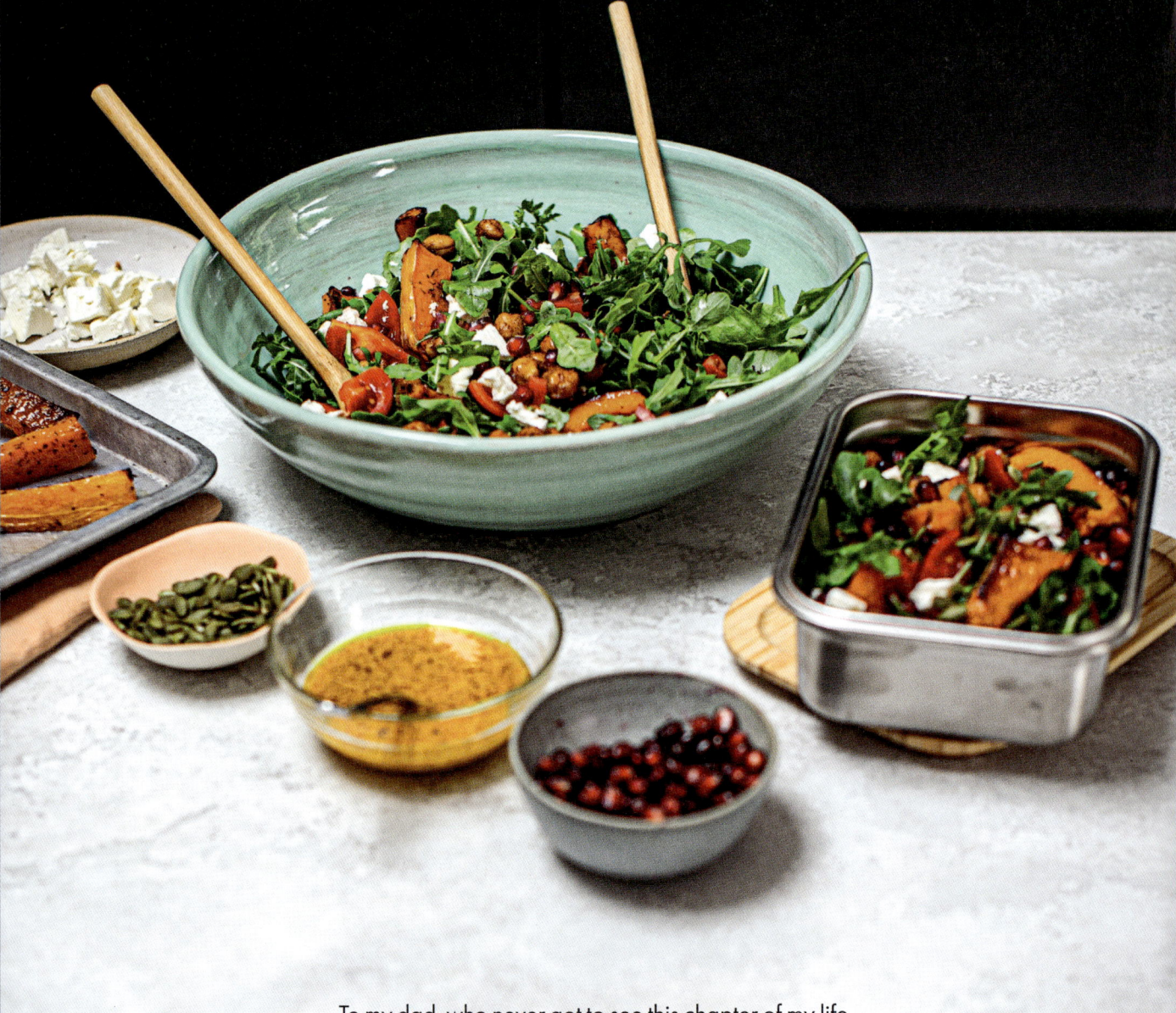

To my dad, who never got to see this chapter of my life.
I know you would have been so proud.

NO-NONSENSE
NUTRITION

The science-based plan to
transform health, lose weight, feel amazing

DOMINIQUE LUDWIG

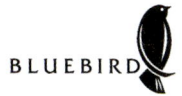

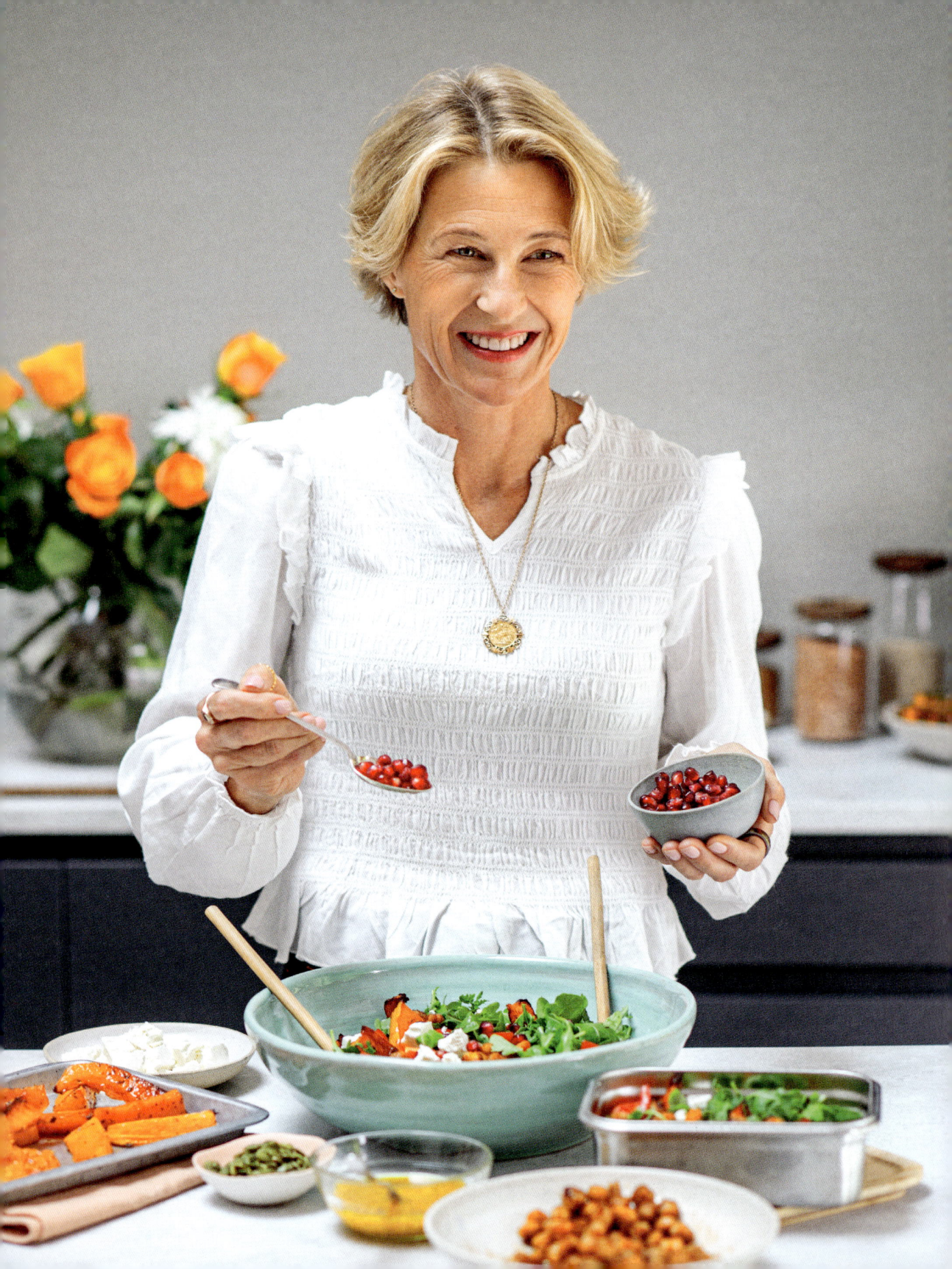

CONTENTS

INTRODUCTION 6

WHY GOOD NUTRITION MATTERS 10

THE SIX PRINCIPLES 26

NO-NONSENSE COOKING
& MEAL PLANNING 78

BREAKFAST 100
LUNCH 154
DINNER 200
BREADS & TREATS 248

NUTRITIONAL INFORMATION 296
HOW TO ADAPT PROTEIN GOALS FOR YOUR BODY 304
REFERENCES 305
INDEX 306
ACKNOWLEDGEMENTS 319

INTRODUCTION

What we eat is the single most powerful tool for taking control over our health and wellbeing. And the good news is that you can make changes immediately, starting with your next meal.

My name is Dominique Ludwig and I'm a nutritionist. For more than thirty years I have worked in the field of nutrition and for the last twenty years in private practice, helping thousands of people at my clinics and on my nutrition programmes achieve better health, with a food-first approach to healthcare.

I love diving into the science and enjoy sharing my knowledge. I distil complex nutritional science into bite-size pieces that are simple to understand and easy to action. Being a King's College London nutritionist as well as a registered nutritional therapist has given me the best of both worlds. I combine my extensive training with the conversations I have every day with people in my clinics, to create easy-to-follow advice and meal plans that will improve their health and wellbeing. I want to take you on a journey, in the same way I do with my clients in clinic, so that you too can feel better and more energised, achieve your health potential now and in the future, and say goodbye to food cravings.

Balanced nutrition is essential for good health. It underpins every single function your body performs every day. I've carefully developed the recipes in this book to optimise your energy, mood and hormones, and to support your cardiovascular system, gut health, weight, skin, sleep and so much more. Good nutrition can improve our health today and plays a vital role in shaping our future wellbeing too, helping to reduce inflammation and the risk of chronic disease.

My clinical work, together with listening to each of my clients' individual experiences, has shown me that while each of us is unique, many of us are facing similar health issues and challenges with our food, and our diet may hold many of the answers.

The most important thing I have learned is that even simple changes can have powerful effects on our health, our mood and our energy.

Perfectly balanced, delicious recipes using fresh ingredients mean you can jump straight into this book and start cooking, almost without thinking, and reap the benefits. My nutrition advice and recipes will help you:

- Increase your energy throughout the day, without the dreaded energy crashes mid-afternoon.
- Say goodbye to sugar cravings by eating food that leaves you feeling nourished and satisfied.
- Experience better digestion with less bloating.
- Feel in tune with your appetite and free up your mind from constant 'food noise'.
- Find weight management easier, in a way that is sustainable in the long-term.
- See improvements to mood, with more stable emotions.
- Enjoy a better night's sleep.
- Clear brain fog to concentrate and focus better.
- Improve your gut microbiome.
- See improvements to your skin.
- Help support natural hormone balance.

There are six easy principles that lie at the heart of my approach to healthy eating. Alongside these, I'll illuminate the science of healthy eating, dispel common myths, and explain why nutrition matters and what really works.

I use a balanced plate approach and my Triple 30 nutrition principles (which means eating around 30g of protein per meal, 30g of fibre per day and 30 or more different plants a week) to create recipes that you'll love and can effortlessly make an enjoyable part of your life. I'll explain why it is the combination of protein and fibre together at every meal that really matters – and how, with this combination, you'll see real benefits.

I'll also explain why it is so important to leave sufficient time between meals and overnight to allow our body to fully digest our food and support our gut health.

You will learn how protein and fibre both positively impact many hormones that influence our hunger and appetite, naturally. These hormones include glucagon-like peptide-1 (GLP-1), which increases our feelings of fullness and is the hormone behind the success of many weight-loss injections. Understanding how food can impact our hormones and affect our appetite and cravings can be revolutionary – even life-changing – for many people. By eating in the right way, we can naturally regulate our hunger and satiety hormones, including our GLP-1. This all helps to reduce cravings and stops the endless food chatter, or 'food noise', in our heads – that voice that affects our food decisions, influences negative thoughts around food and tempts us with 'Should I have this snack or can I wait?' or tries to reason with us: 'If I eat this biscuit, I'll eat less lunch.'

I want to normalise eating properly and reduce food-related stress. Many people feel trapped in a cycle of guilt, restriction and frustration around food, which can feel like a constant struggle. This mental tug-of-war can drain our energy and leave us feeling worse, both physically and emotionally. My approach to eating is one that people tell me feels intuitive and natural. It is a way of eating that allows you to enjoy food, and that aligns with your body's true needs.

With my deep knowledge of nutrition, love of good food and desire to transform the health of every client I see, I have brought together an effective method that sees visible and lasting health transformations.

I hope this book will allow you to achieve greater food confidence, with an abundance of choice, and put an end to deprivation and calorie counting, where food and your appetite no longer rule your life. Most importantly, I want you to be able to feel joy around eating, shopping and preparing food, so that you feel more energised and can live a healthier, happier and more fulfilled life.

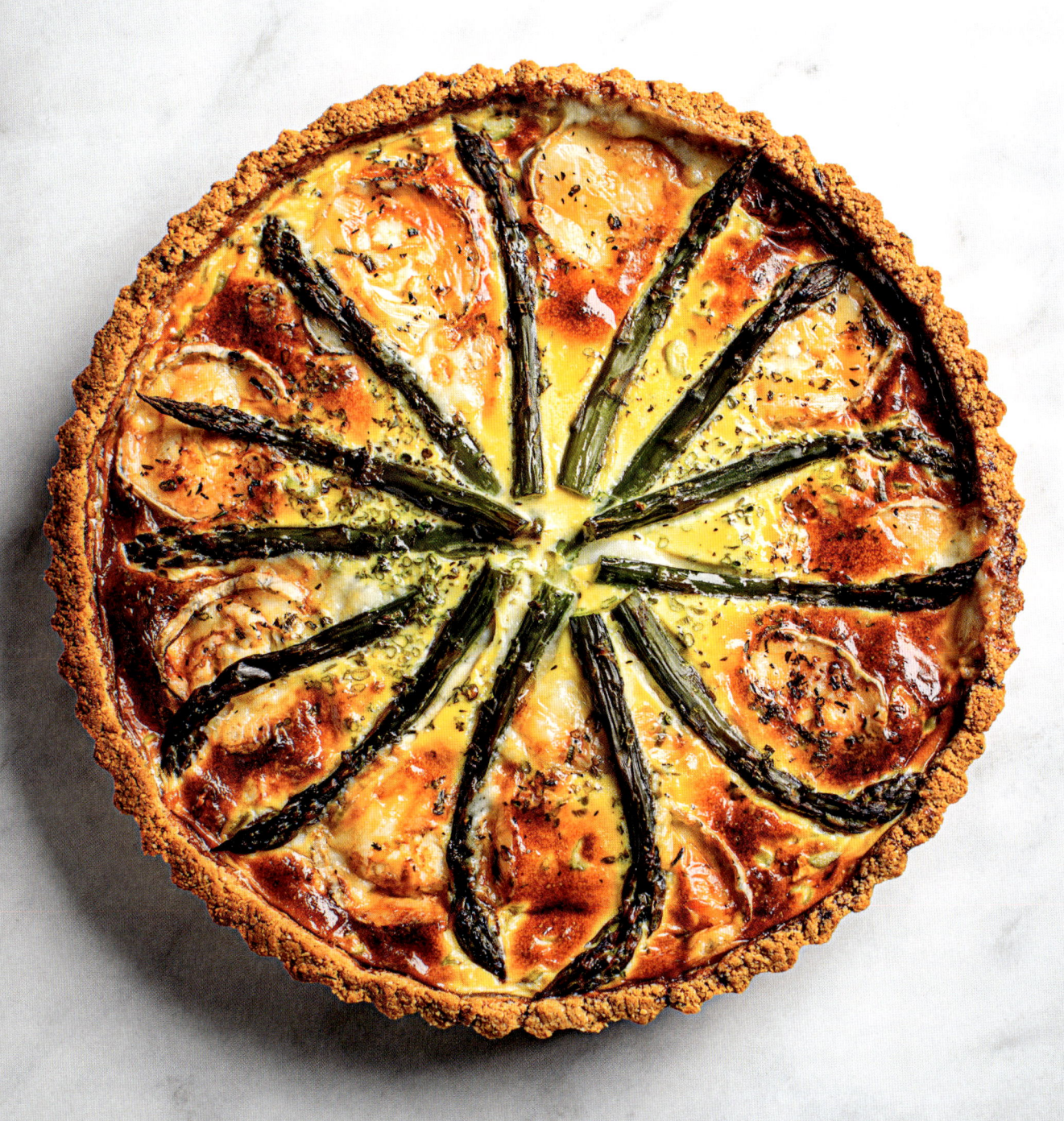

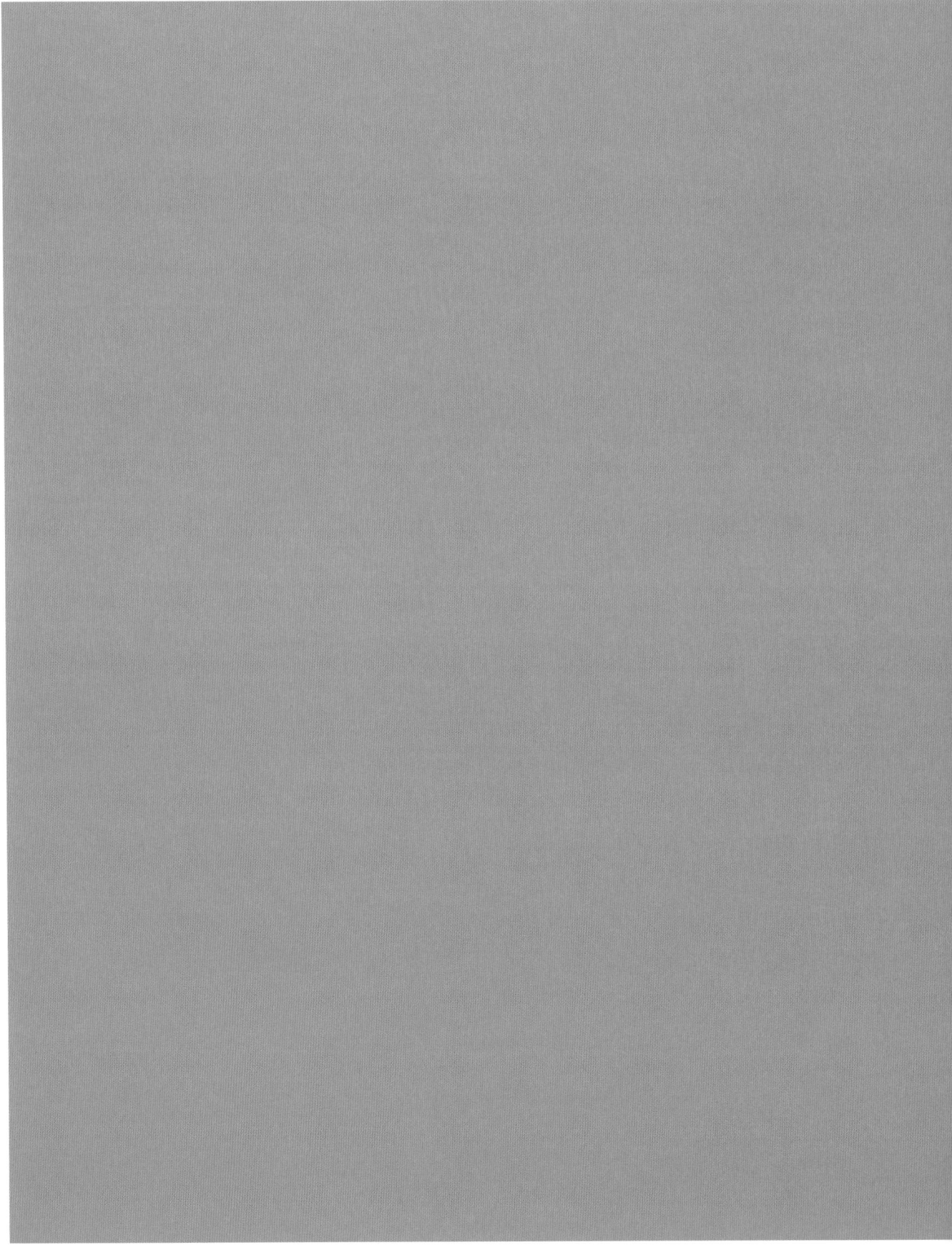

WHY GOOD NUTRITION MATTERS

Nutrition lies at the heart of good health. Our modern-day approach to food can often feel over-simplified, focusing mainly on its immediate effects, such as providing us with energy and satisfying our hunger, but the role of what we eat has a far bigger impact than that.

Food provides us with a huge variety of macronutrients and micronutrients, as well as fibre, that contribute to the way our body functions twenty-four hours a day. If these become out of balance, we might start to see unwelcome changes to our health, such as weight gain, tiredness, low mood, elevated cholesterol, poor digestion, constipation, brain fog, poor blood sugar control and even mental health struggles.

Working with thousands of clients during my twenty years of hands-on clinical practice has given me a wealth of real-world experience, a thorough understanding of the issues that really matter to people, and an insight into the health and nutrition challenges so many of us face.

By combining scientific research and practical application, and by adopting a 360-degree approach that considers our health from every angle, I have devised a nutritional philosophy that I have seen lead to clear results.

Getting our diet back on track means we can often see improved health markers across the board. We all need to eat, so this isn't about making any radical changes to your routine or how you live your life – just choosing what you eat more wisely. Simply making more informed food choices can unlock health benefits that go beyond fuelling our body with energy. When we don't eat the right foods, our body simply cannot function at its best – but when we do, something magical happens.

Meet the macros

Each of us is made up of thousands of different proteins, fats and some carbohydrates. These are our macronutrients. We need to eat foods to supply us with these vital macronutrients in order to maintain our health, supply energy, and also to repair and regenerate every part of our body. Proteins and fats are the building blocks of our body tissues, so eating foods that contain them in the right forms and amounts is paramount.

Meeting our macronutrient targets is usually relatively easy, as they are present in almost every food we eat in varying amounts. Amazingly, the human body also has a skill for biological alchemy and can not only store excess fats to use later, but can also convert excess carbohydrates and proteins into fat for storage. It can also store a small amount of carbohydrate in the form of glycogen in the liver and muscles for instant access. The body does not, however, have a secret compartment for storing proteins, so these need to arrive with our food daily.

Of course, stored excess fats are not always a good thing, and can easily lead to weight gain over time. Our modern lives mean that food is often readily available to us twenty-four hours a day, so we don't need to store fats to the same extent our hunter-gatherer ancestors did, in preparation for a hard winter.

Additionally, in different phases of our life our requirements for macronutrients will differ – for example, as we age, we may need more protein to maintain muscle strength and for bone health. So, we need to be mindful of eating the right amounts of proteins, fats and carbohydrates at the right time.

Say hello to the micros

It is not only the macronutrients, but the smaller micronutrients that our food contains that are essential to our health. Vitamins and minerals such as vitamin C, B12, iron, magnesium, zinc, selenium and calcium all act like individual keys that activate our metabolism and influence every single chemical reaction that takes place in our body, every second of every day. Although required in seemingly small amounts, their absence can lead to serious health issues.

Like a train arriving at the station, healthy food contains a number of carriages that can deliver all these micronutrients to your body, allowing them to get to work at a cellular level. Some minerals we need more of, such as magnesium, where we need around 300mg per day, and calcium, where we might need 700–1,200mg per day. Others are known as trace minerals, which we need only in tiny, but powerful amounts, often just a few milligrams or micrograms – such as iron, where women require around 14.8mg per day and men 8.7mg per day, or iodine, where both men and women require only around 140mcg daily. Depending on our lifestyle, our age and our individual circumstances, we may need slightly different amounts of these essential micronutrients.

Something many people overlook is that micronutrients often work in teams, helping us carry out specific functions. For example, glucose is a fuel source, but it can only be turned into a form of energy our body can use, adenosine triphosphate (ATP), in the presence of vitamins B1, B2, B3 and B5 and the minerals magnesium, iron and manganese. Another example is the thyroid gland, which is a small, butterfly-shaped organ in the front of our neck that produces the hormone thyroxine. Thyroxine plays a key role in regulating our metabolism and how our body uses energy. It can also influence our energy levels, body temperature, growth and development. To make thyroxine, our body needs to join the amino acid tyrosine with the mineral iodine, and it needs selenium, zinc, iron, vitamin A and vitamin D to ensure this entire process runs smoothly.

This means that there is so much more to eating food than simply consuming sufficient energy; we also need to prioritise micronutrients. If we want our body to work like a sophisticated machine, we need to ensure that every part of the machine has state-of-the-art components to help it run efficiently, optimally and smoothly.

Are food supplements the answer?

Food supplements definitely have their place in supporting our health or redressing imbalances, for example, iron supplementation for anaemia, vitamin B12 to prevent deficiencies in people following a plant-based diet, or vitamin D during winter. Supplements can also help support the body at specific times in our life, such as taking folate before pregnancy and during the first trimester. However, we really want to be looking to food for our 'nutritional supplements' rather than relying on a capsule offering a quick fix. When we eat our nutrients as food, the food often naturally contains a combination of nutrients that regularly buddy up and work together. Taking isolated nutrients can overlook how these essential substances function together in the body. (See also page 82 for a few other considerations if you are vegan or vegetarian.)

See results in as little as two weeks

Since food is so vital to every aspect of our health, getting our diet on track is the fastest way to see improvements to our overall wellbeing. Honestly! Your health can improve faster than you think simply by changing what you eat. Moving towards a diet that is rich in plants, proteins, healthy fats and whole-food carbohydrates, and shunning sugars, ultra-processed foods, refined cereal grains and fast foods, can be life-changing. By saying this, I am not advocating this book as a quick-fix diet plan that you follow for a few weeks, before slowly slipping back into more familiar habits. When we start to really focus on our diet and consume nutrient-dense foods in the way that nature intended, it's amazing how we can start to feel better in ourselves.

Common changes that I see in my clinics and across my programmes consistently – in what I like to call the 10-day/2-week phenomenon – are more energy, a reduction in cravings, less bloating, better sleep, weight loss, improved mood and reduced brain fog. But, almost more extraordinary, are those who report additional and somewhat unexpected life-altering benefits from changing their diet. People regularly report a reduction of pain in their muscles and joints, which they had simply put down to getting older, fewer headaches, improved skin conditions such as eczema, rosacea or psoriasis, better hormone balance, reduced perimenopausal symptoms such as hot flashes, and so much more. These transformations are the reason I love practising nutrition and also the reason I want to share this knowledge more widely. Sometimes we simply forget just how powerful our food can be.

Shut down the food noise and gain control of your appetite

One of the main positive results people tell me they experience after following my six principles (pages 28–77) for a while is the reduction or complete silencing of 'food noise'.

Food noise is the constant chitter-chatter between our brain and our stomach, which can feel like a never-ending stream of text messages in which we are constantly thinking about food. These messages can come from hunger, boredom, habit or simply the need to treat ourselves. This can make us become obsessed with our next snack and can lead us by the hand to the fridge, kitchen cupboard or nearest vending machine, looking for a quick fix.

Often, food noise in the afternoon or evening is simply a by-product of our food choices earlier in the day. Maybe we have eaten fewer calories than we need at our meals, or consumed our food in the wrong macronutrient proportions, with too many carbohydrates and sugars, and too little focus on protein, vegetables and healthy fats. These imbalances can heighten our craving for snacks and make it harder for us to make healthier food choices.

What actually helps shut down the food noise is eating more nutrient-rich foods at mealtimes, with more fibre and protein, and cutting back on nutrient-poor snacks in between. In reality, cutting back on calories with your lunch, or skipping meals altogether, might completely backfire on you if all you can think about in between meals is food!

According to the Zoe Predict 1 Study, around 25 per cent of our calories are thought to come from snacks. To put this into perspective, this could mean that as many as 500 kcals of our daily 2,000 kcals are coming from snack foods.

While snacking is not inherently bad for us, can be a way of getting in extra nutrients, and does not necessarily lead to weight gain, it is thought that most of our snacks (potentially up to 75 per cent in the UK) come from unhealthy sources, such as ultra-processed food and drinks. This means that a large part of our diet may actually be coming from poor-quality, high-energy foods that do little to nourish our body, and may in fact be causing us harm. Constant snacking or grazing can also lead to blood sugar highs and lows and sugar cravings, may accelerate our appetite, can interfere with the natural rhythms of digestion, and can often leave us feeling worse, rather than better.

Eating meals with sufficient protein, fibre and healthy fats, however, shuts down this food noise, by keeping us feeling full and positively regulating our hunger and satiety hormones. We genuinely feel more in tune with our appetite, feel nourished, rather than deprived; energised rather than tired.

One of the most important hormones associated with appetite is ghrelin, which is released as our stomach empties and tells our brain that we are hungry. Eating protein and fibre-rich foods that stay in the stomach for longer leads to a delayed release of ghrelin. Another hormone, GLP-1 (glucagon-like peptide-1), is released when we consume sufficient protein and fibre at meals. GLP-1 plays a crucial role in slowing down the rate of gastric emptying and promoting a feeling of satiety. Peptide YY (PYY) is a third hormone, released in the gut in response to proteins, fats and fibre in the diet. This hormone, like GLP-1, helps to reduce appetite and promote fullness, both of which are important for weight regulation. Therefore, by eating the right combinations of food — a balanced plate — we can stimulate the right hormones in a much more natural way.

My experience has shown me time and again that eating well can build a healthier relationship around food, with less anxiety and more food confidence. Around 80 per cent of people on my nutrition programmes report fewer sugar cravings when eating this way.

THE MYTH OF CALORIES IN, CALORIES OUT

We know that eating more calories than we burn can lead to weight gain, and we are all familiar with the simple calculation 'calories in vs. calories out'. But it's really not as simple as this. Our calorie requirements depend on many factors, such as body size, age, activity level, daily energy expenditure and our own metabolism. There is no one size fits all, and our requirements will vary day by day.

Restricting calories can leave us feeling hungry and deprived, and often reaching for a snack between meals. Counting calories also looks at food simply as a number. It doesn't consider its nutritional value, how our body absorbs and utilises the food, and its impact on our blood sugars, appetite and mood. Calories are not created equally: a chocolate bar and a whole avocado each contain around 250 kcals, but how they are digested, the way our body uses the energy, their nutrient composition and how they can affect our appetite later in the day differs dramatically. One will raise our blood sugar levels almost immediately, initiating the blood sugar rollercoaster (page 18), while the other provides a steady stream of energy – as well as a whole host of beneficial nutrients. We absolutely need to consider the nutrients a food contains rather than focusing on just the calories.

Additionally, some foods are easier to break down and absorb, such as high sugar, refined or ultra-processed foods. But when we eat whole foods they take a bit more effort. We use additional energy to process our food through chewing, digesting and metabolising – meaning that some of the calories in our food will actually be used up during this process. In fact, proteins deliver only around 70–80 per cent of their full calories as energy and carbohydrates 90–95 per cent.

Although calories can be a useful guide to how much energy we are consuming, it's far more effective from a long-term sustainable weight-management perspective to focus on how different foods influence our health and appetite. Eating healthy proteins, fibre, beneficial fats, vegetables and fruits as well as wholegrains in the right proportion will create meals that work with our body rather than against it.

Will I lose weight?

This book and my six principles have not been created as a dedicated diet programme. However, since most people describe feeling completely satisfied after meals and less likely to reach for snacks, many people have found that they lose weight in an easier and more sustainable way than before – simply as a welcome side-effect of eating well, and often without even trying.

Choosing a typical breakfast, lunch and dinner from this book would deliver around 1650 kcals per day, which would be an average deficit of around 350 kcals for women, and more for men. This means that if no other foods were consumed, it would be reasonable to expect to see weight loss each week. Those without a weight loss goal are likely to eat slightly more foods, through larger portions or extra sides, and consume additional foods, such as milky drinks, planned snacks (see page 76), extra fruit or a treat after meals to counteract the deficit.

My main focus, though, is sharing with you a toolkit of my principles for better health through balanced nutrition. I want to steer you gently away from calorie counting, and other forms of control over food, towards a more liberating and positive approach to eating. Eating well is like having the magic key to your metabolism, and once you have learned the principles, you can keep them for life.

If weight loss is your goal, though, it's completely possible when following the principles I outline (in the next chapter) and using the recipes in this book.

To give you the best chance on your weight-loss journey, here are my top tips for success.

- Stick to three meals a day and avoid snacking between meals – but make sure to drink plenty of water and herbal teas to stay hydrated. You can also drink green tea, black tea and black coffee, but avoid milky drinks, such as lattes, between meals.

- Fast for 12–14 hours overnight. This might mean finishing your last meal by 7pm and waiting until 7–9am for breakfast. But, again, remember to stay hydrated. Drink water and herbal teas as needed, but if you can, save your milky tea and coffee until after breakfast.

- Don't skip meals! Regular eating helps maintain stable energy levels and metabolism.

- Follow the healthy plate rules in the principles on page 30.

- Prioritise natural, unprocessed foods in your diet and cook from scratch whenever possible.

- Eliminate ultra-processed foods and sugary foods and drinks.

- Slightly reduce portion sizes for weight loss, then adjust as needed once you reach your goal.

- Try eating your wholegrain carbs at just one main meal a day, focusing on proteins and plenty of vegetables at your other main meal.

- Limit alcohol intake as much as possible.

- Stay active! Find an exercise you enjoy, whether it's brisk walking, cycling, swimming or my favourite, mini-trampolining! Exercise should be something fun!

Blood sugars explained

One of the reasons many of us reach for a biscuit mid-afternoon is because we are not eating to support balanced blood sugar levels. Eating balanced, nutritious meals means we should experience less of the dreaded energy crashes, so we won't feel the need to constantly top up our blood sugar levels between meals.

Our blood sugars are designed to gently rise and fall throughout the day as a reflection of our last meal and the types of foods we have eaten. Small fluctuations in our blood sugars are simply the way we, as human beings, process our carbohydrates. Think of your blood sugars gently rising and falling during the day like a wavy line. This undulating curve means our digestion is breaking down the food slowly and keeping our glucose levels steady. When they start to gently dip, the body taps into our natural energy reserves (such as its first-choice, glycogen, or its second-choice, body fat) to keep our energy stable. It can generally do this quietly and without raising our attention or our appetite.

Problems arise when instead of the gentle wavy line, our blood sugars jump on a big-dipper ride, and rather than a gently undulating blood sugar curve, we get taken from high to low blood sugars and then back up high again, in a similar way to a rollercoaster at a theme park. Once we are on the rollercoaster, it becomes hard to get off, as we can get stuck in a vicious cycle of lower energy and sugar cravings. These cravings are a form of 'false' rather than 'true' hunger, as we are craving food to prop up our blood sugars that we may not otherwise have needed. This makes us want to eat more of the high-sugar or quick-fix foods that raised our blood sugar in the first place, and the cycle continues. The trouble with the rollercoaster is that it can take our mood and energy on the ride too, making us more prone to energy crashes and mood swings, and can sometimes cause headaches, as well as influencing inflammation levels in the body. What's worse is that this cycle can be repeated multiple times a day, which can lead to us eating more food than we need, making it harder for us to manage our weight.

So, what foods cause those highs on the rollercoaster? During digestion, carbohydrates are broken down in the gut into their smallest unit, glucose. How quickly this happens is normally determined by how much the carbohydrate has deviated from its natural form – or how sweet the food is. Natural carbohydrates in their whole-food form (such as pearl barley, bulgur wheat, steel-cut oats or quinoa) are all intact or cracked grains. This means they contain more complex chains of glucose and they also retain a lot of fibre, which naturally puts the brakes on our digestion, slowing down the rate at which carbohydrates can be broken down into glucose and therefore how quickly it can enter our bloodstream. When combined with proteins and fats, this process can be even slower.

On the other hand, milling grains into flour breaks down the carbohydrate into tiny pieces, and polishing the grains to make them 'white' removes the fibre and the germ inside, making them even quicker and easier to digest, fast-tracking them into the bloodstream. Sugars, such as white or brown sugar (as well as honey, coconut sugar or maple syrup), are mostly just two sugar molecules stuck together, called disaccharides; alongside glucose, these are fastest to digest. Enzymes – which are like biological scissors – are present in our saliva and get to work from the moment we start to chew our food, unclamping the sugars and carbohydrates into single glucose units. So, with these types of food, much of the hard work has already been done by the time they reach our gut, and the glucose molecules are able to pass into our bloodstream almost immediately. We call these fast-acting carbohydrates, and they come in the form of white bread and other items made from white flour or refined grains, as well as quick-cook oats, fruit juices, soft drinks, crisps, ultra-processed foods and sugary foods, such as confectionery, breakfast cereals and desserts.

Enter insulin. While glucose has an easy job getting into the bloodstream, it can find it harder to exit. Insulin is a hormone released by the pancreas in response to meals containing carbohydrates. It acts like a taxi, scooping up the glucose and taking it to its destination, usually our muscles, cells and brain, where it can be used for energy. Without insulin we could not survive, and its job is to lower circulating blood glucose levels to normal levels again. If we have an excess of glucose in our blood – more than our body requires – these taxis take a diversion and head for the liver, where the excess glucose tops up our glycogen, or it gets stored as body fat. This is a normal process that occurs in everyone and helps us regulate our energy levels evenly throughout the day. However, if we are continually eating more food than we need, excess fat can start to accumulate in our body, particularly in the abdomen and around internal organs, creating what is known as visceral or belly fat. Visceral fat not only leads to weight gain, but also increases the risk of chronic inflammation, cardiovascular disease and Type 2 diabetes. We may think we do not 'feel' when our blood sugars are unbalanced, but in reality, we only start to feel the effects when our blood sugars start to drop rapidly.

The effects can be disguised as:
- Increased appetite
- Poor focus and concentration
- Anxiety and poor mood
- Increased cravings for coffee, sugar and snacks
- Tiredness
- Headaches
- Rapid heartbeat
- Dizziness

In truth, we all process our carbohydrates slightly differently, with some people being more sensitive to the rollercoaster than others. Certain conditions may also affect our ability to process glucose efficiently, such as insulin resistance, obesity and Type 2 diabetes. This can mean that we are less sensitive to the effects of insulin, which allows our blood sugars to stay elevated for longer and can put us at higher risk of longer-term health conditions.

What all this means is that while carbohydrates are an important source of nutrients and fibre, carbohydrates are not created equal. Some are much better for us than others. It also means the amount of carbohydrates we consume at a meal is important, as well as the other foods we consume at the same meal, such as proteins, fats and fibre, which slow down the absorption of glucose into our bloodstream, helping us feel more stable and satisfied between meals. (We'll read more about carbohydrates on page 37.)

Our incredible microbiome

This is still a big buzzword and with good reason. A healthy, well-functioning digestive system is crucial to help us absorb the nutrients we need from our food, but the microbes in our gut can also affect so many other areas of our health and metabolism. As well as helping us digest our food, they produce substances that can reduce inflammation and keep the gut wall healthy, and they can even influence our mood and our hormones, including oestrogen levels.

The microbiome is an incredible ecosystem that resides in our digestive tract. Essentially, the gut is a 7–9m-long tube with different areas performing different functions, but what we are really interested in is our gut microbiome and the organisms it contains. Our gut microbiome is home to trillions of bacteria, as well as viruses, fungi and archaea (another type of single-celled microorganism). We know more about the bacteria than we do about the other residents in our gut, but science is continually enlightening us on the extraordinary relationship that we have with these microscopic organisms.

The small intestine is the upper digestive tract, a convoluted tube, lined with villi, which are small finger-like projections, giving it the appearance of velvet. The villi significantly increase the surface area of the gut, which dramatically increases its ability to absorb more of the nutrients from our food. It is a members-only area of the gut, where only bacteria with the right wristband are welcome. The bacteria in this area of our gut help to educate and regulate our immune cells and are involved in the digestion and absorption of food. After our food has gone through the small intestine and most of the nutrients have been absorbed, the remainder moves to the large intestine for further processing.

Many people assume that bacteria line the entire gut equally, but the majority actually reside in the large intestine, which runs up the right side of our abdomen, crosses the body just under our lower ribcage and then travels down the left side of our abdomen before it exits the body. I like to call the bacteria that live here the 'chompers'. These bacteria are incredibly helpful, fermenting and breaking down the fibre and other plant compounds in our food to make materials that support our gut health, aid repair and regeneration of the gut wall, and lower inflammation in the body. In a healthy gut this process should happen with minimal fuss and gas – however, if our gut is not moving food through at the correct speed or our bacteria are out of balance, we can experience unwanted gas and bloating.

Balance is everything in the gut. Each type of bacteria has a specific function and it's essential that all these roles are filled. In a similar way to a large corporation needing the right number of employees for each department, without too many in one area or too many vacancies in another, our gut depends on us having a balanced mix of bacteria, each performing its own unique task, working together in harmony.

When the microbiome is imbalanced, this is referred to as dysbiosis, indicating that the bacterial composition has shifted away from its optimal state. This generally refers to a gut that has too many or too little bacteria, or a lack of diversity, but can occasionally refer to a gut that has picked up an unwanted guest or even the odd 'hitchhiker' or parasite.

Poor diets, highly processed foods, a lack of fibre, food poisoning, antibiotics and 'hitchhikers' are all factors that can upset the balance in our gut, leading to symptoms such as bloating, discomfort, constipation or loose stools. In response, we may unintentionally restrict our diet in an effort to regain control. But often eating more fibre is the long-term solution rather than the problem, since the bacteria in the large intestine thrive on fibre as their primary food source.

The truth is that our 'good' bacteria generally tend to like healthier foods, so eating in a way that suits our biology and moving away from high-sugar, high-carb, ultra-processed foods and on to a more natural diet is almost always beneficial for our gut health. Over time, eating this way can start to redress the balance in our gut, optimising bacterial numbers and overall diversity and creating an ecosystem that has wider health benefits for our body and wellbeing.

Fermented foods

I like to use fermented foods in many of my recipes as a side dish. Fermented foods are 'live' foods, meaning they contain living organisms that can support our own gut health. We call these beneficial live organisms probiotics, and refer to the foods as probiotic foods. These living organisms mostly comprise beneficial bacteria, such as strains of Lactobacillus and Bifidobacterium, but also some beneficial yeasts. Some of these might take up home in our gut, but many just have a positive effect on our health as they pass through. Common fermented foods include live yoghurt and kefir, fermented vegetables such as sauerkraut and kimchi, miso, and drinks such as kombucha.

Can food affect inflammation?

Yes! Inflammation is a natural mechanism used by our immune system to help protect us from harm and also to initiate healing and repair. It is essential to our survival, but its role should be brief and quickly resolved. Problems arise when our mechanisms for damping down inflammation become impaired, or where our modern lifestyle and diet act as a trigger.

Low-grade, chronic inflammation is now recognised as a key driver behind many modern diseases, including Type 2 diabetes, cardiovascular disease, Alzheimer's and even some cancers. Sometimes chronic inflammation can be silent, other times it can impact our everyday lives, presenting as joint or muscle pain. Lifestyle factors such as our diet, obesity, poor gut health, a sedentary lifestyle, prolonged stress, poor glucose control and lack of sleep are known contributors to chronic inflammation.

Eating foods that are rich in compounds that help to neutralise inflammation, such as fresh vegetables, berries, fatty fish, chia seeds, flaxseeds, fermented foods, spices (including turmeric), extra virgin olive oil, legumes and even dark chocolate, alongside prioritising consuming sufficient fibre to support the gut microbiome can play a powerful role in reducing inflammation.

Ultra-processed foods

Ultra-processed foods (UPFs) are just that: foods that have undergone extensive processing, often using complex industrial methods, and containing additives and ingredients that we are not familiar with using in our own kitchens. Foods that are processed the most tend to have the poorest nutritional quality, but ultra-processed foods have infiltrated every corner of our lives. The trouble with ultra-processed foods is that they are affordable, convenient, profitable and addictive. They include breakfast cereals, many breads, biscuits, cakes, snacks, ready meals, processed meats, ice cream, fruit squashes and soft drinks, and many children's and baby foods.

Although only consumed in small amounts, we are now seeing emerging research questioning how some of the additives used in UPFs, such as emulsifiers, preservatives, colourings, flavourings, sweeteners, stabilisers and thickeners, may affect both the gut microbiome and the protective mucus layer lining the intestinal wall, with certain emulsifiers being associated with inflammation. The job of an emulsifier is to join two substances that naturally repel each other, such as oil and vinegar. In cooking, we might use egg yolk to bind these into mayonnaise. The difference is that the egg yolk is broken down as food in the gut, whereas some artificial emulsifiers may not be broken down sufficiently as they pass through.

The additives in ultra-processed foods are only part of the problem though; the core of the problem is that UPFs are made from poor-quality ingredients that are unable to nourish our body in the same way as natural foods. While UPFs are high in sugars, salt, starches, processed fats and additives which we know are bad for our health, it is their lack of key nutrients, protein and fibre that compounds their negative effects. UPFs also trigger receptors that activate and even overstimulate the brain's reward centres, leading to intense cravings for more and more of these unhealthy foods to chase those rewards – in some instances even resulting in addictive food behaviour. Not only do some of these foods have an addictive nature, but if they upset blood sugar control as well, we will often seek out more of these quick-fix foods to raise our blood sugars again.

Ultra-processed foods have been linked to poor health outcomes across the board, causing concern to doctors, nutritionists, dietitians and other healthcare professionals. Not only are they easy to consume, which can lead to an over-consumption of calories and raise obesity, they have also been linked to higher rates of chronic disease such as heart disease, Type 2 diabetes and dementia.

Shockingly, it is estimated that almost 57 per cent of adult UK energy intake comes from ultra-processed foods, and this figure rises to 64 per cent in children and up to 68 per cent in adolescents. From breakfast cereals, a biscuit mid-morning and a shop-bought sandwich and flavoured yoghurt for lunch, it's easy to see how these foods can quickly add up.

There is a sliding scale for ultra-processed foods though, with some UPFs containing more ultra-processed ingredients than others. This means that while UPFs are mostly not good news for our health, some are potentially more harmful than others, depending on their degree of processing or the amount of ultra-processed ingredients they contain.

We are designed to eat foods in their natural state, or as near to nature as possible. When we eat this way, the body recognises the natural components found in these foods, such as the proteins and fats, as well as the natural vitamins, minerals and trace elements they contain, and ensures that they are absorbed efficiently in the gut and transported to where they are needed in the body.

Are all processed foods bad for us?

No. Processed foods are not the same as ultra-processed foods. Processed foods are those that have undergone a minimal amount of processing, such as milk, cheese or tinned beans. This processing may increase their shelf life, and these foods are mostly not 'bad' for us. Drying, fermenting, freezing and canning are all examples of food processing, but unlike UPFs, this does not change the nutritional content of the food significantly or change the way our body processes them.

UPFs, on the other hand, are often made from finely milled cereals and additives which speed up the way we process them, fast-tracking them through the gut and affecting our blood sugar levels and appetite. Freezing peas still leaves them exactly as peas, but a cheesy puffed crisp is nothing like a corn kernel.

In fact, some food processing can be good for us by making foods available all year round, for example frozen vegetables or berries, or they can increase our ease of use, for example tinned beans. Some methods, such as fermentation, may actually even improve the nutritional properties of certain foods, such as yoghurt, kefir, sauerkraut or kimchi, which contain beneficial, gut-friendly microbes (see page 54).

Typically, the hallmarks of an ultra-processed food are long lists of ingredients, many of which you are unfamiliar with, colourful packaging and often spurious healthy claims. 'Low sugar' does not necessarily mean 'healthy' if the sugar has been replaced with artificial sweeteners. 'Low-fat' foods, where the fat has been replaced by thickeners, stabilisers and emulsifiers, also find themselves crossing the boundary into the category of ultra-processed foods.

Reading the labels is crucial. We don't need to avoid every ultra-processed food all the time, and the odd UPF is unlikely to cause harm. But it is important to be curious about what is in our food and how regular consumption of UPFs might be impacting our health.

It's about being consistent, not militant

This is a mantra that I use a lot in my clinic. When it comes to making any changes to your diet, such as decreasing your consumption of UPFs, increasing the amount of fibre you eat or reducing refined carbs, so often people set the nutrition bar too high. It can put them off from the get-go, as they never feel they are doing enough.

It is the small, consistent changes we make to our diet that become a habit, fifty-two weeks of the year, that are likely to have the most powerful effect on our health, rather than a quick two-week health kick at the start of January.

These habits should be easy and should feel intuitive. It might be that we focus on eating plenty of vegetables, cooking from scratch or moving our body. It is the habits that we implement most days that can start to have a significant effect on our health both now and in the future. And, as we get used to the changes, it can become easier to layer a new healthy habit on top, such as drinking more water, meal prepping on a Sunday or cutting back on sugar.

Eating well shouldn't be overwhelming, rather it should be self-perpetuating, where we notice improvements to our health which gently encourage us to make better choices, simply because it makes us feel better.

No one is expecting us to get it right all the time; it is enough to get most of it right most of the time. This might mean eating well 80 per cent of the time while allowing some flexibility for the remaining 20 per cent when eating out, at celebrations or special occasions.

While we know that some foods are better than others, we also don't need to demonise foods, as this can lead to feelings of deprivation and unhealthy relationships with food. In clinic, I tell my clients that if it's someone's birthday and they are offered cake, they shouldn't feel bad, rather they should enjoy every mouthful – but I might add, 'Maybe just don't do it every day!'

The uncomfortable truth

Without wanting to sound dramatic, I have not yet seen a magic pill or injection that can do all the hard work for us, long-term. What we eat matters because it is something we do multiple times a day. Every day we can start with a clean slate where we can make choices about the foods we put into our body. Alongside breathing in air, sleep and movement, food is the very life-force of health.

It's simple: the fastest way to improve our health involves shunning excess sugars and ultra-processed foods, and focusing on the foods that we know will fuel us, nourish us, facilitate every chemical reaction that takes place in every single cell of our body, and support the health of those incredible organisms that choose to call our gut their home.

However much the people around us love us, they can't do this for us. It has to come from our desire to want to make the changes ourselves, when we feel ready.

THE NO-NONSENSE PROMISE

My promise to you is this: there are no magic wands, but my experience has shown me that food has so much more power over our health than we think. By making some of my recipes, consistently, you will find that your energy improves, your sugar cravings decrease and your digestion calms. You will likely find yourself thinking less about food and feeling excited about cooking and mealtimes.

You will notice your tastes change, and that you find yourself wanting less sweet food, and that you start to notice the subtle flavours in your food again. Firm favourites in your old diet may start to lose their appeal and you might surprise yourself with the foods you long for.

This book is not asking you to eliminate food groups, but rather it is about bringing in more diversity by adding vibrantly coloured vegetables, legumes, nuts, seeds, fruits, fermented foods and oily fish to your plate.

Each of you will be coming to this book with a different base-line diet, different health concerns, different genetics and, of course, different microbiomes. While everyone is different and some people do require more specialised support than others, what I see in my clinic is that the vast majority of people I work with, or who join my programmes, see improvements across a wide range of symptoms from doing exactly the same thing . . . improving their diet.

Nutrition can't solve every issue, but food is so much more than just energy. It is nutrients, it affects our mood, our sleep, our digestion, inflammation, our stress levels, our cardiovascular health and countless other functions in our body, which in turn are all important in having a healthier, happier life. Changing how you eat, one meal at a time, is easy with my six principles . . .

THE SIX PRINCIPLES

The most powerful health advice I can give you is: go back to basics. This is the simplest but most effective strategy I have used in my clinics for the past twenty years. When we reconnect with how our body is actually designed to eat, everything else starts to fall into place. Getting back to basics means focusing on eating natural foods that resemble their original form in nature as closely as possible, or that are minimally processed – essentially, they are foods you can grow, pick or catch.

It doesn't have to be complicated, but preparing home-cooked meals lies at the heart of eating well. Opting for fresh ingredients like tomatoes instead of ready-made pasta sauces, or choosing rolled oats and seeds over sugary breakfast cereals, can have an immediate and significant impact on our health. Simplicity is the key here; this isn't about creating elaborate recipes. It can be as quick as assembling healthy ingredients on a plate – and you'll find plenty of easy assembly ideas in the recipe chapters later on. To make things even easier for our busy modern lives, we can incorporate some minimally processed foods, such as grabbing a tin of cooked beans, a tub of fermented yoghurt or a piece of filleted fish. These are all still great options and tick the boxes for a healthy diet.

If it still feels overwhelming at first, start with just one meal a day and build from there. (But if you're going to change just one meal, make it breakfast! A nutritious breakfast lays the foundations for better food choices throughout the day.)

Going back to basics means prioritising natural, higher-quality ingredients for your home-cooked meals – but it's not only about the ingredients we eat; it's also about how we combine them at mealtimes and throughout the day to give our bodies exactly what they need to function at their best. And that's where my six principles come in . . .

In this chapter, I'll show you how to put together a plate of food, combining proteins, fibre and fats in just the right proportions to optimise their benefits and your health. I'll explain how to eat to support your gut microbiome, and how the timing of your meals can have incredible benefits, too.

PRINCIPLE 1: IT'S ALL ABOUT PROPORTION

When you're deciding what to cook for your evening meal, I know how easy it is to think 'let's have pasta tonight' or 'something with a jacket potato' or 'noodles'. But when we approach meal planning like this, it's easy to overlook all the necessary components and forget about balance. Focusing too heavily on the carbohydrate element first often leaves little room for vegetables and healthy fats, and the protein portion can end up being too small. After eating, you're likely to feel unsatisfied and hungry again within a couple of hours. You'll be aware of that constant 'food noise' going on in the background – and you can't override those cravings, they're too powerful. That's why many of us end up reaching for a chocolate biscuit or another quick high-energy snack to fill the gap, usually leaving us feeling worse, emotionally as well as physically.

But when we eat food in the right proportions, that's when we start to see something extraordinary happen! By maintaining the right balance of proteins, fibre and fats from breakfast to dinner, we can increase our satiety and decrease hunger hormones. We feel fuller for longer, and are more energised and more in tune with our bodies. Amazingly, it can also completely switch off the 'food noise', so you no longer have to deal with those annoying food cravings – because your body isn't craving anything, it has everything it needs. As a hidden benefit, eating a balanced plate of food means we're also more likely to be getting all the micronutrients we need for our body to operate at its best.

Why have our meals become so unbalanced?

Modern Western diets – or the Standard American Diet (SAD) – have moved away from primarily home-cooked meals toward convenience-driven eating, leading to increased consumption of sugar, refined carbohydrates and unhealthy fats, while reducing fibre, vegetables and whole foods. The dominance of supermarkets for our grocery shopping and the rise of ultra-processed foods have further changed the way we cook and eat. There is an incredible availability of convenience foods today, of which the majority is often refined carbohydrate based. Even if we are cooking our meals from scratch, we are likely to include too much carbohydrate in proportion to the other food groups.

Modern eating habits also place a huge emphasis on snacking, and this can easily throw us off track. Done right, snacking can be a great way of getting in extra nutrients, but more likely than not we will be grazing on poor-quality energy boosters rather than well-planned, balanced options.

So, what is the right balance?

We often see recipes boast that they are 'high protein' or 'high fibre', but the real power comes from combining protein with fibre. It's this synergy that has the greatest impact, because

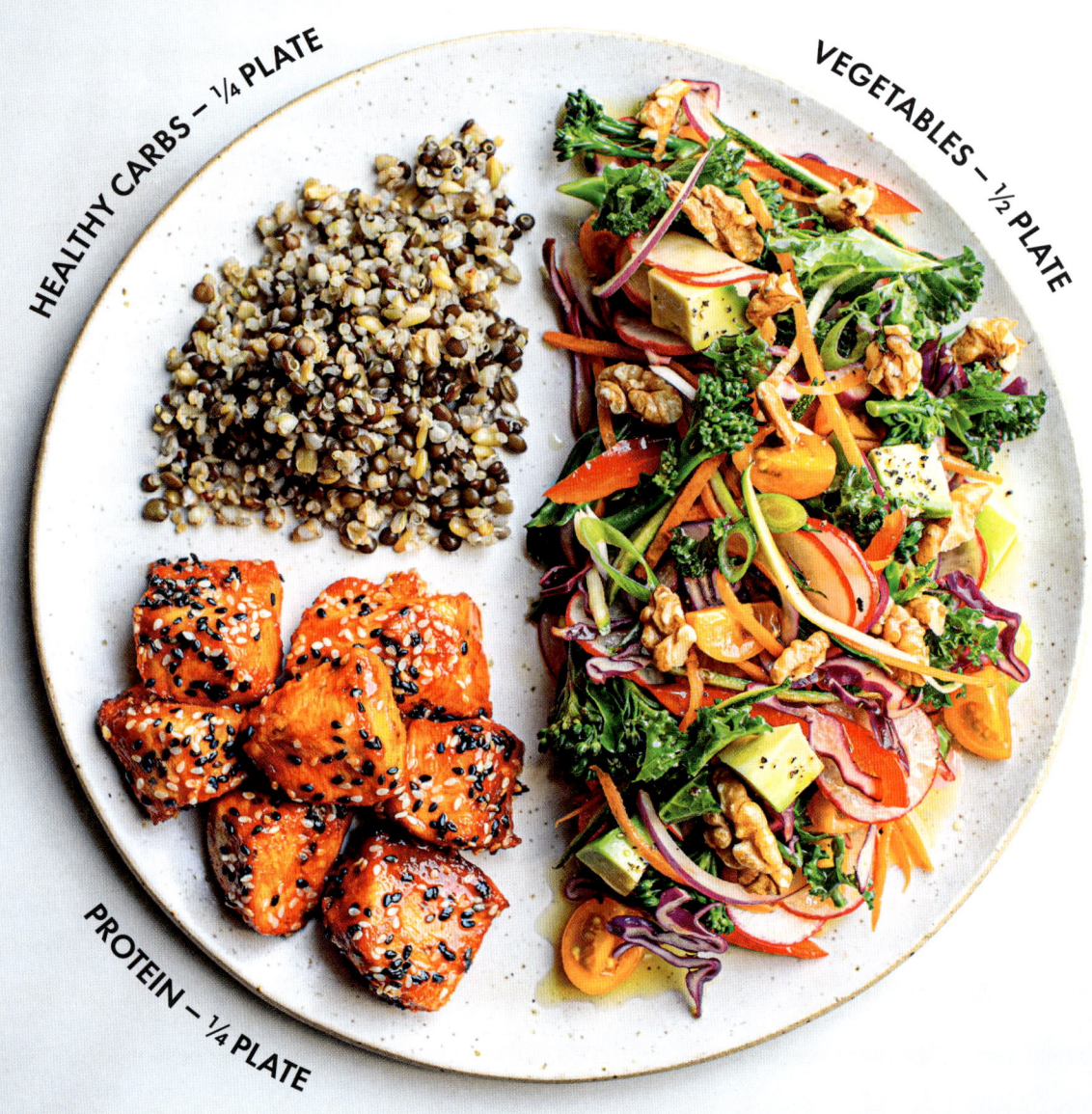

Plus added HEALTHY FATS
eg. Seeds, avocado, walnuts or olive oil dressing

both protein and fibre play a vital role in supporting our health, regulating our appetite and reducing cravings.

To keep things simple, I follow a system I like to call my Triple 30 approach. This method lies at the heart of how I create all my meals and recipes to help people reap the benefits of adequate protein, fibre and plant diversity, so they can feel their best every day. All my balanced plate recipes have been designed to include ¼ plate protein, ½ plate plants and ¼ plate healthy carbs, as well as meeting my Triple 30 guidelines.

The Triple 30 approach simply means that we are aiming for:

- 30g of protein per meal (or thereabouts)
- 30g of fibre per day (around 10g per meal)
- 30+ plant points from eating 30+ unique plants per week (often more)

Fibre is lacking in most people's diets, so I pack as much fibre into each meal as I can, to help balance our recommended 30g of fibre per day over our three meals. This means that an average recipe will have 25–35g of protein per serving, around 10g of fibre, and plenty of plant points. (You can read more about how to get more protein, fibre and plant points into your diet, as well as their benefits, on pages 42, 51 and 68.)

The healthy plate (see opposite) is a great visual that we can use every day in most situations to help us easily get close to the Triple 30 principles. However, it's a little more nuanced than simply dividing the plate into food groups.

In reality, foods are a combination of macronutrients, overlapping in a similar way to a Venn diagram.

The foods we eat are a mixture of proteins, carbohydrates and fats in varying amounts. This means that when we class a food as a carbohydrate or a protein, for example, we are simply saying that food contains more of that macronutrient than others. Carbohydrates are found in grains, vegetables, fruits and legumes. We get our fibre from a wide range of different plant sources, such as starchy carbohydrates like grains or potatoes, vegetables and fruits (which are predominantly made up of water), legumes (which can be classed as healthy carbs as well as a protein source), and nuts and seeds (which might be classed as a fat or a protein, depending on how they are being used in a recipe). So, in truth, the total fibre in your meal will come from all these components which make up different areas of your healthy plate!

I know that this sounds as though it could get complicated, but rather than weighing everything or having to do lots of calculations, following the plate method (see also pages 92–95 for how to put together a perfect plate in any situation) means you can easily assemble a meal which balances optimum macronutrient levels. By following these proportions, healthy fats typically take care of themselves. Of course, you don't need to separate out the elements with all your veg on one side of your plate – my recipes usually combine them together, for example in my healthy Firecracker Chicken or Sticky Tofu Noodles (page 208 or 211).

What about calories?

This focus on nutrient-dense, natural foods in balanced proportions removes the need for calorie-counting, helping restore our body's natural appetite regulation and teaching us to trust our hunger cues to guide how much we should eat. It's almost impossible to eat too many calories when you're following the balanced plate method, as the food is so filling. (See also page 16 where we discussed the myth of calories in, calories out.)

The science: why a balanced plate matters

A balanced plate means balanced nutrients. And when we arrange food on our plate in a certain way, it makes it easier to reach our protein and fibre targets, almost without trying.

The gastrointestinal tract contains specialised cells that sense the chemical composition of the food we eat – in real time. Equipped with chemoreceptors, these cells act like mini laboratories, detecting nutrients and other

SAME INGREDIENTS, DIFFERENT APPROACH

When we pour out our granola in the morning, it's easy to load 60–80g into your bowl, which, along with milk, yoghurt and berries, could lead to consuming almost 20g of sugar (about 5 teaspoons) before the day even starts. Adding a small glass of fruit juice could contribute another 4½ teaspoons of sugar, quickly surpassing the recommended daily sugar intake of 6 teaspoons (25g) from the World Health Organization, or 7 teaspoons (30g) according to NHS England.

Now, let's flip the bowl. Start with a generous serving of thick, strained Greek yoghurt, which has more protein to keep us full for longer. Add a large handful of berries and just 2 tablespoons of one of my delicious homemade granolas: rich in nuts and seeds, lower in oats and only around 2g of sugar per serving (pages 107 or 119). Though both bowls contain broadly the same ingredients, they can have vastly different effects on the body. While having similar calories, one has significantly more free sugar, much less protein and would inevitably lead to a sugar crash by 10.30am – while the other should see us through until lunch.

It's not just about the sugars, it's about balancing foods for optimal health. The extra fats and proteins in the yoghurt, the protein and fibre from the seeds, combined with the fibre from the berries, work together to slow down our digestion. Protein and fibre act like the brakes on the digestive process, slowing the release of sugar into the bloodstream, helping keep blood sugars stable and providing more sustained energy. Better blood sugar control can also lead to improved focus, energy and mood, with fewer cravings between meals. (See page 18 for more on the blood sugar rollercoaster.)

chemical signals as they pass through the gut. In response, hormones are released that communicate with the brain to help regulate appetite and satiety. By eating good-quality proteins, healthy fats and an adequate amount of fibre, alongside healthier whole-food carbohydrates, we can start to reset the mechanisms that control appetite to reduce food cravings and feel fuller for longer.

Ultra-processed foods, however, often contain a 'bliss point' ratio of fats, sugars, salt and food additives that can upset this process. Some ultra-processed foods can activate reward centres in the brain by stimulating the release of dopamine, leading to us experiencing higher levels of pleasure, and leaving us craving more (see page 22 for more on UPFs). These foods are also soft, low in fibre and quick to digest, meaning that they can flood the bloodstream with energy before the gut has had time to release its satiety hormones.

Lead with your protein — ¼ plate

Healthy proteins are the essential building blocks of a balanced plate. Although many foods, including vegetables and grains, provide some protein, certain foods are officially considered better protein sources due to their higher concentration of essential amino acids (see page 42). Protein, as we know, plays a vital role in almost every function in our body, but it also affects our appetite, slowing digestion and contributing to feelings of fullness. A common reason why we may feel hungry after a meal is that the protein content was too low.

So, instead of planning a meal around pasta or noodles, think about the protein first. Centre your supper around chicken or fish or tofu, then add half a plate of vegetables, and the rest of your plate can comprise healthy fats and carbohydrates. It's a subtle shift in how to approach what you're eating, but it makes a huge difference.

Mix and match

Rather than relying on a single protein source, one of the best ways to boost protein is by combining different protein sources at each meal. Topping up animal proteins with a range of plant proteins also adds more fibre — and helps support the environment too. I love to find easy ways to top up my protein, for example, sprinkling nuts and seeds on soups and salads or making a dressing from tahini. See page 45 for more quick ideas.

If you are vegetarian or vegan, or follow a dairy-free diet, it's still perfectly possible to meet your protein targets — see pages 82–85, where I discuss swaps and additions you can make in your cooking.

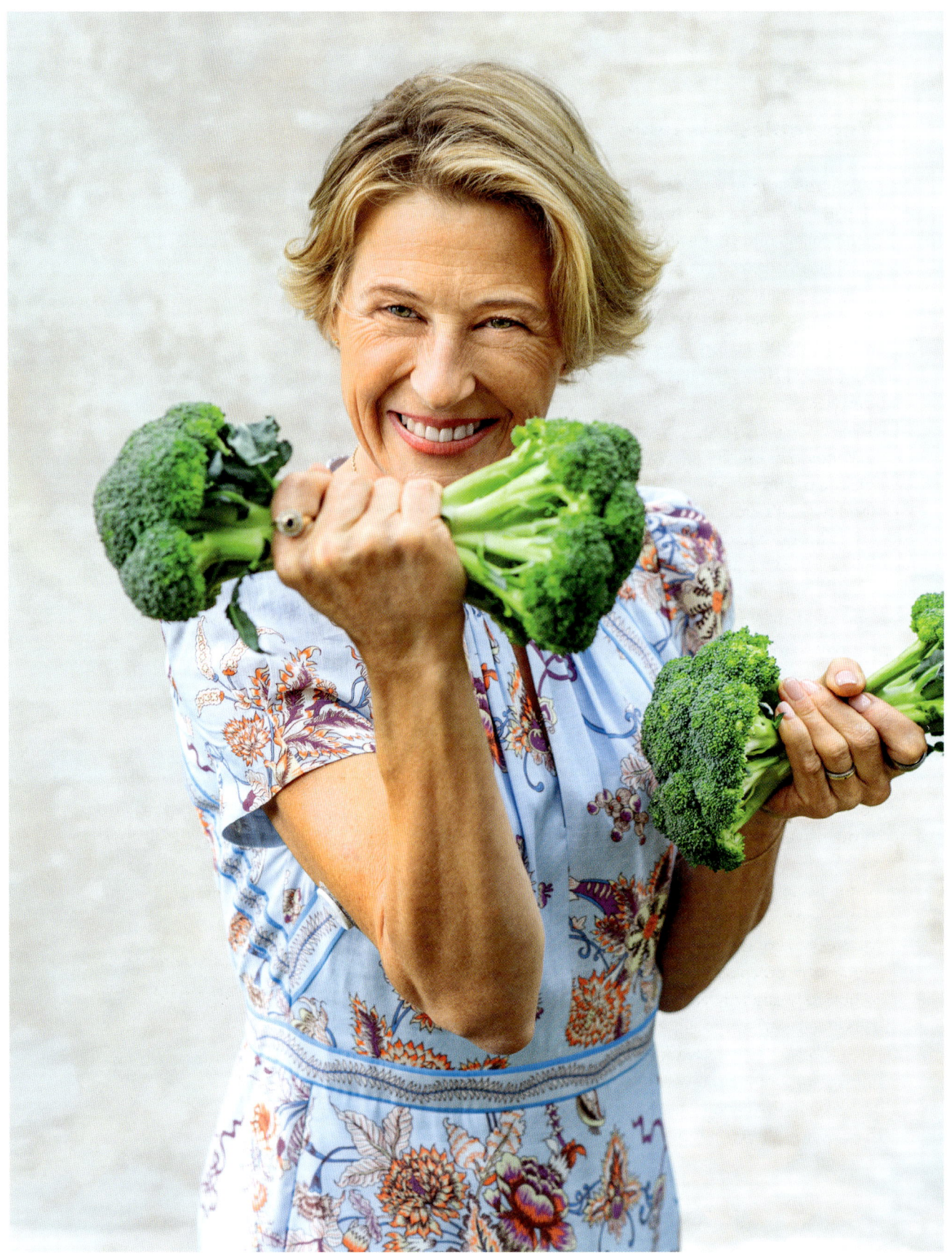

Vegetables – ½ plate

Vegetables are essential for our health, and ideally, they should fill half your plate at lunchtime and your evening meal. Two clenched fists or two cupped palmfuls is a good way to visualise the quantity of vegetables to aim for on your plate. This can easily amount to around 200–250g per meal, although the right amount for you varies based on your height and body-frame. 150g may be enough for some people; others may need more than 250g.

Vegetables are key in helping us meet our 30g of fibre per day. Fibre is what your gut microbes feed on, so it's vital for supporting and maintaining a healthy gut microbiome. They are also packed full of important minerals and vitamins, as well as special phytonutrients (or plant compounds) that are found only in plant foods – around 10,000+ have already been identified and research is continuing to discover new ones and to reveal more about their benefits to human health.

Fruit also contains many important vitamins and phytonutrients, as well as fibre, but fruit also tends to be higher in natural sugars. I tend to focus on veg in my meals, and allow for us to eat around three servings of fruit per day, best eaten with a meal (see page 36 for more on fruit).

Your vegetables can be chopped, grated, cut into crudités, eaten as soup, stir-fried, roasted, added to a casserole or pasta sauce, boiled, steamed or eaten as a simple or complex salad – basically any way you like to eat them!

Note: If you're not used to eating a lot of vegetables, it's a good idea to increase your intake gradually to allow your body to get used to the extra fibre and reduce any symptoms such as bloating or discomfort.

My Top 20 healthy vegetables

- Asparagus
- Artichokes
- Beetroot
- Broccoli
- Brussels sprouts
- Butternut squash
- Carrots
- Cauliflower
- Fennel
- Garlic
- Green beans
- Kale
- Kohlrabi
- Mangetout
- Mushrooms
- Onions
- Peppers
- Radishes
- Spinach
- Watercress

Bonus points

Cruciferous vegetables Try to include at least one cruciferous vegetable each day, e.g. cabbage, broccoli, cauliflower, kale, radishes, watercress, rocket or Brussels sprouts. These vegetables are rich in plant compounds that support liver detoxification and act as powerful antioxidants.

Alliums Try to include at least one allium each day, e.g. onions, garlic, leeks, shallots or spring onions. Their sulphur compounds not only bring great flavour, but they also support liver detoxification by enhancing key detox pathways that help process and eliminate toxins from the body.

Brightly coloured vegetables Aim for at least three different-coloured vegetables on your plate, e.g. purple cabbage, green kale and orange carrots. This helps you get a wider range of phytonutrients into your diet.

HOW MUCH FRUIT?

I love to add fruits to my diet. Contributing to our 30+ plant points each week, fruits, like vegetables, are a fantastic source of beneficial bioactive plant compounds, such as polyphenols, and prebiotic fibre, as well as vitamins and minerals. The more colourful they are (e.g. cherries, blueberries and strawberries) the more polyphenols they are likely to contain (see pages 68–69). Some fruits, such as apples, are rich in a soluble fibre called pectin, which can promote more regular bowel movements and has also been linked to lowering cholesterol.

Fruit counts towards our five a day, but it's important to prioritise vegetables over fruit in our diet because fruits contain natural sugars that can impact our blood sugar levels if consumed in large amounts. Pairing fruit with a meal or a source of protein can help minimise spikes in blood sugar. For example, you might choose berries with your yoghurt at breakfast, pomegranate seeds in a salad at lunch, and an apple after dinner. Combining fruits with yoghurt, cheese or nuts can help maintain a more stable blood sugar response.

Some fruits have a lesser impact on our blood sugars than others. This is because fruits contain different types of sugars, which impact our blood sugars in different ways. The combination of different sugars can also affect how quickly we are able to absorb them. Fruits with a lower sugar concentration, and a higher polyphenol and fibre content, are also mostly slower-acting. This is why mango has a different glycaemic effect (its effect on blood sugar levels) to strawberries. Green bananas also contain more resistant starch and less sugar than ripe or brown bananas, where more of the starches have turned into sugars.

- Lower glycaemic fruits include: blueberries, blackberries, raspberries, strawberries, apples, pears, kiwi, cherries, plums, orange, pomegranate and peaches.

- Higher glycaemic fruits that may have a higher glucose response include: bananas, mango, grapes, pineapple, watermelon, dates and dried fruits.

Eating whole fruit provides the most benefit for our health. While fruit juices still contain nutrients, they lack the pulp and skins, which are rich in fibre. Once the fibre is removed, the sugars in fruit juices are considered free sugars, which can cause higher blood glucose levels compared to eating fresh fruit. When drinking a glass of orange juice, it is likely to contain the juice of 3–4 oranges, with more free sugar, and we will feel less satisfied than if we were to eat a single piece of fruit. Smoothies still contain the fibre from the fruit, but blending disrupts the food matrix – the structure of the food – meaning that the sugars are more freely available. Smoothies made from vegetables, such as spinach or kale, with fruits such as avocados or seeds to thicken them, and just a little apple to sweeten, are a better option.

Healthy carbs – ¼ plate

Eating healthy carbs is also essential if we are to meet the 30g of fibre we need to aim for each day. Studies show that, eaten in the right proportion and in the right form, carbohydrates are an important source of fibre, energy, vitamins and phytonutrients that support our metabolic health, and may help to reduce the risk of chronic disease, such as heart disease and obesity. In contrast, excessive consumption of refined carbohydrates and added sugars is associated with an increased risk of diseases, such as Type 2 diabetes, obesity and heart disease as well as cognitive decline. I never advise eating ZERO carbohydrates, even when aiming for weight loss: in clinic, I see how cutting back on healthy carbs inevitably cuts back on fibre. Low-carb diets can slow down our gut motility, leading to fewer bowel movements, or worse still, constipation. Low-carb diets can also deplete and alter the balance of our gut microbiome. Instead, eating the 'right carbs' has been associated with better long-term health outcomes, sustainable weight loss, better mood and increased energy.

Because our foods are a combination of different macronutrients, sometimes your carbs might look like lentils or butter beans, other times cooked bulgur wheat, butternut squash or sweet potato. You will see that the carbs appear in different forms in my recipes, but they are almost always present – although they might appear to be hiding in the recipe or on your plate!

What exactly are carbs?

All carbohydrates are made up of chains of glucose molecules. In their natural state these chains are long and branched and are harder to digest. When a carbohydrate is processed (i.e. refined to remove the outer husk or milled into tiny fragments), this reduces its fibre content and increases the surface area, allowing it to be digested and absorbed more quickly into the bloodstream (see pages 18–19).

Issues arise when high-carb foods – even healthy carbs – are eaten in large amounts or in isolation, without the correct balance of protein, fibre and healthy fats to act as the 'brakes'. This leads to rapid absorption in the small intestine, which can trigger the blood sugar spikes and dips that can exacerbate food cravings. Serving baked potatoes or pasta without sufficient protein-rich toppings, vegetables or healthy fats, or simply serving up too much rice, naan or garlic bread on the side, can also unbalance a meal. It is not that these foods are inherently bad in themselves, but they can be quite pushy and can quickly start to take over the plate, nudging out the protein, vegetables and other healthy foods and affecting the balance and our overall nutrient intake.

What carbs should we be eating?

As with everything, then, it is a balancing act. We need to eat some carbs, but the right carbs, and we also need to not eat too much or too little of them – which I realise sounds more complicated than Goldilocks's bowl of porridge, so let me simplify it.

- Eat your carbs as they are found in nature (whole-food, complex carbs) and reduce your consumption of processed (refined or simple) carbs. Whole-food carbs are those that have not had their outer fibrous coating and germ removed and have not been finely milled.

- Make carbs a side dish and not centre stage. Sometimes just a few tablespoons may be sufficient, but if you are younger, taller or more active, you will probably need a bit more.

Reduce refined or simple carbs. Refined or white carbohydrates are higher in available starches but lower in fibre and nutrients. Most of the nutrients in our carbohydrates sit just under the husk and can be lost through refining. By 'white' carbohydrates, I mean foods that have been processed, such as white bread and flour, white pasta, sugar, white rice and most breakfast cereals. These are known as quick-energy release carbohydrates, and they can wreak havoc with your blood sugar and insulin levels if eaten regularly. Rather than supplying your body with added fibre, refined carbohydrates are broken down quickly in the stomach and small intestine and are more likely to flood your body with simple sugars that make you feel hungry again soon after you have eaten them.

Eat more whole-food, complex carbs.
In contrast, wholegrains, beans and lentils and some starchy vegetables provide us with a wealth of nutrients and are digested more slowly in the gut, giving us a steadier supply of energy as they pass through the small intestine, and feeding the gut bacteria as they enter the large intestine.

It would be difficult to consume 30g of fibre from fruits and vegetables alone, as most only contain 1–3g of fibre per 100g. You might need to consume somewhere in the region of 1.25kg–1.5kg of vegetables every day to reach your target! This is where healthy carbs, including wholegrains and legumes, really step up and add some weight to the fibre game.

Beans and lentils

When talking about healthy carbohydrates, we also need to bring in the legume food group. Legumes can be interchangeably called pulses and include all peas, beans and lentils. Legumes are a hybrid food that can be classed as a protein or as a healthy carbohydrate, having a foot in both camps. I like to use them as proteins to give structure to vegetarian and plant-based meals, but they can also be used in the quarter of your plate designated for healthy carbs.

Legumes are also gentler on our blood sugars than some other carbs, which might make them a better form of carbohydrate for those with sensitive blood sugars, insulin resistance or Type 2 diabetes.

THE GLYCAEMIC INDEX

How carbohydrates affect our blood sugars is what determines how 'healthy' they are – as well as the nutrients they contain. Those with the lowest glycaemic response (those that have the least effect on blood sugar levels) are considered the healthiest – often because they contain more fibre, which makes them kinder to our blood sugars – while those with a high glycaemic response are considered the least healthy.

The glycaemic index gives us a broad idea of how different foods might affect our blood sugars. The index runs from 0–100, where zero would have no effect on our blood sugars and 100 would have a very significant effect. It has its limitations, as there is a huge personal difference in how carbohydrates affect us individually, but it is based on an average response to consuming around 50g of carbohydrate in a food. However...

It does not take into account... how much of the food you are going to be eating. A few croutons in your soup will have a smaller effect on blood sugars than a large bread roll. To consume a 50g serving of carbohydrate from a watermelon (which is a high glycaemic food) you would need to consume around 700g, which is unrealistic, whereas you might only need to consume a 60g bowl of cornflakes (another high glycaemic food).

It does not take into account... the way you cook the food – fried or roasted potatoes will have a higher GI, as will overcooked grains.

It does not take into account... the foods you will be eating alongside, i.e. the effect of the proteins, fats or fibre eaten at the same meal.

Low glycaemic <55
- Edamame beans
- Peas
- Lentils
- Beans
- Split yellow/green peas
- Chickpea/green pea pasta
- Pearl barley
- Freekeh
- Bulgur wheat
- Whole rye
- Whole farro
- Red lentil pasta
- Black rice
- Buckwheat groats
- Black rice
- Soba noodles (100% buckwheat)

Medium glycaemic 56–69
- Rye pumpernickel
- Red rice
- Quinoa
- Whole spelt (spelt barley)
- Rolled oats
- Wholegrain pasta
- Seeded sourdough
- Brown rice
- Parsnips

High glycaemic >70
- Couscous
- Sweet potato, boiled
- Potato, boiled
- White rice
- Cornflakes
- Potato chips

Healthy carbs to enjoy (in proportion!)

When it comes to carbohydrates, there are three important things to remember:

Quality: Whole or cracked grain carbohydrates are higher in nutrients, higher in fibre and are harder for us to break down. This means more sustained energy and better blood sugar control.

Quantity: Even if we are eating healthier carbohydrates, a small portion will contain less glucose and have a smaller blood sugar response than a large portion, which will contain more glucose and have a bigger blood sugar response. Therefore, the amount or serving size matters! Eating the right amount of carbohydrates might be just a few spoonfuls that fit neatly into one cupped palm.

What you are going to eat with it? Eating carbohydrates in proportion to proteins, vegetables, fibre and fats helps to keep the portion size in check and also slows down the rate that we break them down and absorb them.

The carbs we should be eating less of

We know we should be eating less of the white, fluffy, processed, sugary or sweet carbohydrates, such as white bread, white rice, white flour, biscuits, cakes, breakfast cereals, crisps, white crackers, confectionery, pizza bases, table sugar, honey, maple syrup, sweets, desserts, ice cream, sugary soft drinks, fruit smoothies and ultra-processed food and snacks. And it's not that rice and potatoes are bad for us in moderation, it's just that there are better options available to us from a fibre perspective – bulgur, freekeh, rye and spelt contain around 13g fibre per 100g (dry weight), whereas brown rice contains only around 3.5g.

Simple swaps are easier than you think!

Couscous ➜ bulgur wheat or freekeh

White rice ➜ quinoa or green lentils, or swap rice for frozen peas

Potato mash ➜ white bean mash

Potato chips/fries and roast potatoes ➜ sweet potato wedges with their skins

White pasta ➜ wholegrain pasta, red lentil, chickpea or green pea pasta

White potato ➜ lentils or cooked beans

White bread ➜ my Red Lentil Bagels or my Seed and Nut Loaf (pages 267 or 253)

Rice noodles ➜ black bean, edamame or soba noodles

Potato crisps ➜ roasted nuts, Chilli and Lime Cashews (page 279), Crispy Edamame Beans (page 276) or seaweed thins

White crackers ➜ Rosemary and Sea Salt Seeded Crackers (page 261) or wholegrain sourdough crackers

Include some healthy fats

Healthy fats are a key component of our meals and will already be present if you're enjoying foods like fatty fish or you have used extra virgin olive oil to sauté vegetables or in a salad dressing. But adding avocado, olives or a sprinkle of nuts and seeds will make sure you have some healthy fats on your plate.

It's often easier to incorporate foods into your meals that naturally contain beneficial fats, rather than feeling the need to add them on top. Since fats carry flavour, meals without them can feel much less satisfying. Using a delicious dressing for your salads, or cooking with toasted sesame oil, can make a big difference to both your healthy fat levels and your enjoyment of your meal!

While this doesn't mean you should go overboard (since fats are calorie-dense), don't shy away from including them – they help keep you fuller for longer and are vital for our brain, nervous tissue and cell membranes. If you are watching your weight, try to keep added fats in dressings or in cooking to around 1 tablespoon per meal (15ml). See pages 60–67 for more on why healthy fats are essential, and how to include them in our diet.

PRINCIPLE 2: PRIORITISE PROTEIN

Proteins are made up of chains of amino acids. The human body uses twenty different amino acids to build proteins, nine of which are 'essential', meaning that the body cannot produce them itself and so we must consume them in our food. The other eleven are called 'non-essential', meaning our body can make them from other amino acids. The specific order and shape of these 'chains' allow the body to create thousands of different proteins that support many areas of our health and wellbeing.

Proteins are essential for almost every function in our body. They build the muscles that hold us upright, burn energy and enable us to move with ease. They form enzymes, hormones and antibodies, transport substances around the body, support our immune system, and are needed for building structure, for example in our hair, skin, nails and joints. Proteins are also the building blocks of chemical messengers called neurotransmitters, which regulate our nervous system, mood and sleep and are vital for brain signalling. Without all these chemical reactions taking place, our body and health would be compromised, affecting our liver detoxification, energy production, digestion, thyroid health and so much more.

The human body is excellent at recycling proteins, by breaking them down into their individual amino acids and rebuilding them; in a similar way to how we might take apart and reassemble LEGO bricks, to form a new structure or shape. However, the human body does not have an efficient way of storing excess amino acids and so coverts them into glucose or fats to be used as energy – or stored as body fat – meaning we need a constant supply of protein.

It makes sense to split our protein across three meals to get the most benefits. Eating sufficient protein at breakfast ensures we bring in a fresh supply of amino acids for the body to use and to stabilise our blood sugars from the get-go.

The science: why protein matters

I've frequently observed the benefits of prioritising protein at mealtimes in my work with clients. The key benefits are:

Strong muscles and bones. Protein is essential for maintaining healthy muscles and bones. It provides the building blocks that are needed to repair and grow muscle tissue and can help reduce age-related muscle loss. Protein is also an integral part of our bone matrix, which affects its structure and framework.

Stabilised blood sugars. Proteins take longer to digest compared to carbohydrates, staying in the stomach for an extended period, and slowing down the release of sugars (carbohydrates) consumed during the same meal. Food is therefore absorbed over a longer timeframe and results in a more regular blood sugar curve. Slower digestion and more consistent blood sugar levels keep us feeling fuller for longer and can significantly reduce cravings. More stable blood sugars can also positively impact our mood, sleep, concentration and energy levels.

Improved appetite and hunger signalling. Keeping off the blood sugar rollercoaster helps prevent snack-attacks between meals! Protein also triggers a series of hormones that increase satiety and decrease hunger, helping to reduce the desire to snack.

Easier weight management. Protein is therefore a crucial cogwheel in weight management. Controlling cravings and staying satisfied between meals can greatly improve our metabolic health by reducing the urge to snack on high-sugar or high-carbohydrate foods – making weight maintenance a piece of cake!

Improved mood. With blood sugar levels stabilising into a more consistent pattern, we are less likely to experience the dreaded post-lunch energy slump or the crashes that can leave us feeling fatigued and low. In my clinic, people report that when their protein intake is adequate, they feel calmer, more resilient and more emotionally balanced.

Back in charge. When the focus is on adequate protein, many people feel that they regain control of their diet and eating patterns, and develop a true sense of food confidence. We start to make better, healthier food choices when our appetite feels more stable, without any feelings of deprivation. We start to eat better because we start to feel better.

Plant protein

Eating more protein does not have to mean eating more animal protein. I have included plenty of plant-based and vegetarian protein sources in my recipes. This not only enhances diversity in your diet but also boosts fibre and plant intake. Plant proteins also come with added benefits, such as beneficial phytonutrients and antioxidants, and nutrients including folate and magnesium. Providing we are eating a wide range of different plant proteins, it's still possible for us to obtain all the amino acids in the correct amounts we need for our body, even if we are following a plant-based, vegan or vegetarian diet. (Also see page 41 for my simple swaps.)

DO YOU NEED TO EAT A HIGH-PROTEIN DIET? FACT OR MYTH?

Protein is vital for life, and the word comes from the Greek 'proteios', meaning 'taking first place'. But prioritising protein does not mean following a high-protein diet. Rather, it's about ensuring that each of our three meals contains adequate amounts of protein to support our health.

Aim for around 30g protein per meal

Our protein needs naturally vary due to our size and activity level: if you are tall and active you will need more protein daily than someone who is petite and sedentary. Protein is also important in helping to prevent muscle loss, so we may need to eat a bit more protein as we get older to retain our strength and help us remain active as we age. Although there's no exact number to aim for, we do have ways of estimating requirements.

We know that we need to be eating at least 0.8g protein/kg body weight in order to obtain sufficient amino acids to cover our body's daily requirements. This level equates to an average amount of 46–56g per day. Most people achieve this amount, but since requirements can vary between individuals depending on factors such as age, exercise and training goals as well as general health, it means there is no one-size-fits-all approach. Current thinking suggests that the optimal intake may exceed 0.8g/kg body weight, with many experts recommending around 1–1.4g/kg body weight, as a more realistic or even optimal baseline.

A good aim is 1.2g protein/kg body weight each day. Following my Triple 30 approach, each recipe in this book has around 30g of protein per serving or around 90g per day. (To help you, on page 304 I have put together a chart to show what optimal protein might look like for you.) You know your body best, though, so adjust the portions to what feels right for you. If you need more than 90g/day, simply add more nuts, seeds, eggs, cheese, chicken, fish, tofu, edamame beans, quinoa, beans, sourdough and other foods, or enjoy a larger portion size! (See pages 48–49 for more on quality protein sources.) If you need less, reduce your portion size accordingly.

I don't suggest weighing food, but rather that we learn to visually gauge what our portion sizes should look like. When you consume sufficient protein and fibre at meals – by following the balanced plate – you should be able to feel the effects on satiety for yourself.

Eating very high-protein diets is seen as an easy weight-loss trick used by many to help achieve faster weight loss, because protein is extremely filling and converting excess protein into body fat is inefficient. However, while it may be an effective short-term strategy, it is unsustainable and unnecessary in the long term and could lead to deficits in other areas of your diet.

Sometimes we see recommendations of 2g protein/kg body weight, particularly in the fitness industry. While eating this amount of protein is unlikely to cause harm (provided it comes from a balanced variety of sources rather than solely from animal proteins, which contain more saturated fats), this probably isn't necessary and does not consider other factors that affect our health, such as fibre intake and the nutritional value of other foods consumed.

Excess protein will also mostly be converted into fats by the body, so while consuming sufficient protein contributes to the promotion of lean muscle mass, the benefits do not continue to increase proportionally the more protein we consume, and may diminish above 1.6g protein/kg body weight. There is a natural cut-off with most people where more protein is not associated with greater muscle mass, or better health, even if they are very active.

Easy 10g protein top-ups

This list can help you add an extra 10g protein to your plate! Some of these might be more than you would eat in one sitting, however they should give you an idea of how you can incorporate more protein in your meals throughout the day. Try to make sure that your plate includes some plant-based protein. (See photo overleaf.)

- 170g frozen peas
- 40g nuts or seeds
- 120g cooked beans
- 40g dried lentils (add to a soup)
- 80g cooked red lentil pasta
- 100g cottage cheese
- 100g Greek yoghurt
- 60g feta cheese
- 2 small, boiled eggs or 1½ large
- 80g edamame beans, shelled
- 30g Parmesan cheese
- 60g cooked prawns
- 70g tofu
- 40g cooked chicken breast
- ½ tin of sardines (around 45g drained weight)
- 1 thick slice of sourdough
- my Red Lentil Bagel (page 267)
- 30g hemp seeds
- 15g nutritional yeast
- 50g tempeh

EASY 10G PROTEIN TOP-UPS

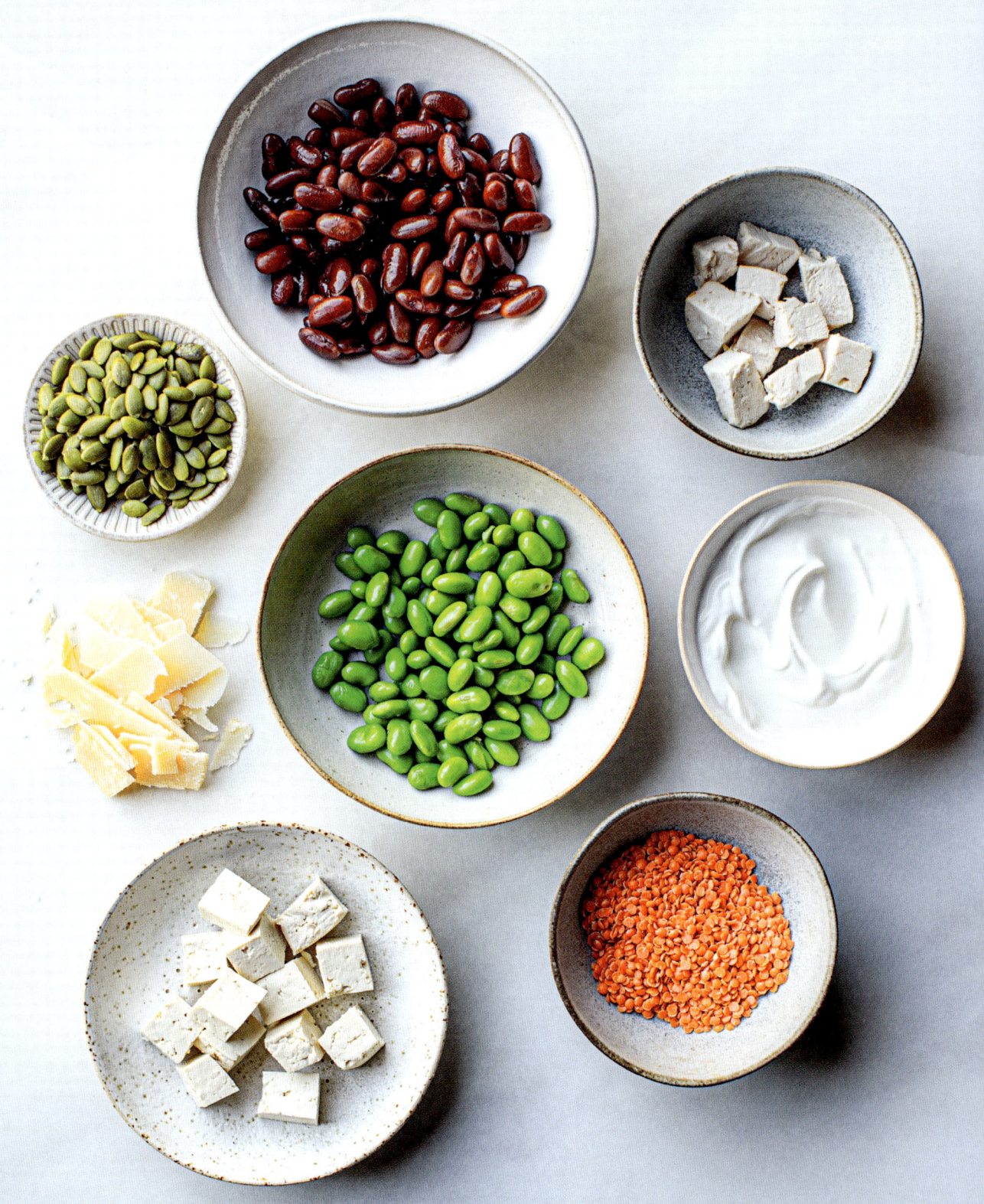

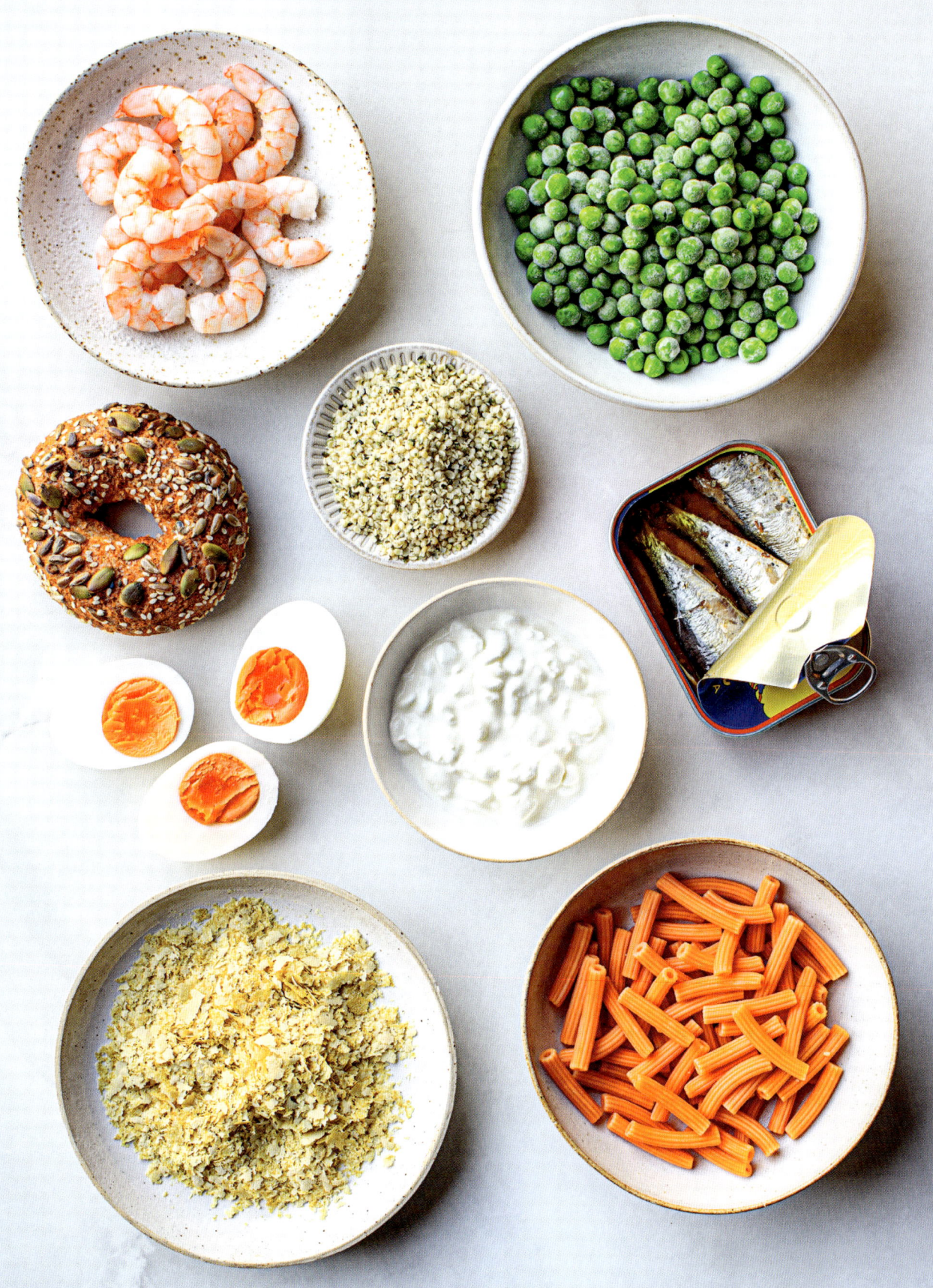

PROTEIN SOURCES

The lists below show the average amounts of protein found in our most commonly used ingredients. Whether you eat an omnivorous diet, are plant-based, vegetarian or pescatarian, there are plenty of proteins to choose from. Aim to include plenty of plant-based proteins in your diet for their added health benefits.

Meat
g protein/100g (raw)

- Beef (10% fat mince) 20g
- Chicken breast 23g
- Lamb (lean) 21g
- Pork (lean) 23g
- Turkey breast 24g
- Venison 23g

Fish
g protein/100g (raw)

- Calamari 20g
- Mackerel 21g
- Prawns 18g
- Salmon 24g
- Sardines 22g
- Scallops 18g
- Tuna 26g
- White fish 20g

Dairy and eggs
g protein/100g

- Eggs (per medium egg) 6g
- Cottage cheese 10g
- Cream cheese 5g
- Feta cheese 16g
- Full-fat natural yoghurt 3.5g
- Greek yoghurt 10g
- Goat's cheese 20g
- Quark 13g
- Kefir 3.5g
- Halloumi cheese 23g
- Hard cheese, e.g. Cheddar 25g
- Whole milk 3.5g
- Mozzarella 17g
- Parmesan 32g
- Paneer 21g
- Blue cheese 21g

Plant proteins
g protein/100g

- Almond cheese 7g
- Almond milk 1g
- Almond yoghurt 3g
- Coconut yoghurt 2g
- Oat milk 1g
- Tofu 16g
- Seitan 23g
- Tempeh 21g
- Quorn 14g
- Soya mince (cooked) 17g
- Soya mince (dried) 52g
- Soya milk 3.3g
- Soya Greek yoghurt 6g
- Vegan feta 0g
- Vegan hard cheese 0–3g (depending on brand)

Nuts and seeds
g protein/100g

- Cashew nuts 17g
- Chia seeds 21g
- Flaxseeds 20g
- Nut butter 25g
- Pecans 9g
- Pumpkin seeds 24g
- Sesame seeds 18g
- Sunflower seeds 24g
- Walnuts 15g

Pulses
g protein/100g

- Butter beans (cooked) 7g
- Chickpeas (cooked) 8g
- Edamame beans 12g
- Green or black lentils (dry/cooked) 21g/10g
- Green pea pasta (dry) 22g
- Green peas (petits pois) 5g
- Kidney beans (cooked) 7.5g
- Red lentil pasta (dry) 26g
- Red lentils (dry/cooked) 24g/9g
- White beans (cooked) 7g

Other
g protein/100g

- Brown rice (dry) 7.5g
- Buckwheat (dry) 13g
- Bulgur wheat (dry) 13g
- Freekeh (dry) 13g
- Oatcakes (per oatcake) 1g
- Oats (dry) 11g
- Pumpernickel bread 6g
- Quinoa (dry) 13g
- Sourdough bread 9g
- Spelt barley (dry) 13g
- Wheat pasta (dry) 12g

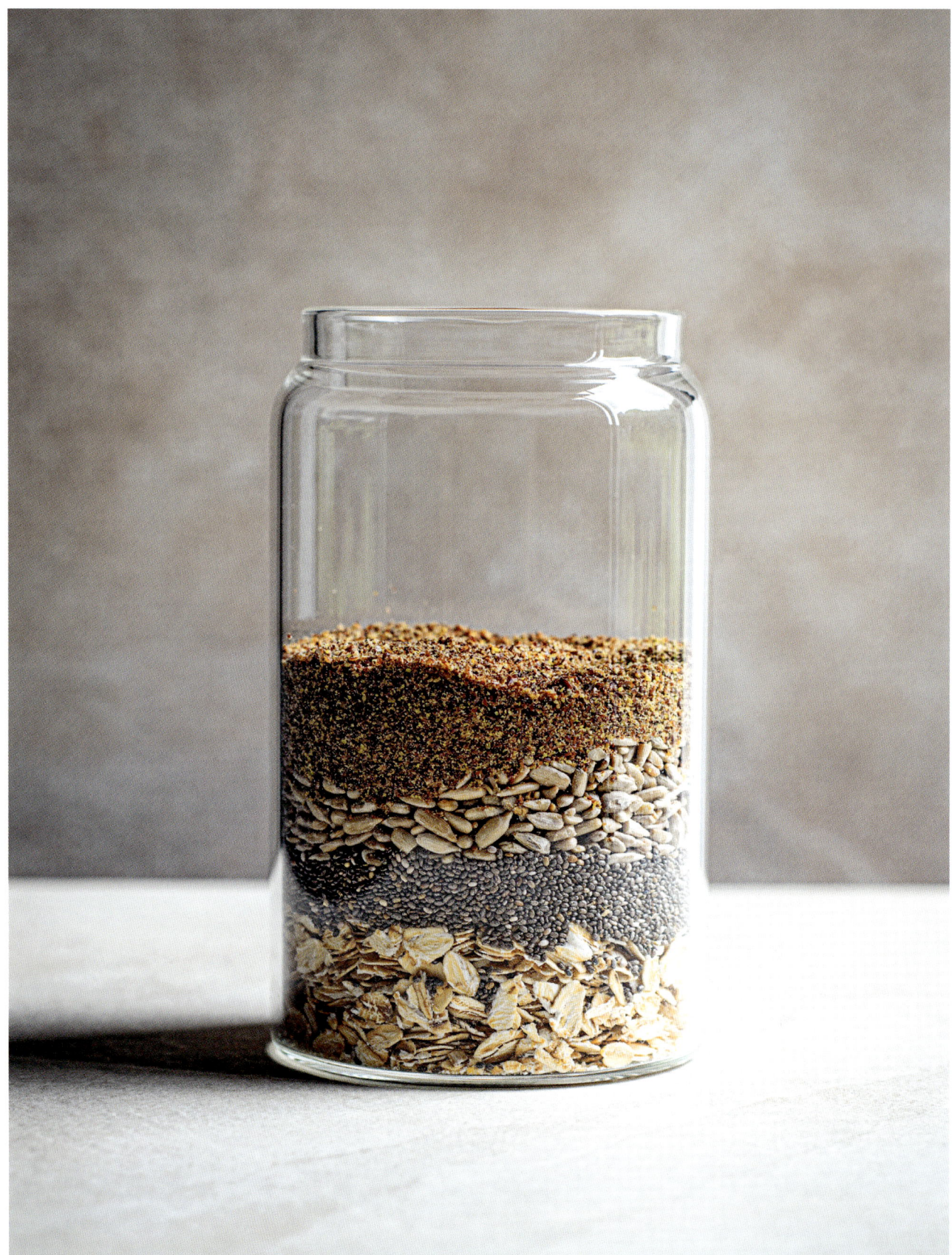

PRINCIPLE 3: FOCUS ON FIBRE

Dietary fibre is the name given to the non-digestible parts of plants that our digestive enzymes cannot break down. While fibre may pass through our body undigested, it has many functions as it completes its journey through the gut. Fibre is found in all plants and provides structure and rigidity to their cell walls, allowing the plants to stand upright. Fibre is found in fruits, vegetable, nuts, seeds, grains, legumes, cacao and even coffee beans.

It is estimated that approximately 90 per cent of adults are not consuming enough fibre, a deficiency that is a contributing factor to chronic health conditions, such as digestive issues, heart disease, Type 2 diabetes, certain cancers and obesity. Until recently, fibre was primarily seen as something our gut needed to ensure healthy bowel movements. However, research has significantly advanced in recent years, revealing the full scope of the benefits of eating more fibre.

Fibre acts as a food source to the trillions of bacteria that live in our gut, helping support and maintain a healthy microbiome. These bacteria perform a huge range of essential functions crucial to almost every aspect of our wellbeing.

Most health guidelines suggest aiming for 30g of fibre per day, though this amount can vary between 25–35g, depending on factors such as your height and body composition. My balanced plate recipes contain around 10g of fibre per portion – sometimes more – made up of vegetables, fruits, legumes, grains and seeds, which can make these recommendations easier to achieve.

The three main types of fibre:

Soluble fibre
Soluble fibre dissolves in water and has a gel-like texture. It is very important for the health of our gut microbes, as it slows down the absorption of sugar and carbohydrates in the small intestine, adds bulk to the stool and can help lower cholesterol.

We can find soluble fibre in grains – especially oats – beans, lentils, seeds (such as chia and flaxseeds), psyllium husk, and in the soft leaves and fleshy part of fruits and vegetables.

Insoluble fibre
This is the type of fibre that does not dissolve in water. Insoluble fibre absorbs water and so adds bulk and volume to the stool, promoting regular bowel movement as well as exercising the walls of the intestine and keeping them toned.

It is found in the peel, skin and inedible seeds of vegetables and fruits, and the husk of wholegrains and legumes, but is also found in tougher leafy greens, seeds and nuts.

Resistant starch
This type of fibre can be found in green or underripe bananas, but it also forms in some foods when they have been cooked and cooled, or even frozen, in a process called retrogradation. These foods include rice, potatoes, pasta, bread, beans and lentils. As these foods cool after cooking, some of the starches are converted into resistant starch which, as the name suggests, is 'resistant' to our

own digestion and behaves like fibre in the body. It is not absorbed as energy, but instead can be used as energy by the microbes residing in our gut. Even when reheated, studies have shown that the starches that have become resistant mostly remain in this indigestible form.

The science: why fibre matters

The science is clear: a fibre-rich diet is linked to improved health markers in almost every area:

Improves digestive health. Fibre can help prevent both constipation and diarrhoea, by keeping our internal train moving! Adding bulk to the stool helps to exercise the gut wall and aids the contractions that are necessary for this muscular movement, known as peristalsis.

Supports a healthy microbiome. The prebiotics in fibre are essential for a healthy microbiome – read more about this on page 54.

Reduces the urge to snack. Fibre fills us up and slows down digestion. The more slowly the energy from our meal is released, the longer we stay satisfied, warding off cravings between meals and reducing the desire to reach for less healthy foods. Like protein, fibre also regulates hunger hormones, especially GLP-1, helping to control appetite and promote satiety.

Helps with weight management. By reducing snacking and preventing over-eating, fibre makes us less likely to overconsume. Eating sufficient fibre makes it easier to lose or maintain our weight, almost without trying.

Regulates blood sugar control. Fibre creates an obstacle course in our digestive tract. This makes it harder for glucose molecules to reach the bloodstream as they become tangled in the fibrous mesh, helping to reduce blood sugar spikes.

Improves heart health. Soluble fibre is thought to lower cholesterol levels by keeping food and cholesterol moving through the gut for excretion as well as reducing its reabsorption back into the bloodstream.

Supports oestrogen balance. When oestrogen has completed its work in the body, the liver packages it up and sends it to the gut for excretion. Soluble fibre is thought to help escort these packages out of the body. Science suggests that eating more fibre can have a positive effect on circulating oestrogen levels. This may be due to increased transit time allowing for better excretion of oestrogen, but it may also influence the gut microbiome directly and, in particular, by helping to rebalance certain beta-glucuronidase-producing bacteria that may affect the recirculation of oestrogen.

May reduce the risk of certain cancers. A higher fibre intake has been associated with a reduced risk of developing certain types of cancers, such as colorectal and breast cancer.

Increases the nutrient density of our diet. Plant foods that are rich in fibre are also an abundant source of vitamins, minerals and beneficial plant compounds. By increasing fibre, we automatically improve the quality of our diet.

6 tips to increase fibre

Switch to whole-food carbohydrates. Wholegrains are higher in fibre, protein and nutrients, so choose heavier, darker rye or seeded breads, add quinoa, bulgur wheat, freekeh, buckwheat and barley, and reduce refined grains and flours such as couscous, white rice, white flour, white flour and white bread.

Eat the skins! Not all vegetables and fruits need to be peeled. Peeling carrots, parsnips, potatoes and apples, for example, leads to a reduction in fibre and also in the nutrients, which are most concentrated just below the skin. Just give them a good wash and a scrub first.

Add nuts and seeds to your salads, soups, breakfasts and bakes. These are not only a rich source of vitamins, minerals, proteins and healthy fats, but are also a rich source of fibre.

Eat more legumes. Include beans, chickpeas, split peas and lentils in more of your meals. Add them to soups and stews. Green or black lentils can be used to bulk out your mince in Bolognese, chilli or lasagne – see my Beef Chilli with Lentils on page 219.

Aim for around 200–250g of vegetables in your main meals! (See page 31 for more on Proportions and pages 68–71 for my section on Plant Points.)

Snack smarter! If you do need a snack, include vegetables sticks, hummus, seeds, nuts, avocado, roasted chickpeas, edamame beans, chia pudding or savoury popcorn! See page 76 for more ideas.

Slow and steady

If you're not used to eating large amounts of fibre, start slowly. Speak to your GP first if you have a condition where fibre may need to be limited, e.g. inflammatory bowel disease. Listen to your body, as we all respond differently to fibre. If you do not tolerate beans or lentils well, go easy on those recipes, try starting with a smaller amount, or substitute with another form of fibre. If you are not used to eating chia seeds, start by eating 1 teaspoon and see how you get on before you go all-out with a larger portion. Side-effects of increasing fibre too quickly are gas, bloating, stomach cramps, diarrhoea, constipation, nausea or feeling overly full.

Hydration

Fibre needs to stay hydrated. Keeping our stools soft decreases the risk of constipation and cramping and helps expel waste from the body. We need 1.8–2.5 litres of water a day (6–8 300ml glasses), depending on our body size, activity level and the weather. Some people may need more than this. Observe the colour of your urine. It should be light yellow. If it's a darker yellow, you're probably dehydrated and need a glass of water! Be aware that vitamin B2 (riboflavin) can colour urine bright yellow and some medications can also affect urine colour. Most of our water intake should come from plain water or herbal teas. Small amounts of black tea and coffee can count, but should only make up a minimal amount of your fluid intake.

MICROBES: THE DJS IN YOUR GUT!

Fibre is crucial for the health of our digestive tract, but also in supporting the trillions of beneficial bacteria that inhabit our gut – the gut microbiome. The remarkable activity of these microbes means that the positive effects of eating more fibre extend far beyond the gut alone, influencing many systems in the body – and we're discovering more about the wide-ranging ways it impacts our health and wellbeing all the time. Think of your microbiome like a DJ turning up or dialling down various pathways in the body. This might influence the delicate balance of our hormones and our neurotransmitters, but it can also affect levels of inflammation in the body, both positively and negatively.

The main functions of the gut microbes are:

• Gut microbes produce short-chain fatty acids (SCFAs), which have a number of roles. They nourish the cells lining the gut, helping to keep the intestinal barrier (the gateway between the gut and our bloodstream) healthy and resilient. This barrier acts as the body's border control, and when it's working correctly it allows essential nutrients and water to pass into the bloodstream while blocking other molecules, such as microbes, chemicals, and undigested food particles, from entering. SCFAs, such as butyrate, acetate and propionate, are also thought to help to dampen down certain types of inflammation in the body, particularly low-grade or chronic inflammation, by regulating the immune system and helping to reduce the release of compounds, such as pro-inflammatory cytokines.

• Assisting in the digestion of beneficial plant chemicals, such as polyphenols (see page 68).

• Digesting our food and producing B-vitamins and vitamin K. While this can be helpful as a top-up, vitamins are only made in small amounts in the gut and are not sufficient to meet our daily needs.

• Natural crowd control! Beneficial bacteria act like natural crowd controllers, deterring the colonisation of harmful bacteria and parasites. They do this by out-competing unwanted guests for resources, producing antimicrobial compounds, and training the immune system to hunt down and eliminate potential threats.

• Supporting brain health and mental health (see opposite).

The gut-brain axis

You may have heard the headline that 90 per cent of serotonin is produced in the gut and not, as we might imagine, in the brain. This could lead us to believe that happiness could be achieved by nourishing the gut microbes. However, the gut uses serotonin differently from the brain (mostly to support peristalsis or gut motility). It is now thought that serotonin made in the gut is unable to cross the highly selective blood-brain barrier, but actually has a more indirect influence on our mood in other ways, for example via the gut-brain axis and via the production in the gut of other metabolites, which may be used in the manufacture of brain neurotransmitters, including those linked to mood.

Although this is a relatively new area of research, we know that the gut and brain have developed a unique two-way communication system via a connection called the vagus nerve, which runs from our brain to our gut, allowing messages to be transmitted between the gut and the brain and vice vera.

The diversity of our gut microbiome is directly associated with how much fibre we consume, which in turn is thought to influence this internal text-messaging system. While research is still emerging, growing evidence suggests that supporting a healthy gut microbiome could have profound effects on mood, mental health and positivity.

Easy 5g fibre top-ups

Choosing just two of these to include in each of your meals will easily help you reach 10g of fibre per meal. (See photo overleaf.)

- 75g cooked beans or cooked chickpeas
- 75g cooked lentils
- 100g frozen peas
- ½ avocado
- 80g edamame beans
- 80g raspberries
- 1 large apple
- 1 ½ oranges
- 120g broccoli
- 150g mixed berries
- 150g green beans
- 60g almonds/peanuts/pistachio nuts
- 1 heaped tablespoon flaxseeds
- 1 tablespoon chia seeds
- 1 tablespoon whole hemp seeds
- 15g raw cacao powder
- 50g dark chocolate
- 50g lentil pasta (dry weight)
- 200–250g mixed vegetables
- 50g dark rye bread/pumpernickel bread
- 80g seeded sourdough
- 45g bulgur wheat or whole spelt (dry weight)
- 50g pearl barley (dry weight)
- 40g freekeh (dry weight)
- ½ slice of my Seed and Nut Loaf (page 253)
- 100g hummus
- 150g sweet potato (with skin)
- 6g psyllium husk
- 60g rolled oats
- 25g nutritional yeast

EASY 5G FIBRE TOP-UPS

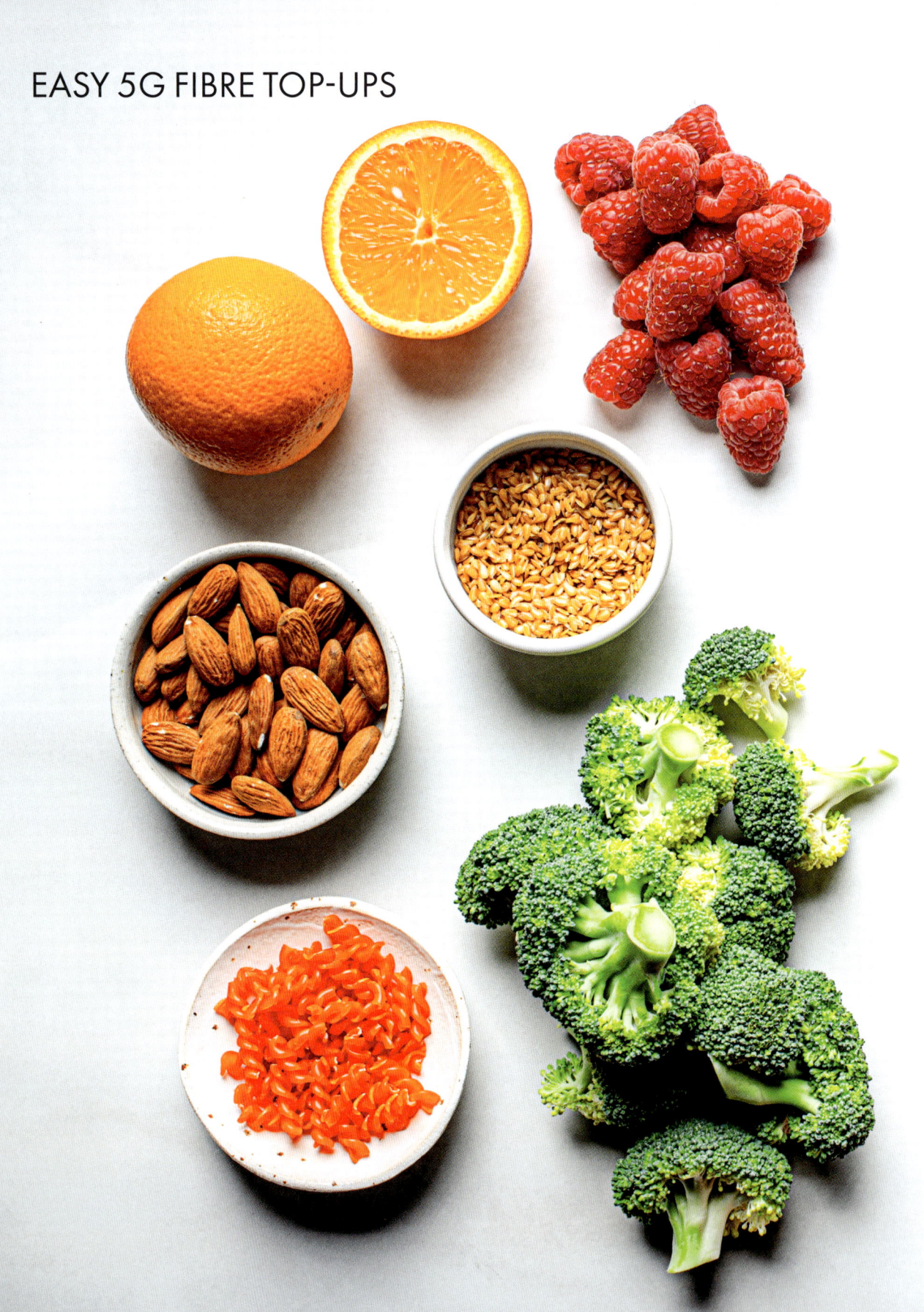

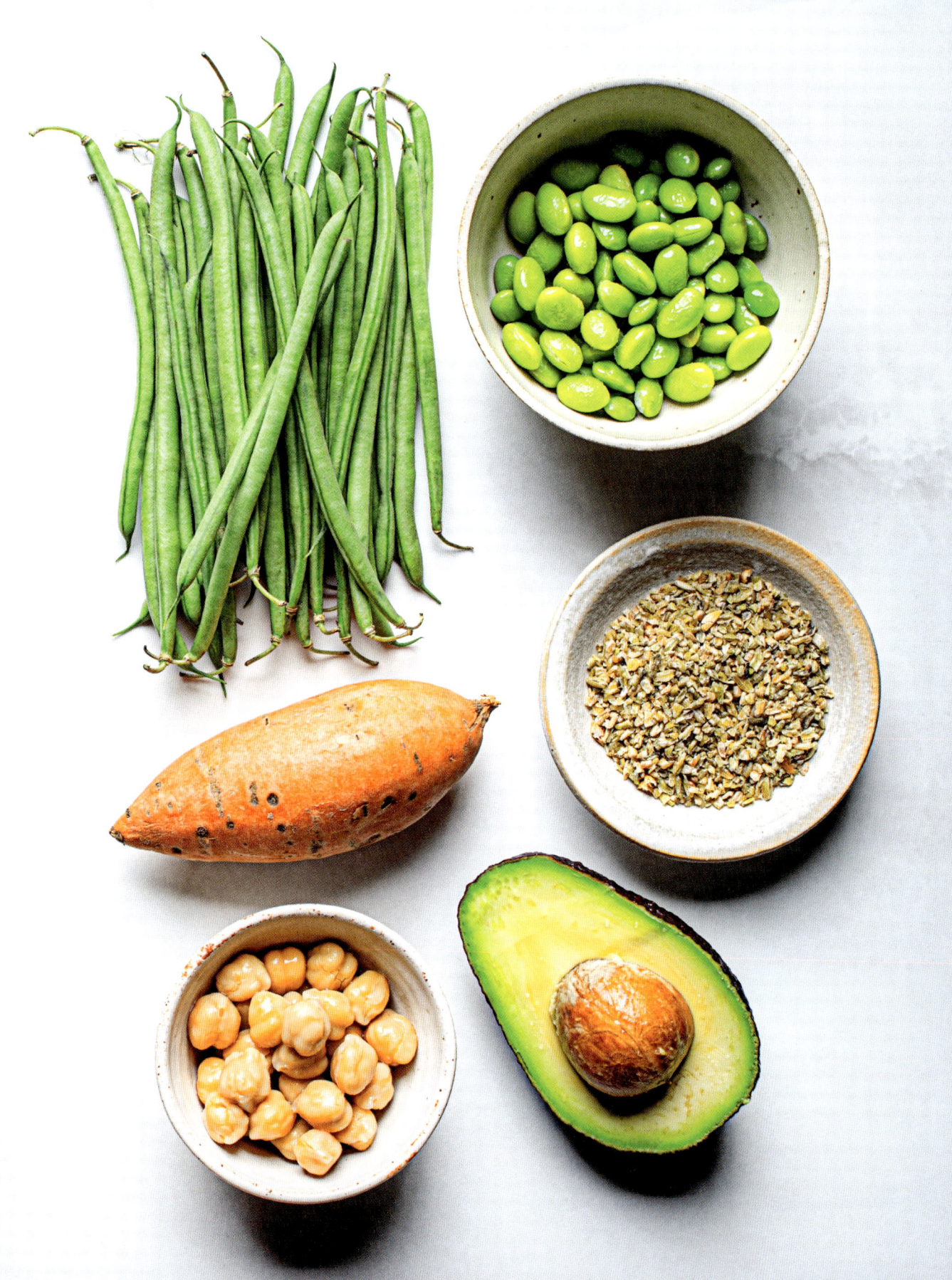

FIBRE SOURCES

The lists below show the average amounts of fibre found in our most frequently used ingredients. Aim to include a diverse range of fibre sources in your meals, to benefit from a wider range of nutrients. See page 303 for more on how I have calculated these quantities.

Vegetables
g fibre/100g raw

- Artichoke hearts 5g
- Aubergine 2g
- Beetroot 1.9g
- Broccoli 4g
- Brussels sprouts 4.1g
- Butternut squash 1.2g
- Cabbage 2.3–4g (depending on type)
- Carrot 2.4g
- Cauliflower 1.8g
- Celery 1.1g
- Courgette 0.9g
- Cucumber 0.7g
- Fennel 2.3g
- Green beans 3.4g
- Kale 3.1g
- Leeks 2.2g
- Lettuce 1.3g
- Mange tout 2.1g
- Mixed vegetables 2.5g
- Onions 2.2g
- Parsnips 4.7g
- Peas 5g
- Peppers (red/green) 2.2g
- Potato 2g
- Radish 0.9
- Rocket 1.7g
- Sauerkraut 2.5g
- Spinach 2.1g
- Swede 0.7g
- Sweet potato 3.5g
- Tomato, cherry 1.3g
- Watercress 1.5g

Fruit
g fibre/100g raw

- Avocado 5g
- Apples 2g
- Banana (mid-ripe) 2g
- Blackberries 3.4g
- Blueberries 1.5g
- Berries, mixed 3.5g
- Cherries 1.6g
- Dates 4g
- Figs 3g
- Kiwi 1.9g
- Melon (cantaloupe) 1.8g
- Nectarine 1.5g
- Oranges 2g
- Passion fruit 3.3g
- Peach 1.5g
- Pears 1.6g
- Plums 1.6g
- Pomegranate 3.4g
- Raspberries 6g
- Strawberries 3.8g
- Watermelon 0.1g

Legumes and pulses
g fibre/100g

- Black beans (cooked) 5.7g
- Chickpeas (cooked) 6g
- Cannellini beans (cooked) 5.6g
- Chickpea pasta (dry) 9.2g
- Edamame beans 7g
- Hummus 5g
- Kidney beans (cooked) 6g
- Lentils (dry) 10–18g (depending on type)
- Lentils (cooked) 6–8g (depending on type)
- Split peas (dry) 20g
- Tofu 1.9g

Grains, breads and whole-food carbohydrates
g fibre/100g

- Bulgur wheat (dry) 8–12g
- Barley (pearl) (dry) 9.6g
- Freekeh (dry) 12g
- Gluten-free bread 8g
- Gluten-free wholemeal bread 10g
- Green pea pasta (dry) 8.8g
- Pasta, wholemeal (dry) 8g
- Pasta, white (dry) 2.5g
- Polenta (dry) 4g
- Porridge oats (dry) 9g
- Quinoa (dry) 7g
- Rye pumpernickel bread 10g
- Rice, black (dry) 3.8g
- Rice, white (dry) 1.1g
- Rice, wholegrain (dry) 3g
- Sourdough bread, white 2.5g
- Soba noodles (100% buckwheat) 3.5g
- Spelt (whole) 11g
- White bread 2.5g
- Wholemeal bread 10g
- Wholemeal sourdough 7g

Nuts and seeds
g fibre/100g

- Almonds 11g
- Almond butter 11.8g
- Brazil nuts 6g
- Cashew nuts 4.3g
- Chia seeds 34g
- Coconut (dried) 13g
- Flaxseeds 22g
- Hazelnuts 6.9g
- Macadamia nuts 8.6g
- Peanuts (roasted) 8.7g
- Pecan nuts 6.3g
- Pistachios 9.8g
- Pumpkin seeds 6.5g
- Sesame seeds (unpolished) 10g
- Sunflower seeds 10g
- Tahini 8g
- Walnuts 5.5g

Other
g fibre/100g

- Cacao powder 30g
- Coffee 0.5-0.75g
- Dark chocolate 10g
- Nutritional yeast 20g
- Popcorn (air popped) 8–12g
- Psyllium husk 85g

PRINCIPLE 4: EAT FATS – BUT THE RIGHT FATS!

There are few food groups that have experienced as much criticism and caused as much confusion as fats. Fats are one of the most important elements of a healthy diet, but we need to focus on eating the right ones. Healthy fats found in oily fish, nuts, seeds and extra virgin olive oil play a crucial role in brain function, heart health and overall wellbeing. However, some saturated fats and those found in ultra-processed foods should be consumed in moderation, as they can have less favourable effects on our health, including increasing cholesterol and our risk of heart disease. Prioritising natural, nutrient-rich sources of fat helps support long-term health and vitality.

Most of the fats we eat form part of our food itself, such as the fats contained in meat, oily fish, eggs, nuts and seeds, cheese, yoghurt, avocados and olives. This means that it is not only the oils we cook with or what we spread on our bread that we need to think about, but also the foods themselves.

Fats, often called lipids, can occur in many forms in our food – some are liquid, others solid. There are three main types of fats: saturated, monounsaturated and polyunsaturated.

In the same way that foods contain a mix of macronutrients, fats also contain a mix of the different fat types. Therefore, almost all foods contain a combination of saturated fats, some monounsaturated fats and some polyunsaturated fats in differing amounts. We tend to classify them by the type of fat that is predominant.

Saturated fats

Saturated fats are primarily found in animal products, including meat and dairy, but they are also present in coconut oil. These fats are solid at room temperature because their structure allows them to pack closely together, making them denser.

The quality of animal fats can vary depending on the animal's diet, welfare and environment, with wild meats often having a more favourable fat profile than farmed alternatives. Wild or grass-fed meats and, to some extent, organic meats, are generally lower in total fats, lower in saturated fats and contain higher levels of omega-3 fatty acids compared to farmed meats.

Since our individual response to saturated fats may differ, there is no one-size-fits-all guideline for intake, with some people being more sensitive than others. Not all saturated fats affect the body in the same way, and their impact depends on the specific fatty acids they contain. It is also important to note that saturated fats may not be created equal! For clarity, it would make sense to reduce our intake of saturated fats found in processed meat products, red meats, tallow and lard, to enjoy butter in moderation, and to reduce cream in our cooking.

Moderate amounts of grass-fed, organic red meat can still be beneficial, though, providing a good source of protein as well as iron, zinc and vitamin B12. Good-quality fresh meat differs nutritionally from processed meats, such as smoked meats, salami and sausages. These are often made using poorer-quality meat and are mostly higher in salt, highlighting the importance of food quality and context.

Fermented dairy products such as yoghurt, kefir and cheese, as well as egg yolks and cacao butter, also contain saturated fats but these are believed to have a smaller effect on our cholesterol compared to red meat, butter or cream. These foods also bring benefits of probiotic gut-friendly bacteria, protein, calcium, vitamin D and even, in the case of eggs, special fats known as phospholipids that support our brain health.

Monounsaturated fats (MUFAs)

These are found abundantly in olive oil and avocado oil, olives and avocados, and many nuts and seeds, such as macadamia nuts, pecans and almonds and sesame seeds. Monounsaturated fats have been associated with lower cholesterol and, in the case of olive oil, are a rich source of antioxidants that protect our cardiovascular system. Olive oil is a rich source of the MUFA oleic acid and is thought to help the liver remove cholesterol more efficiently from the bloodstream. Monounsaturated fats are generally liquid at room temperature, but can solidify slightly when chilled.

Polyunsaturated fats (PUFAs)

PUFAs are mostly found in plants, all nuts and seeds, and their oils, for example sunflower, soya, walnut or rapeseed oil, but are also present in some animal foods, such as eggs and oily fish. Polyunsaturated fats have double bonds in their structure, which create kinks in their chains preventing the molecules from packing tightly together and making them liquid at room temperature. Polyunsaturated fats are also considered heart-friendly, in that they improve the rate that the liver is able to remove cholesterol from the bloodstream. They also contain some plant sterols which may have a small cholesterol-lowering effect.

Omega-3 and omega-6 fatty acids

Omega-3 and omega-6 are forms of polyunsaturated fats that are essential to our health and crucial for our cell membranes and brain tissue. We cannot make these fats ourselves and so they must be eaten as part of our diet.

Omega-6 fats are present in high amounts in nuts and seeds as well as in seed oils, such as rapeseed and sunflower oil. Omega-6 fats are essential for cell membrane structure, energy production, growth, development and skin health. Most modern diets contain an abundance of omega-6 to meet our needs, so we tend to focus more on omega-3, which can become deficient in the diet without care.

Omega-3 fats have been linked with many health benefits, including lowering triglycerides (a type of fat that circulates in our blood) and blood pressure, reducing blood viscosity, as well as forming an integral part of all our cell membranes. They are abundant in our brain and nervous tissue and are vital for brain development, mental health and skin health, as well as for foetal development during pregnancy. They also play a vital role in reducing inflammation in the body.

Deficiency of omega-3 can often go unnoticed but can present as dry, flaky skin, poor memory and focus as well as poor mood, depression and anxiety.

Omega-3 fatty acids can be harder to obtain from our diet, as they are not found in as many foods. The richest source is oily fish, such as sardines, mackerel, anchovies, salmon and herring, where they are in their active forms – eicosapentaenoic acid (EPA) and docosahexaenoic acid (DHA). These active forms arrive in the body ready for action, are easy for the body to utilise and have the most powerful effects. DHA and small amounts of EPA are also present in some algae, making them a plant-based source of these essential fats. Fish at the bottom of the food chain consume algae, which is why their fatty flesh is a good food source of both EPA and DHA.

Plants, such as nuts and seeds, especially chia and flaxseeds, contain a form of omega-3 – alpha linolenic acid (ALA). Although it is still an omega-3, our body needs to convert it into its active forms, EPA and DHA. The human body is an extremely poor convertor when it comes to converting ALA into its active forms, so we need much more from plants to have the same effect in the body. Estimates vary, but studies highlight that possibly only around 5 per cent of the omega-3 we consume from plants is converted into EPA, and even less into DHA.

If you follow a plant-based diet or avoid or dislike oily fish, you may want to consider taking a good-quality vegan algae omega-3 supplement with both DHA and EPA.

CHOLESTEROL

Cholesterol is a waxy, fat-like substance that is essential for our health and is found in all our cell membranes. It also forms the base to many of our hormones, such as cortisol and oestrogen, as well as vitamin D.

When our cholesterol is tested at the doctor's, they are looking at total cholesterol as well as the ratios of high density lipoproteins (HDL) and low density lipoproteins (LDL). We usually refer to our cholesterol as being 'good' (HDL) or 'bad' (LDL), but in reality it is much more nuanced.

Cholesterol and triglycerides (fats) are transported by LDL and HDL, which effectively act as 'taxis'. LDL mostly transports cholesterol from the liver to the rest of the body, whereas HDL mostly carries it back to the liver for removal. So, the more cholesterol and triglycerides we have in our bloodstream the more lipoproteins we will likely need to shuttle them around our body.

Elevated cholesterol has many causes, including our genetics, our lifestyle (e.g. smoking, physical inactivity and obesity), and also our diet, and has been associated with increased risk of heart disease and strokes.

The liver contains LDL receptors (or docking stations) which can act like mini vacuum cleaners, sucking the LDL cholesterol out of the bloodstream. Some foods, such as butter, red meat, tallow and cream, are thought to 'dull' these receptors (a bit like having a sock stuck in the Hoover), whereas foods such as MUFAs and, in particular, PUFAs, are thought to increase the suction power of these receptors.

Diets high in refined carbohydrates and sugars can also impact our cholesterol. This is because excess carbohydrates in the diet are converted into fats (such as triglycerides), and those extra fats will, therefore, also be wanting to grab a LDL taxi to transport them where they need to go.

Some people are genetically more sensitive to the effects of saturated fats and cholesterol in the diet than others. These hyper-responders are less able to regulate their cholesterol levels in response to their diet and can also be more sensitive to foods such as butter, eggs, dairy and meat. This means that there is not simply one approach for everyone, but rather best-practice advice for most people.

The science: why fats matter

We need healthy fats, and a low-fat diet is not sensible or advisable for most people. In fact, many supermarket low-fat alternatives are actually less healthy than their full-fat versions. To restore the creamy, smooth texture lost when reducing fat content, manufacturers often add starches, sugars, stabilisers or emulsifiers to the foods, making them more processed. We do not need to reduce fats, but instead we need to ensure we are eating the right fats.

Fats are an important energy source. Fats contain around 9 kcals per gram as opposed to proteins and carbohydrates, which contain 4 kcals per gram. This often gives them some bad rap, but fats are essential structurally in the body and for so many other reasons listed below.

Fats fill us up. Healthy fats help fill us up and can help regulate our appetite by influencing several hormones in the body that are involved in satiety, as well as potentially slowing gastric emptying. However, the high-fat content and extreme palatability of many UPFs can override this system, so the quality of fats is very important. Skimping or using low-fat products might cause you to reach for a biscuit with a coffee later on, which would be a false economy.

Fats contain fat-soluble vitamins, such as vitamins A, D, E and K, required for our immune system, bone health, blood clotting and skin health, and some act as antioxidants. Fats also facilitate the absorption of fat-soluble plant compounds in our food such as beta-carotene and lycopene, so eating an olive oil dressing with your carrots or tomatoes is beneficial.

Fats support brain and nervous tissue. Fats form the building blocks of our brain and nervous system. Fats are also found in every single one of our 30 trillion cell membranes. These fats give support and structure to our cells, helping to maintain flexibility and facilitate the movement of molecules in and out of the cells. Some lipids, such as omega-3, found in the cell membranes, can help us regulate inflammation. Others make up part of the myelin sheath which surrounds our nerves, acting like the protective plastic coating on electrical wires.

Fat support hormones. Cholesterol is the main building block for a number of steroid hormones in the body, such as cortisol, oestrogen, testosterone and progesterone.

Fats increase flavour and palatability. Fats carry flavours in our food and make them more satisfying to eat, providing that much desired 'mouth feel' and increasing our enjoyment of our meals. If we are satisfied at our mealtimes, we are less likely to snack in between.

Fats are packed with antioxidants. Some oils contain antioxidants, such as polyphenols, which offer numerous health benefits. The most notable and well studied is extra virgin olive oil. Olive oil has been linked to heart and brain health, better blood sugar control, weight management, longevity and reduced inflammation, mostly due to its high concentration of polyphenols.

A balance of healthy fats

We should be eating mostly monounsaturated and polyunsaturated fats. When it comes to saturated fats, some are still a healthy choice, and others require moderation.

The healthiest fats in our diet include:
- Olives
- Avocados
- Nuts, e.g. almonds, Brazils, cashews, hazelnuts, macadamias, pecans, pine nuts, walnuts
- Seeds, e.g. chia, flax, hemp, pumpkin, sesame, sunflower
- Nut butters and tahini
- Fatty fish: sardines, mackerel, anchovies, salmon and herring – think SMASH!
- Oils: extra virgin olive oil, avocado oil, flaxseed oil, hemp oil, cold-pressed rapeseed oil, pumpkin seed oil, sesame oil, walnut oil, cold-pressed sunflower oil

Many animal-based products, despite containing saturated fats, are a rich source of nutrients and so can still have benefits for our health – including eggs, which are a good source of protein, choline, vitamin B 12, iron and zinc; fermented dairy, such as kefir or yoghurt, which contains calcium and beneficial bacteria; as well as poultry and small amounts of good-quality red meat, which contain a wide range of other valuable nutrients, including B vitamins, zinc and iron. I therefore still recommend including these foods as part of a balanced diet.

Fats to eat more sparingly:
- Processed meat, e.g. bacon, sausages, salami
- Butter
- Ghee
- Cream
- Lard
- Tallow
- Coconut oil
- Manu ultra-processed foods, e.g. packaged biscuits, pastries, fried snacks, ready meals, chocolate spreads, and ultra-processed cheese products
- Deep-fried foods

Easy ways to add healthy fats to your plate

- Sprinkle seeds or nuts over meals and salads.
- Aim to eat omega-3-rich fatty fish a few times a week.
- Serve half an avocado on the side of your plate.
- Include olives in your salads and pasta sauces.
- Use extra virgin olive oils or cold-pressed oils in dressings, sauces and dips, or drizzle over roasted vegetables.
- Add almond butter or hazelnut butter to your breakfast or tahini to your dressings.
- Stir chia, flax and hemp seeds through your porridge or yoghurt at breakfast.

THE QUEEN OF OILS: EXTRA VIRGIN OLIVE OIL VS OTHER OILS

One of the healthiest fats we can add to our diet is **extra virgin olive oil**. Extra virgin olive oil contains powerful antioxidant plant compounds called polyphenols, which benefit our body in a number of ways. The more peppery the olive oil tastes, the higher the level of polyphenolic compounds. Olive oil becomes lighter in colour and contains fewer polyphenols the more it is processed and refined. Extra virgin olive oil is the highest quality olive oil, gleaned from the first oil pressing – so it really is the QUEEN of oils in the kitchen. I use it in almost all my cooking, as well as in dressings and sauces. Olive oil also contains vitamins E and K.

Some people still believe that you cannot cook with extra virgin olive oil, but it actually has as high a smoke point as most other oils, with added benefits. Although the healthy polyphenols in extra virgin olive oil may reduce slightly on cooking, those same polyphenols offer added protection to both the oil itself and the food you are cooking, helping reduce heat damage and oxidation. This means that it is the perfect oil to cook with, and it's safe to roast or fry vegetables in extra virgin olive oil at moderate temperatures. If you're cooking at higher temperatures though (for example, searing meat), then you may want to opt for ghee or avocado oil which do have higher smoke points.

Ghee is clarified butter that has been heated to remove much of the water and milk solids, making it more stable at high temperatures, and it is less likely to splutter and burn than butter. Both butter and ghee contain a beneficial substance called butyric acid. This is a short-chain fatty acid (SCFA) like the ones produced by our gut microbes that support the health of our gut lining. **Butter** also contains some vitamin A and D. This means that even though it's a saturated fat, small amounts in the diet can still have benefits.

Coconut oil is high in saturated fats and can raise cholesterol in many people. Some liquid coconut oil is sold as MCT oil or medium-chain triglyceride oil. MCT oil contains shorter-length chain fatty acids which makes it liquid at room temperature and may affect cholesterol less than solid versions.

Avocado oil is a mostly monounsaturated oil, like olive oil. It contains less of the heart-healthy polyphenols than olive oil but is another good choice to cook with, as it has a slightly higher smoke point than olive oil. It also has a more neutral flavour for using in dressings or homemade mayonnaise.

Cold-pressed oils such as **hemp** or **flaxseed oil** are best used in salad dressings and in cold dishes. These are a rich source of ALA and can be a way of topping up our omega-3s.

Cold-pressed rapeseed oil has the slight edge over other vegetable oils (such as sunflower or corn oil), as it has slightly higher levels of omega-3. This can be used where a more neutral flavour is required, e.g. in cakes or mayonnaise.

Aromatic oils, such as **sesame oil**, **pumpkin seed oil** or **walnut oil**, contain mostly polyunsaturated fats and can be used to add flavour to our food. Aside from their deeper, more distinctive flavours, these oils are naturally richer in bioactive plant compounds, such as polyphenols and other antioxidants that support overall health. Sesame oil is great in stir-fries and pumpkin seed oil can be drizzled over soup.

Sunflower oil, **corn oil** and **soybean oil** are all polyunsaturated oils that are widely available. They can support healthy cholesterol and be cardioprotective. Cold-pressed versions are less processed and usually of higher quality.

Oil top tips

- Always buy and store your oils in glass bottles (dark glass if possible), to protect the oils from oxidation or damage. Additionally, glass does not react with the oil, making it a safer option than plastic.

- Oils are sensitive to sunlight and heat, so keep your bottles in a dark place and away from your oven and warm hob. Avoid keeping in direct light, such as on a windowsill.

- Use flaxseed and hemp oils for salads and cold food, as heating them can damage their delicate fats.

- Take care not to reheat oils for deep frying, as this will lead to more oxidation and damage to the fats.

PRINCIPLE 5: PLANT POINTS – 30 IS THE MAGIC NUMBER

Eating at least 30 different plants a week isn't just a trend; it is backed by scientific research. Plants provide fibre, vitamins, minerals, trace elements and phytonutrients essential to our overall health. And our gut microbes don't just like to eat fibre, they thrive on different plant foods. Different microbes enjoy different plants too, so in order to keep all the microbes happy and support the many different strains of bacteria in our microbiome, we need to be eating a lot of different plants. A balanced and flourishing gut ecosystem is critical to our health.

Eating a Mediterranean-style diet, packed with colourful vegetables, herbs, spices, fruits, legumes, nuts, seeds and whole grains, makes it easy to meet your goal. Every time we consume a different plant food, we earn 'plant points', and over the week we are aiming to reach 30 or more. Studies show that those who consume more than 30 different types of plants per week have a healthier, more diverse gut microbiome than those who consume less than 10 types of plants per week. Remember, 30 is just a number. You can always eat more than this!

The science: why plants matter

We don't need to go completely plant-based to reach these goals, but we do need to make plants a big feature on our plate. They provide so many of the vital nutrients and vitamins we need every day.

Plants provide prebiotics. By far the most important reason to add more plants to our diet is the prebiotic fibre they contain. Fibre aids digestion and prevents constipation, but eating a wide range of different plant fibre also supports the diversity of different bacteria, creating a more stable and resilient gut microbiome. A varied gut microbiome supports improved digestion, a stronger immune system and a lower risk of chronic diseases.

Plants contain phytonutrients, including polyphenols. Plants contain thousands of known plant compounds. These can be antioxidant, anti-inflammatory and even antibacterial. One of the most important groups of phytonutrients is called polyphenols. Polyphenols are bioactive plant compounds. Some can act as antioxidants or have anti-inflammatory properties, and many scientists now think some may also promote the growth of certain beneficial gut bacteria, such as Lactobacillus. Polyphenols are found in abundance in colourful fruits and vegetables, olive oil, cacao and berries.

We might recognise some plant phytonutrients as the colours, flavours and smells in our food. Beta-carotene is the orange pigment found in foods like carrots, pumpkins and sweet potatoes. Purple-coloured plants, such as beetroot and blueberries, contain anthocyanins, while lycopene gives foods like tomatoes and watermelons their red colour. Plant compounds that influence the flavour of foods include glucosinolates, which are sulphur-containing compounds in cruciferous vegetables such as broccoli and cabbage that taste bitter or pungent; while oleocanthal in olive oil gives a peppery flavour; and chlorogenic acids in coffee contribute to its bitter astringency. Allicin in garlic is a sulphur-containing compound that gives garlic its distinct smell and taste.

There's magic in plant synergy! Many of the benefits from plants are thought to be amplified when they work together, improving nutrient absorption or enhancing antioxidant effects. A well-known example is where extra virgin olive oil is cooked with tomatoes. This improves the absorption of lycopene, a potent antioxidant in the tomatoes. Similarly, pipirine in black pepper can increase the bioavailability of curcumin from turmeric by up to 2,000 per cent, significantly boosting its anti-inflammatory effects when added to recipes and in our food. Eating healthy fats such as olive oil or avocado with carrots can also increase the absorption of the beta-carotenes they contain. And vitamin C is believed to be more effective when consumed alongside naturally present polyphenols called bioflavonoids found in fruits, which may enhance its benefits.

How to eat more plants

Just a few tweaks to what you are already doing will help you to load up on extra plants with minimal effort. No need to track plant points (see over the page) on a fridge chart, we can make it easier by adjusting how we shop, plan and assemble our meals. Top tips for adding more plant diversity:

- Add a few more fresh herbs to your recipes. Use bunches of chopped herbs in salads.

- Experiment with more spices and mix them into dishes – try cumin, coriander, chilli, turmeric and paprika.

- Sprinkle seeds and nuts on your food, or try my Sunrise Sprinkles and Savoury Seed Mix on pages 110 and 136.

- Use a range of beans and lentils – remember that different beans and different colours of lentils all count as different plants.

- Aim for at least three different vegetables with your main meals.

- Try using different grains as a side dish or in your salads. Freekeh, bulgur wheat, buckwheat and quinoa are all nutrient dense.

- Add new vegetables and fruits to your shopping trolley each week that you may not normally have picked up. Or order yourself a seasonal vegetable box!

HOW TO COUNT YOUR PLANT POINTS

As this is a relatively newer area of science, there's no set way (yet) of calculating exactly how much of each plant makes up a plant point, but the key message is that when we talk about plant points, we're referring to the *variety* of unique plants we consume, rather than quantity.

All plants count towards your plant points – fruits, vegetables, wholegrains, pulses, nuts and seeds, herbs, spices, coffee and even chocolate (see opposite).

We tend to count any amount that we consume of fruits, vegetables, wholegrains, pulses, nuts, seeds and fresh herbs as one point. This means, if you add a few walnuts and some sunflower and pumpkin seeds to your salad, you have successfully added three plant points! But you do need to put your 'no-nonsense hat' on when counting plant points: although technically one raspberry will count as one point, a larger portion will obviously have more benefits. For this reason, dried herbs and spices, coffee and cocoa powder tend to be counted as ¼ point as we eat less of these.

Plants also only count towards your total points the first time you eat them in a given week. If you were to add more walnuts to another salad later in the week – or if you consume broccoli five times or have blueberries for breakfast every day – these will only count as one of your plant points. Eating different versions of the same food, such as a red pepper and a green pepper, would count as two plant points though.

I've calculated the plant points in all my recipes and you'll see them marked at the top of each page – but bear in mind that if you have already eaten one or more of the ingredients that week, the total plant points will be less. I don't actually recommend you count the points in all your meals though, as it is unnecessary if you are eating a balanced diet. And I can assure you that in the recipes in this book, I have the diversity covered for you!

Foods that don't typically count as plant points:

- Plant milks, unless homemade and non-strained.

- Typically, refined grains such as white bread, couscous, white flour, cornflour, white rice and ultra-processed breakfast cereals, as these are usually lower in nutrients and fibre.

- Fruit jams and vegetable chutneys.

- Milk or white chocolate.

Increase your plant diversity

The lists opposite show the six major plant groups that count towards our plant points – plus a few bonus foods. Plant points can include fresh, frozen, tinned or dried foods, but aim for ones that do not contain added sugars. Each of the items listed are counted as 1 plant point per serving, unless stated otherwise.

Vegetables
- Artichokes
- Aubergines
- Bell peppers
- Broccoli
- Brussels sprouts
- Cabbage
- Carrots
- Cauliflower
- Cavolo nero
- Chicory
- Courgettes
- Cucumber
- Endive
- Fennel
- French beans
- Iceberg lettuce
- Kale
- Kohlrabi
- Leeks
- Mangetout
- Marrow
- Mushrooms
- Onions
- Parsnip
- Peas
- Radicchio
- Radishes
- Rocket
- Salsify
- Spinach
- Swede
- Tomatoes
- Turnips
- Watercress

Fruits
- Apples
- Apricots
- Blueberries
- Blackberries
- Cherries
- Dates
- Figs
- Grapefruit
- Kiwi
- Lemons
- Limes
- Melons
- Nectarines
- Oranges
- Peaches
- Pears
- Pomegranates
- Pomelo
- Plums
- Raspberries
- Strawberries

Pulses
- Aduki beans
- Black-eye beans
- Black beluga lentils
- Borlotti beans
- Broad beans
- Cannellini beans
- Chickpeas
- Edamame beans
- Flageolets
- Green lentils
- Haricot beans
- Lima beans/butter beans
- Mung beans
- Pinto beans
- Red lentils
- Puy lentils
- Soya beans
- Tofu

Wholegrains
- Barley
- Black rice
- Buckwheat
- Bulgur wheat
- Freekeh
- Oats
- Quinoa
- Red/black rice
- Rye
- Whole wheat
- Wholegrain bread
- Wholegrain rice
- Wholegrain spelt

Nuts and seeds
- Almonds
- Brazil nuts
- Cashew nuts
- Chia seeds
- Flaxseeds
- Hazelnuts
- Hemp seeds
- Macadamia nuts
- Pine nuts
- Pistachio nuts
- Poppy seeds
- Pumpkin seeds
- Sunflower seeds
- Sesame seeds

Herbs and spices
Large handful of fresh herbs: 1 plant point
Small serving of dried herbs: ¼ plant point
- Basil
- Cardamom
- Chilli
- Chives
- Cinnamon
- Coriander
- Cumin
- Curry powder
- Fenugreek
- Nutmeg
- Oregano
- Parsley
- Rosemary
- Saffron
- Sage
- Thyme

Bonus foods
- Tea, coffee (including decaffeinated), miso, soy sauce = ¼ plant point per serving
- Dark chocolate and unsweetened popcorn – a few squares of dark chocolate eaten a few times a week, or one large handful of unsweetened popcorn = 1 plant point

PRINCIPLE 6: MIND THE GAPS – WHY THE TIMING OF YOUR MEALS MATTERS

The science tells us that spacing out meals and incorporating regular fasting periods may be linked to numerous health benefits, including improved blood sugar regulation, better metabolic health, better weight maintenance, improved sleep quality and a healthier gut microbiome. Time-Restricted Eating (TRE) is an approach to nutrition that has gained widespread recognition for its potential health benefits. Our hunter-gatherer ancestors were only too familiar with feast and famine, and the theory is that if we restrict our eating periods, it allows us to mimic the way we have always eaten and evolved as humans.

TRE involves consuming all our meals within a specific daily eating window, typically ranging from 8 to 12 hours. This means that the remaining hours of the day are dedicated to fasting, allowing the body time to rest and digest. I often recommend a 10–12-hour eating window combined with a 12–14-hour overnight fast, as this rhythm aligns well with the body's natural biological clock – but I also like to go one step further and put more emphasis on healthy balanced meals, less emphasis on snacking and leaving 4–5 hours between each meal.

Following these guidelines, a typical day may look like:
- **Breakfast: 8–9am**
- **Lunch: 1–2pm**
- **Dinner: 6–7pm**

Why gaps are important

My clinical experience has shown me that most people feel better, experience less bloating and find it easier to manage their weight when they leave a longer gap overnight without food and reduce snacking between meals during the day. This might make sense for a number of reasons.

First, it means that we naturally cut back on excess snacking calories between meals, and it prioritises the quality of our meals, which generally become more nutrient-rich.

Additionally, it takes around four hours for food to fully pass through our stomach, which should mean that we can easily go without food between meals – providing we have got our proportions right!

If we focus our attention on eating nourishing, nutrient-rich meals, even sometimes eating more than we currently do at our mealtimes, we are likely to eat fewer nutrient-poor snacks in between. Over the course of a day this could mean we swap the estimated 500 kcals a day we dedicate to snacks (see pages 14–15) for higher-quality foods containing more nutrients, fibre, protein and healthy fats. This means that we are fuelling and nourishing ourselves better over a 24-hour period and bringing in more of the macro and micronutrients that fire up our body.

It can support weight management. Benefits are often seen in terms of healthier weight management and improved metabolic health, including blood sugars control. When the body is not digesting food, it looks for other sources of energy. Initially, the body draws on its glycogen reserves, but as these deplete it can start moving on to the fat stores, which release ketones that the body can use as an alternative fuel.

Supports a diverse microbiome. Having a break overnight can improve microbial diversity and composition by allowing a beneficial shift in our microbiota. It is thought it can promote the growth of certain bacteria, for example species like Akkermansia muciniphila, which as their name suggests are important for the health of the mucus (mucin) layer that protects our gut lining, and are also important for our metabolic health.

Helps support gut lining integrity. The gut lining (epithelium), which is just one cell thick, undergoes constant renewal. Animal studies suggest that this regeneration speeds up when the gut is at rest. Alongside regeneration of the protective mucus layer, this helps to maintain the integrity of both the gut barrier and the mucus layer. This process ensures the gut barrier is able to select exactly which substances it absorbs and prevents larger 'unwanted' molecules from reaching the bloodstream.

Promotes better-quality sleep. Eating late in the evening can not only disrupt our sleep quality and our natural circadian rhythm, but may also disrupt our blood sugar control overnight.

Inflammation and snacking

It might surprise you, but every time we eat food, we initiate a mild inflammatory reaction in our gut. This is a normal reaction, because eating food is quite a risky business for the gut: a game of roulette where we unwittingly invite bacteria, viruses and fungi along with our food into the body, requiring our immune system to decipher and make decisions about what is friend and what is foe. But our choice of food can also initiate inflammation.

In a healthy body, inflammation subsides between meals, and overnight too; but it is now thought that constant grazing on unhealthy foods has the potential to disrupt these resolution periods, especially in those with poor gut health or obesity, contributing to longer states of inflammation.

It is an area of science that we are still learning about, but it appears that specific dietary fats, ultra-processed foods, and to a slightly lesser extent sugar, appear to drive this inflammatory response the most. In contrast, fibre-rich vegetables and lean protein foods are associated with less inflammation. Eating a colourful, natural, whole-food diet and reducing snacking on convenience foods could be one of the simplest ways to support gut health and lower inflammation in the body.

YOUR STOMACH IS LIKE A WASHING MACHINE

I often compare the stomach to a washing machine because they function in remarkably similar ways. When we load clothes into the drum, the machine fills with water and detergent to help break down dirt. It then churns the clothes, thoroughly cleaning them before moving on to the rinse cycle.

Our stomach operates in much the same way. It fills with hydrochloric acid and digestive enzymes, which work together to break down food over the course of 2–4 hours. Once digestion is complete, the food moves into the small intestine, where nutrients are further broken down and absorbed, followed by a clever 'rinse cycle' which I will explain in a moment.

Just as we wouldn't keep opening a washing machine mid-cycle to toss in a dirty towel and expect everything to come out clean, our stomach functions best when given the time to digest a meal properly. Constantly adding more food before the previous meal has been processed can overload the system, making digestion less efficient. Allowing the stomach to complete its work before introducing more food may support a smoother digestion with less bloating.

The dance of the small intestine – the rinse cycle

Did you know that your small intestine loves it when we leave gaps between meals? It takes around 90 minutes to 3 hours after a meal for our small intestine to set up for a deep clean and rinse cycle once the stomach has emptied. We call this the migrating motor complex, or MMC for short. The MMC is where the small intestine and the villi start to rhythmically pulse in a downward motion, sweeping all unwanted food debris, bacteria and waste matter through to the large intestine. This is the body's way of cleaning up after our last meal, and also occurs at night. Constant snacking can interfere with this process, delaying this important part of our digestion.

The problem with frequent snacking

Many people turn to snacks to boost energy levels, but frequent snacking may be a sign that the previous meal lacked sufficient calories or was not properly balanced. As we know, grazing can upset our blood sugar regulation, and quick-fix snacks are often high in refined carbohydrates and sugars but low in fibre and essential nutrients. Relying on these foods to meet our nutritional requirements may mean that we are short-changing our body, making it harder for us to meet our nutritional goals over the course of a day.

Reducing snacking can be something that a lot of my clients struggle with at first, or they believe eating little and often is a healthier way to eat. Many people also believe that reducing calories at meals will help them stay in shape, but what I have seen in clinic is the opposite! When we consume insufficient calories or nutrients at mealtimes, we are more likely to feel deprived, which can lead to us eating more later in the day. By focusing on balanced, nutrient-dense meals and reducing unnecessary snacking, you can support stable energy levels, improved digestion and better metabolic health.

Choosing a healthy, balanced snack isn't harmful to our health in itself, but constant grazing on high-calorie, low-nutrient foods can be – and those extra grazing calories can quickly add up. Regular snacking interferes with the body's natural hunger cues, increasing the likelihood of over-eating, while also leading to stronger food cravings, mood swings and energy crashes, creating a cycle of dependency on fast-digesting, low-nutrient foods.

Does snacking always lead to weight gain? Not exactly . . .

Ultimately, weight gain occurs when we consistently consume more calories than we expend. Technically, someone who snacks frequently but still maintains a calorie deficit will lose weight. However, snacking makes over-eating more likely due to its effects on blood sugar control and hunger regulation.

How to leave more space between meals

The most important step is to find timings that work for you. In an ideal world, we want to aim to finish eating at least 2–3 hours before we jump into bed. This allows time for our food to have left our stomach and for our digestive tract to have a well-earned rest while we sleep.

If you finish your evening meal at 7pm, try not to eat your breakfast before 7am or, better still, 9am the next day, to give you a full 14 hours – but see what feels intuitive to you.

Don't worry if you don't manage this every night – the art is to start forming habits that we stick to most of the time. Making a conscious effort not to eat after our evening meal also helps to reduce those late-night snacks.

What can you have between meals?

Ideally, we should aim to not snack between meals, most of the time. If you typically have a snack around 4pm, try shifting your snack to immediately after lunch to see if it helps reduce the need for additional snacks later in the day. Focus on eating enough at mealtimes so that you feel satisfied and energised between meals.

Don't forget to stay hydrated throughout the day: water, herbal teas, black tea and green tea are great options to enjoy at any time between meals – but save the frothy lattes or other milk-based drinks for with your breakfast or as an after-lunch treat. Remember that decaffeinated coffee offers almost all the same health benefits as caffeinated.

When a snack is the right thing!

Not everyone responds to fasting or snacking in the same way. Individuals with higher energy needs, such as athletes, pregnant or breastfeeding women, those with poor blood sugar control or those with physically demanding jobs, or who are underweight, may benefit from incorporating nutrient-rich snacks into their routine, so listen to your body. If you have specific needs, such as a weakened immune system or chronic fatigue, your nutritional approach may need to be different too. If you have Type-1 diabetes, a pre-existing condition, or take medications that affect blood sugar, always consult your doctor before making dietary changes.

Also, if your gaps between meals are too long, or you are having a busier day than usual, of course have a snack! If you are feeling dizzy or light-headed this could be a sign that your blood sugars are lower than normal, in which case a healthy snack would be the right approach.

Remember, health and nutrition are all about consistency and doing the right things most of the time. As soon as things get restrictive, we are more likely to give up. In this case, choosing a balanced snack which is low in sugar and rich in proteins and fibre might be what you need.

If you do need a healthy snack – here are some of my favourites:
- A slice of seeded bread with cream cheese and grated radish
- Greek yoghurt and berries
- Vegetable sticks with hummus (page 269)
- Chia pudding (page 125) or a small portion of one of my breakfast recipes
- A handful of nuts with an apple
- Celery filled with almond butter
- See page 88 for more ideas

THE SIX PRINCIPLES, AT A GLANCE

Principle 1: It's all about proportion
A balanced plate means balanced nutrition. Aim for your main meals to comprise ¼ protein, ½ vegetables and ¼ healthy carbs, and include some healthy fats. By maintaining the right proportions, you will feel fuller for longer and shut down the food noise.

Principle 2: Prioritise protein
Build your plate around the protein and aim for 30g with every meal. Proteins are essential for almost every function in the body, and eating adequate protein triggers hormones that increase satiety and keep us from snacking. Include plenty of plant-based proteins too, to benefit from their added health benefits.

Principle 3: Focus on fibre
A fibre-rich diet is linked to improved health markers in almost every area, and our microbiome thrives on the prebiotics in fibre. Aim for 10g fibre with every meal, from a combination of vegetables, fruits, pulses, nuts and seeds, and whole-food carbohydrates.

Principle 4: Eat fats – but the right fats!
Fats often get a bad rap, but we need fats in our diet to support our brain health, heart health, hormones and so much more! They need to be mostly healthy fats though, so aim to include extra virgin olive oil, nuts and seeds, avocados and oily fish in your meals.

Principle 5: Plant points – 30 is the magic number
Plants provide fibre, vitamins, minerals, trace elements and phytonutrients essential to our overall health – and our gut bacteria love diversity. Aim to consume 30+ different plants each week. Vegetables, fruit, nuts and seeds, pulses, wholegrains, herbs and spices, and even coffee and chocolate, all count!

Principle 6: Mind the gaps – why the timing of your meals matters
Aim for three meals a day, spaced 4–5 hours apart, without snacking, and 12–14 hours fasting overnight. Having proper gaps between meals is linked to numerous health benefits, including less bloating, improved blood sugar regulation, better metabolic health, better weight maintenance, improved sleep quality and a healthier gut microbiome.

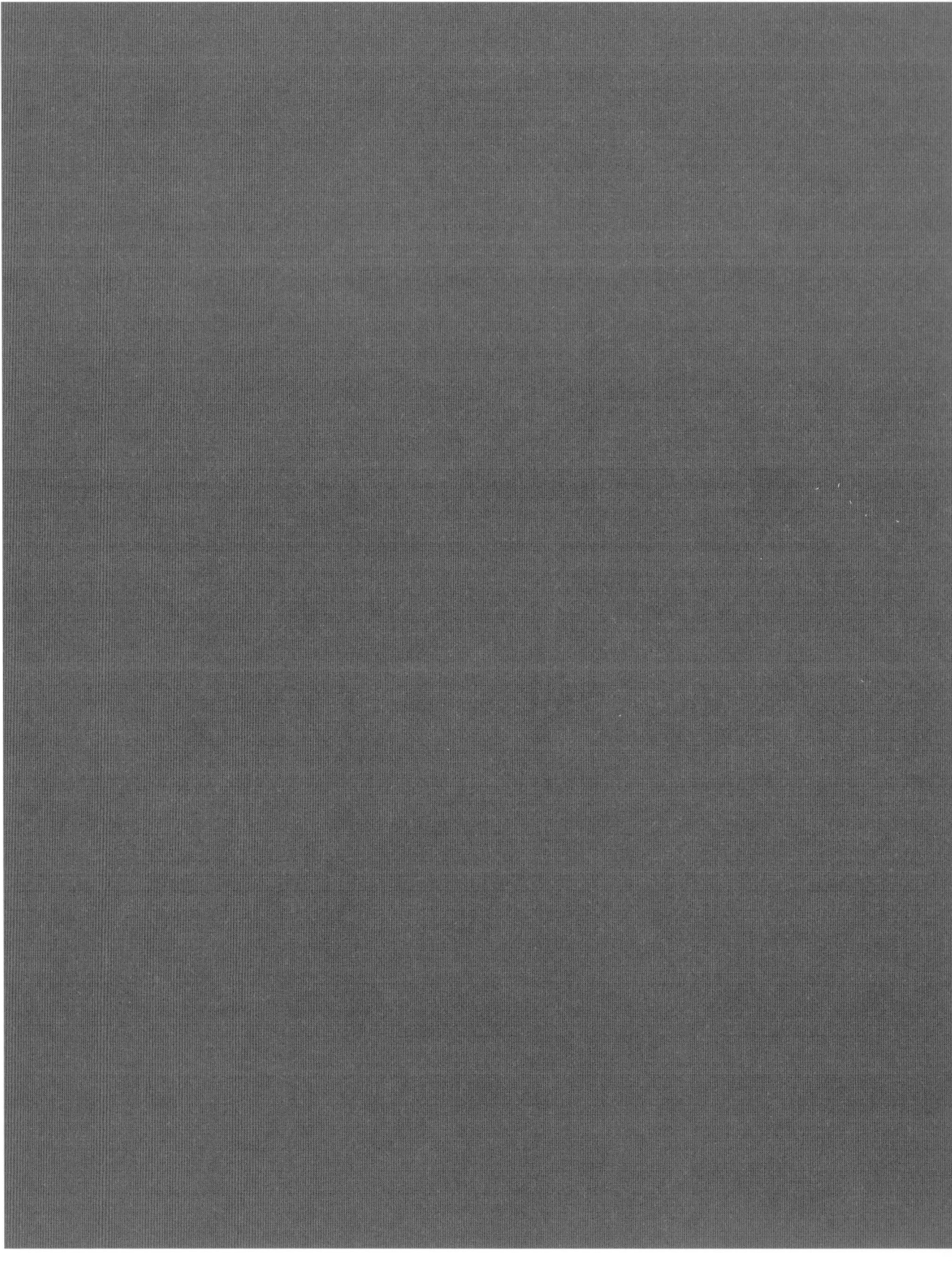

NO-NONSENSE COOKING & MEAL PLANNING

'Don't try to eat the elephant all in one bite' is a metaphor I often share with clients who are beginning their journey towards healthier eating. Diving in headfirst can work for some but, more often than not, we can quickly return to our old habits once the initial enthusiasm has faded.

While the word 'longevity' might feel overused, it simply means that the choices we make today shape the story of how we age. There are no guarantees, but what we eat, how we move, the quality of our sleep, and how we manage stress are all powerful indicators of our long-term health. Prioritising these things now can help us stay healthier, stronger and more vibrant for longer.

When it comes to implementing the advice in this book, you can move freely through the recipes, choosing any breakfast, lunch or dinner knowing that they will all work well together every day. Each recipe (apart from the breads and treats in the final chapter) is perfectly balanced to help you reach your daily protein and fibre goals, as well as including healthy fats and carbohydrates, and they will more than meet your 30 plant points per week.

There are no medals for cooking all the recipes in record time or following my meal planners (on pages 96–99) to the letter. Go at your own pace.

Making healthy eating part of your life

One of the most common reasons people say they struggle with eating more healthily is that it takes more time. I know that eating well needs to fit in with our busy lives, otherwise it won't stick. That's why most of my recipes are very quick to prepare – some take just 5 minutes to put together! I also have a few tricks that I use in my own kitchen to save time.

Make-one-take-one

My 'make-one-take-one' philosophy is a way of maximising leftovers and means I only need to cook once each day. When I'm preparing a recipe and the oven or pan is already hot, I might cook an extra salmon fillet to use in a salad the next day, or I make more of my hard vegetable salads than I need (such as the Broccoli, Hazelnut and Cranberry Salad on page 171), knowing that they will last for up to three days in the fridge. This simple habit makes it easier to maintain a healthy lifestyle, especially on busier days, and means I always have something healthy in the fridge ready to eat. You would be surprised how many meals you can create around your leftovers, padding them out with fresh foods into a whole new meal. (See also how to put together a perfect plate, on pages 92–95.)

Batch cooking

Batch cooking is perfect for keeping in the fridge or freezing portions of soups, chillies, curries and casseroles – you can double-up quantities and/ or prepare them in advance when you have more time. Often on a Sunday – or whenever

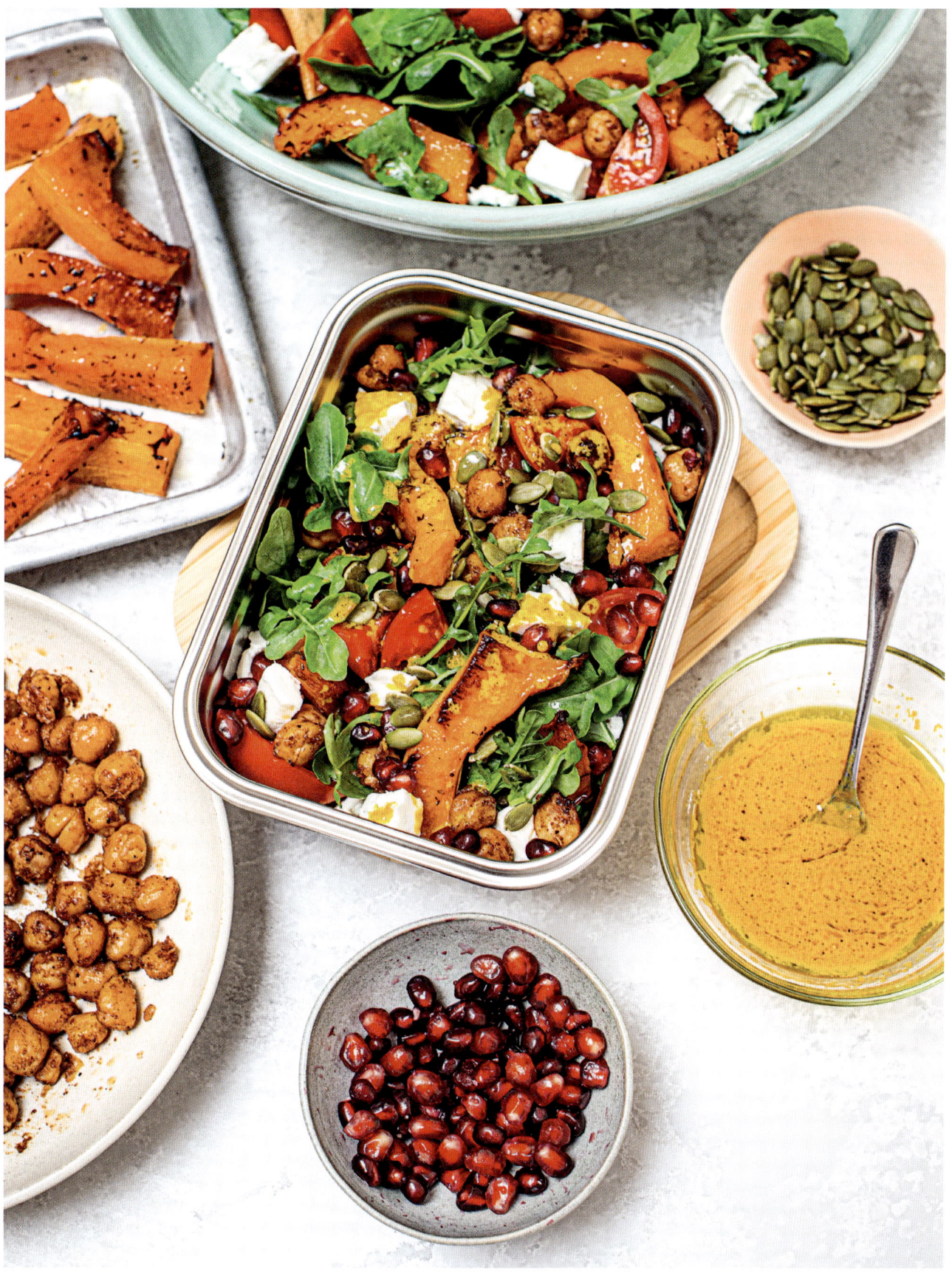

the oven is already on – I love to throw in a couple of trays of vegetables drizzled with olive oil, sea salt and herbs. Red onions, carrots, beetroot, butternut squash, Brussels sprouts and Mediterranean vegetables all work well. They can become the base for a salad with feta or mozzarella cheese, or a side with leftover meat or fish, beans, lentils or tofu. As with make-one-take-one, it's another great way of always making sure you have food that can be put on the table in a flash, especially when you don't have the time or energy to cook from scratch.

Storage

I use stainless steel or glass containers to store my food in the fridge or freezer or to pack up and take with me. Glass and stainless steel are non-toxic, making them healthier and more sustainable choices than plastics. If you use heat-resistant glass containers, you can also pop them straight into the oven to reheat your food. On cooler days, I love taking a food flask with me too, so that I can enjoy a warm, home-cooked meal even when I am on the go.

Save your jam jars!

Jam jars and old glass bottles are ideal for mixing dressings and storing small amounts of leftovers. I keep leftover cooked grains, mayonnaise, sauces and soups in glass jars that have once been home to pickles, beans or jams.

Vegetarian, vegan and dairy-free diets

One thing the science makes clear is that the more plants we include in our diet, the better it is for our health. Although my recipes mostly contain all food groups, since no-nonsense nutrition is centred around fibre and protein, it naturally features plenty of plant-based foods. If you are following an exclusively vegan or vegetarian diet, then it is still possible to meet all your dietary requirements, but it is a good idea to consider certain nutrients to make sure they are not lacking. Below is the advice I give to my clients, but always consult with your own doctor if you are worried about your vitamin and mineral levels, or to discuss the specifics of your diet.

Vitamin B 12 is a B vitamin that is found only in animal foods, such as meat, fish, eggs and dairy. I recommend it is supplemented on plant-based and vegan diets – and it is still advisable on a vegetarian diet. Vitamin B 12 is necessary for a healthy nervous system, brain health, DNA synthesis and mood, and a lack of B 12 can result in a form of anaemia called megaloblastic anaemia, where the red blood cells become enlarged, leading to fatigue and muscle weakness.

Vitamin D. We manufacture most of our vitamin D in response to sunlight under our skin, and for this reason it is recommended that everyone in the northern hemisphere takes a vitamin D supplement throughout the winter, when the sun's rays are mostly too weak to stimulate its production. We can obtain limited amounts of vitamin D from some foods, including butter, egg yolks, mushrooms and oily fish – however, it would be very unlikely to be enough to meet our daily needs. Many people need to take vitamin D all year round to keep levels in a healthy range. Our genetics, skin tone, our clothing and the amount of time we spend outdoors can all impact our natural vitamin D production. Vitamin D is necessary for our bone density, as it helps us to absorb and utilise calcium and phosphorus, but it also plays a role in our immunity and mental health.

Selenium is essential for our thyroid gland and our immune system, and it protects our cells from oxidative damage. It can be found in legumes and wholegrains – but it can usually be covered by adding just one Brazil nut to your diet daily!

Iodine plays a key role in our energy metabolism, growth and development. It is mostly found in animal foods such as dairy, meat, eggs, fish and shellfish. Vegetables are not a reliable source of iodine, however it is found in significant amounts in some seaweed, such as nori or kelp. Iodine may require supplementation on plant-based diets, up to 140mcg daily. Dairy is a key contributor to iodine in the UK diet, yet with more people switching to plant-based milks (which are mostly not fortified with iodine), more people, especially adolescents, may be vulnerable to developing a deficiency.

Iron is an essential nutrient and a key component in our haemoglobin, found in our red blood cells. Meat and fish contain good amounts of iron that is easier for us to absorb and utilise in the body, but some plant foods are also a source. Women in particular, due to their menstrual losses, can become depleted on plant-based diets if they are not eating sufficient beans, lentils, nuts and seeds, tofu and dark leafy vegetables. As a bonus, iron is also found in dark chocolate.

Zinc is key to over 300 enzyme reactions in the body, and is essential for a healthy immune system, cellular repair, DNA synthesis and fertility, and a times of rapid growth, such as in children or during pregnancy. Zinc from plant foods may be less well absorbed by the body than zinc from animal sources, so people following plant-based diets may need to consume slightly more zinc to cover requirements. Plant-based sources of zinc include seeds, nuts, wholegrains and legumes.

Calcium is a main component of our bones and teeth and is essential for our muscle contractions and nervous system. Tofu, fortified plant milks, green leafy vegetables, nuts, seeds and legumes are good plant-based sources.

Omega-3 fatty acids. If you aren't eating oily fish, such as sardines, mackerel or salmon, you will need to find different ways to meet your omega-3 fatty acids requirements. Flaxseed or hemp oil can help support levels of omega-3 in our body – however, these may not be sufficient as your sole dietary source. Plant algae supplements can be a more reliable form of omega-3 fats, as they can be found in algae in the forms EPA and DHA, which we know are the easiest forms for the body to use. (See page 62 for more on omega-3.)

Protein. People often worry that they won't be able to meet their protein goals while following a plant-based, vegan or vegetarian diet. It is absolutely possible to obtain all the protein we need without consuming animal products – and many of the recipes in this book are entirely plant-based – however, we cannot afford to be complacent. It is vital that we (all) include plenty of protein-rich plant foods, such as beans, lentils, tofu, seitan, nuts and seeds in our diets. While it is always better to get protein from whole foods, protein powders can be a helpful and convenient way of topping up protein too, but it is important to look at the formulation carefully to check that it is a high-quality formulation, and I generally don't recommend these as a protein source unless your diet is likely to be low, you need a quick breakfast or snack, or you have higher protein requirements (e.g. you do a lot of sport). Remember, too, that sourdough bread, oats, freekeh, quinoa and wheat pasta also contain some protein, which all counts towards daily goals. You can mix and match any of the plant-based foods shown in the protein lists on page 49, and you're welcome to make additions and swaps to any of my recipes. See also page 45 for my quick 10g protein top-up ideas.

Non-dairy yoghurts are usually made from coconut or almond milk and can be lower in protein than their dairy alternatives. Soya milk yoghurts often have slightly more protein. Plant-based yoghurts are also generally more processed than cow's milk yoghurts, so it is advisable to read the labels and opt for those with fewest additives. These can still be good options, though, for those who avoid dairy.

Vegan cheeses can add flavour and texture to a dish; however, their quality can vary greatly. Some fall under the label of ultra-processed foods, due to the way they are made and the ingredients they contain. Soft cheeses made from cashew nuts or almonds fare better, and some are fortified with nutrients such as calcium, vitamin D and vitamin B12. Many vegan hard cheeses, though, are made from a combination of coconut oil and starches, and some contain virtually no protein at all. This means that while they might offer flavour or texture, they may be of little nutritional value.

Plant-based milks. As a rule of thumb, plant milks are fine to use as an alternative to dairy. Soya milk is the most similar nutritionally to cow's milk, but really it is down to personal preference. Try to choose one with added vitamins and minerals, such as vitamin D, calcium, iodine, and vitamins B2 and B12. Look for plant milks with minimal ingredients; try to avoid ones that contain emulsifiers, stabilisers, thickeners and added sugars.

Vegan meat products. The levels of food processing and the increased number of ingredients necessary to make meat-like products can mean that some can be highly processed, so read the ingredients list carefully as some are better than others. Healthier choices might be tofu (see more on tofu opposite), seitan, tempeh, beans and lentils, as these are minimally processed and can be great sources of protein.

Swapping meat or fish for cauliflower steaks, jackfruit, oyster mushrooms or watermelon steaks is a creative way of using vegetables, but it is still important to add the protein from other food groups at the same meal, otherwise you may find yourself feeling hungry again two hours after eating.

A word on tofu. Tofu is made from soya beans and has high levels of protein (around 16g protein/100g). Soya beans are special because they contain all nine of the essential amino acids, making tofu a complete protein and a great addition to the diet. Some tofu is calcium-set and provides significant amounts of calcium per serving, which is important on a plant-based diet without dairy. If calcium is a priority, check for calcium on the label.

Tofu takes on the flavours of a dish and lends itself beautifully to Asian cooking. It crisps up when marinated and fried in cubes and can be used in curries and stir-fries and added to soups. Tofu can also be used to replace cheese, chicken and fish in recipes. See my recipes for Sticky Tofu Noodles (page 211) and Tofu Scramble (page 122). Silken tofu can be blended into smoothies.

Vegetarian labels. I have added a label (V) to my recipes that are suitable for vegetarians. Please note, though, that traditional Parmesan cheese is made using animal rennet, however vegetarian Parmesan-style cheeses are available, made with vegetarian rennet. Although many supermarket cheeses are now made using vegetarian rennet, some cheeses are still made by traditional methods – including some goat's cheeses, Manchego, burrata, mozzarella, halloumi and feta. Always check that the cheese you are using is 'suitable for vegetarians', as animal rennet may not be included in the ingredients list.

Simple plant-based swaps

- Instead of halloumi cheese, use crispy tofu, tempeh or seitan.
- Swap chicken for tofu in curries and stir-fries.
- Mince can be replaced in recipes with Puy or green lentils.

Remember to ADD more foods when following a plant-based approach, to compensate for any foods you have taken out!

- Add beans and lentils to dhal, curries and even stir-fries.
- Add chickpeas and lentils to salads and soups and use them freely in dips.
- Use beans to thicken sauces for pasta, and replace pasta with beans in recipes.
- Have crispy beans, edamame beans, nuts and seeds as healthy snacks (see my Crispy Edamame Beans and Chilli and Lime Cashews on pages 276 and 279).
- Add nuts and seeds to your breakfasts and salads, and sprinkle them over your main meals (see my Sunrise Sprinkles and Savoury Seed Mix on pages 110 and 136).
- Add a handful of nuts and seeds or nut butter to your yoghurt or porridge.
- Add sunflower seeds to rice dishes.
- Make crispy tofu as a topping for your beans and soups.

Gluten-free? No problem

Almost all the recipes in this book can easily be adapted to become gluten-free, simply by swapping out one or more of the ingredients. I've labelled some of my recipes as gluten-free (G) if they can be made gluten-free with a simple switch, which I have included in the ingredients list.

For example, many of my breakfast recipes use oats, but choosing gluten-free oats instantly makes these recipes completely gluten-free. In the same way, all my bread recipes can be made gluten-free by switching the oats to gluten-free oats. Some are already gluten-free, such as my Red Lentil Bagels (page 267), Naked Loaf (page 258) and Gluten-free Flatbreads (page 264). If you cannot tolerate oats in any form, buckwheat, millet or quinoa flakes may be used instead.

When it comes to grains, there are plenty of gluten-free grains you can choose, such as quinoa, buckwheat, millet or amaranth which can be used in my Grain and Lentil Healthy Carb Mix (page 159). Buckwheat, despite its name, is gluten-free and is classed as a pseudocereal. It forms the base of soba noodles, which I serve with my Prawn Fishcakes (page 206) and in the Sticky Tofu Noodles (page 211) – do check they are 100% buckwheat and gluten-free though, as brands vary.

It's important to be aware that some naturally gluten-free grains (such as oats) may be grown, harvested or processed alongside other gluten-containing grains, which means they can become cross-contaminated. If your sensitivity to gluten is severe (such as in coeliac disease), look for a gluten-free certification on the packets.

For clarity, gluten-containing grains include wheat, barley, rye, spelt, emmer, einkorn (farro), Khorasan wheat and freekeh, as well as kitchen staples made from them, such as regular bread, breakfast cereals, pasta, semolina and couscous. Also flours, and any foods containing them, including many processed and ultra-processed foods, such as biscuits and cakes.

Naturally gluten-free alternatives:
- Gluten-free oats
- Gluten-free flour/chickpea (gram) flour/cornflour
- Green pea or red lentil pasta/gluten-free wholegrain pasta
- Quinoa
- Amaranth
- Millet
- Black, red and wholegrain rice
- Edamame/black bean noodles
- Soba noodles (100% buckwheat)
- Buckwheat groats
- Lentils
- Tamari sauce (a naturally gluten-free alternative to soy sauce)
- Dijon mustard is mostly gluten-free, but most English mustards contain gluten so do check

Organised snacks vs constant grazing

My no-nonsense philosophy focuses on properly balanced healthy meals to reduce the need to snack in between. But I also want to make it clear that there is a difference between mindless snacking and organised snacking. Organised snacking is like a balanced mini meal to keep us going from one meal to the next. It can help us get through from lunch at 1pm to dinner at 7pm – this six-hour window might just be too long if you have had a busy day or want to go to the gym after work. Organised snacks can help keep our energy and mood more stable – and can help top up our nutrients, too. Rather than simply hitting us with a rush of sugar or carbohydrates, an organised snack can keep our energy on an even keel, without sabotaging our good intentions.

Mindless snacking – or grazing – on the other hand, catches us out when our energy is low or cravings are high. Or maybe we are just feeling a little jaded or under-stimulated, and a snack may lighten our mood. It makes the sugary snacks and higher-carb convenience foods seem more appealing, and we end up eating them to give us a quick energy boost. It's not necessarily about eating more food than we need; it is that the foods we choose may not leave us feeling our best, and it can form a pattern of eating that is hard to break.

Case study 1: Emma starts the day with a bowl of cereal and a cup of coffee but is ravenous mid-morning at work and can't resist the pastries at the meeting and an extra cappuccino. This fills her up for a while, but by lunchtime she is feeling unsatisfied and hungry again and buys herself a lower-calorie sandwich and drink (as she thinks she might have eaten too much earlier). Again, the cravings set in a couple of hours later, and she finds herself grabbing a hot chocolate from the vending machine and a packet of crisps. On the way to the train station, she picks up a small bag of chocolate raisins (partially healthy, she figures) to keep her going. She cooks a balanced, nutritious meal, but finds herself nibbling on some snacks while she is watching TV. Does this sound familiar?!

Case study 2: Claire starts the day with her gut-boosting breakfast (page 118), with 30g of protein and 10g of fibre, and sets off to work. Feeling energised and satisfied, the biscuit selection at the meeting looks less appealing. Four hours later and still thriving from her breakfast, Claire is happy to wait in the queue to get her healthy falafel salad bowl (with the most amazing dressing), which she takes back to the office, allowing herself a lovely cup of tea and finishing off her meal with an apple. She knows she is going to the gym after work, so she has planned a snack to keep her going, as she knows she won't eat dinner until 7.30pm, six hours after her lunch. She has packed herself a snack pot containing some chopped carrots and peppers and a couple of hard-boiled eggs, which leaves her feeling powered-up for exercise. She comes home to make a stir-fry with chicken and the veggies she has in her fridge. After a couple of squares of dark chocolate, her treat straight after her meal, she doesn't feel the need for any more snacks.

By not getting on the blood sugar rollercoaster in the morning, Claire manages to dodge some of the energy slumps and cravings that could have upset her energy and general wellbeing throughout the day. She still made space for a snack, but as she was less driven by the quick fix, she was able to make healthier choices.

20 SNACKS THAT WILL BOOST YOUR ENERGY AND PRODUCTIVITY

- Greek yoghurt with a handful of nuts and blueberries
- Strawberries and cottage cheese (with a grind of black pepper!)
- Two oatcakes with avocado and cheese slices
- Half an avocado with prawns and dressing
- Crispy Edamame Beans (page 276)
- Two hard-boiled eggs with vegetable sticks
- Leftover veggies with hummus
- Celery sticks filled with cream cheese or peanut butter
- Hemp and Chocolate Shake (page 147)
- Creamy Chocolate Chia Pudding (page 125)
- Rosemary and Sea Salt Seeded Crackers with Whipped Feta and Bean Dip (pages 261 and 175)
- A slice of Super Green Bread (page 254) with smoked mackerel and cucumber
- Apple slices with cheese squares or almond butter
- Apple, Carrot and Walnut Flapjacks (page 274)
- A handful of roasted pumpkin and sunflower seeds
- Mini mozzarella balls with cherry tomatoes, Green Pesto (page 205) and Rosemary and Sea Salt Seeded Crackers (page 261)
- A small bowl of soup with beans
- Egg Muffins (page 272)
- Chilli and Lime Cashews (page 279)
- Rosemary and Sea Salt Seeded Crackers with hummus and vegetable sticks (pages 261 and 269–271)

Snacking rules

If you're having a snack immediately after lunch or dinner, this is when you can go sweet – dark chocolate or a bliss ball (page 290), chocolate fudge (page 284), Salted Caramel Bars (page 282) or dates with chocolate hazelnut spread (page 289) can be eaten here. If you consume them directly after your meal, the sweeter snack will have a duller effect on our blood sugars than if we were to eat it mid-afternoon on an empty stomach. If you are snacking between meals, go savoury and you will probably feel better for it.

Let's go shopping!

When you start making my recipes, you'll probably find yourself hanging out in the veg aisle more than you used to, and reading the backs of labels on the items in your basket. There's an incredible amount of healthy ingredients available to us today, and it makes shopping and cooking healthily so much easier – and more enjoyable!

All forms of cooking, soaking, transport and storage can affect the nutritional quality of our food. Some losses are inevitable, but storing our food carefully and eating it while it's as fresh as possible can help to maximise the nutritional value. Here are my tips for next time you go shopping.

Meat and fish. My approach is always to try and eat less meat, but with higher welfare quality where possible. Not only is this better for the animals, but their food and living conditions also impact the quality and nutritional content of their meat. If you can, go for grass-fed, organic meats and wild-caught fish; otherwise, choose the next best to suit your budget. Tinned sardines and mackerel are great cost-effective ways of bringing healthy food into your diet.

Vegetables and fruits. Eating your veggies and fruits in season can make it easier to eat a diverse diet and it can also be kinder to our pockets, especially if you are shopping at markets. If there is a cost-effective organic choice, go for it, otherwise always wash your produce well.

Frozen produce is usually picked and frozen at peak ripeness, meaning that it can be excellent quality and involves less wastage. Frozen vegetables tend to have a softer texture when cooked but are a good alternative in soups and casseroles. Frozen peas, edamame beans and berries are some of my top choices that I usually have in my freezer.

Cost-effective proteins. There are plenty of protein foods that are priced more reasonably than meat, and are great, sustainable options for our health. Tofu, beans, lentils, eggs, cheese, tempeh and yoghurt are all foods that we can be eating more of in our diet. To save costs, use dried lentils rather than buying them pre-cooked in pouches. When it comes to nuts and seeds, source them from health food stores to get the best value. Small supermarket packages are expensive, but buying from health food stores can make these an economic protein source, especially for sunflower seeds. As a tip, if you are buying in bulk, store them in an airtight container in a cool, dark place – you can even store them in the freezer to keep them extra fresh!

Eggs are a food where for a small upgrade we can enjoy far better quality. Choose free range or organic, if funds allow.

What's in my yoghurt?

It sounds like it should be simple, but there are four things to check for when you're buying yoghurt.

Protein. Most yoghurts contain around 3.5g protein per 100g, but a properly strained Greek yoghurt contains in the region of 10g protein per 100g. This is because more of the whey (liquid) is strained off, leaving a thicker yoghurt that is more nutrient-dense. You will notice that I use quite a lot of Greek yoghurt in my cooking, as it is a great way of boosting the protein content of recipes and adding a creamy texture. Many Greek-'style' yoghurts are generally not strained as well as traditional Greek yoghurt, meaning they are less creamy, have a higher water content and have less protein per 100g. Greek yoghurt also contains slightly less lactose than regular yoghurt which means some people find Greek yoghurt easier to digest.

Probiotic bacteria. Not all yoghurts contain live bacteria, so always check the label to see if your yoghurt contains beneficial strains such as Lactobacillus or Bifidobacterium, which are good for our gut health.

Low fat vs full fat. Some low-fat yoghurts have added ingredients such as modified starch to make them thicker. This is more common in flavoured, sweetened yoghurts than in natural yoghurt. For regular natural yoghurt, I recommend choosing full fat. But with Greek yoghurt the fat content is less important. Greek yoghurt is thicker than other yoghurts, so is much less likely to have thickeners, even if low fat, so you can choose the one you like best (both have a similar protein content).

Keep it plain. Yoghurt should have just one ingredient listed: milk. Flavoured yoghurts usually contain added sugars and sweeteners and more unnecessary additives. Flavoured yoghurts are mostly classed as ultra-processed foods and are not ones that I would recommend. It is healthier to add your own fruit or even some honey to your own plain yoghurt than to choose flavoured yoghurts.

What about kefir?

Kefir is a fermented milk drink made using a starter culture of gelatinous kefir grains. It contains a wide range of beneficial bacteria and yeasts. Kefir can be added to your breakfast or consumed on its own, and is prized as it contains a wider range of bacteria than yoghurt. It has a thinner consistency and a tangier flavour.

What to consider when buying bread

I have included several of my healthy homemade bread recipes on pages 253–258. However, if you don't have time to make your own bread (although I really recommend it and it doesn't take as long as you think!), here are a few things to look out for:

Real bread should contain just four ingredients: flour, salt, a starter culture (e.g. sourdough) and water. These are the ingredients that have been used for centuries to make our bread, but due to the commercialisation of the bread industry, some supermarket breads have ingredients that we would not use in our own kitchen, such as preservatives which keep the bread fresher for longer or emulsifiers to add softness or to improve the stability of the dough.

The addition of extra seeds would be seen as beneficial when choosing your breads, but it is important to read the label carefully to check for unnecessary other ingredients, such as emulsifiers which hide under the cover of E-numbers such as E471, E481 and E477.

Many white milled flours, by law, still have added nutrients such as calcium, iron, thiamine (vitamin B1) and niacin (vitamin B3), which is considered to be a good thing if you see them on the ingredients list. These measures were introduced during wartime to help prevent deficiencies and add back some of the nutrients that were lost during the refining process. They are still added to most white, but not wholemeal, flours today. Folic acid will soon to be added to this list in the UK.

Sourdough bread is a superior type of bread because it contains a sourdough starter which is made up of numerous wild yeast strains with lactic acid bacteria, as opposed to just one strain in commercial yeast. The bacteria give the loaf its distinct tangy flavour and they are vital for the fermentation process. The longer fermentation time allows for some of the harder-to-digest carbohydrates (known as fructans) as well as some of the gluten proteins to be broken down, which can make it easier for us to digest and can cause fewer digestive issues, such as bloating.

Equipment

Eating healthily is easier with the right equipment! I try to keep things simple in the kitchen. For this book I recommend the following:

- Knives (ask any chef and their most important tools will be their knives)
- Vegetable peeler
- Chopping board (try to avoid plastic if you can)
- Weighing scales
- Measuring spoons
- Mixing bowls, varying sizes
- Garlic crusher
- Grater with coarse and fine sides
- Silicone spatula
- Wooden or silicone spoons
- Colander and fine sieve
- Food processor with a large bowl
- Stick blender for soups and dressings
- Heavy-based frying pan
- Various sizes of saucepan
- Ceramic oven trays
- Silicone mat or non-stick baking paper
- Glass containers to store leftovers and for freezing
- Food flasks for transporting foods
- Stainless steel or glass packed-lunch boxes
- Jam jars and glass bottles for storing leftovers (see page 82)

Optional but helpful
- Vegetable dicer
- Microplane
- Julienne vegetable peeler
- Mandoline slicer with hand guard
- High-speed blender such as a bullet blender or Vitamix
- Air fryer

HOW TO PUT TOGETHER A PERFECT PLATE – IN ANY SITUATION!

Not every meal needs to be perfect. What we are looking for is building some consistency that becomes a habit. All my recipes in this book are balanced (apart from the breads and treats, which are meant to be accompaniments), but knowing how to put together your own balanced plate is easier than you think!

Breakfasts

Most people are creatures of habit and tend to eat the same breakfast every day on repeat.

I recommend you choose three or four recipes from this book and mix them up throughout the week. As well as keeping things more interesting, it will also increase diversity of nutrients. Remember, we want to bring IN different foods and not limit the number we are eating.

As a rule, always make sure that your breakfast has 1–2 portions of vegetables or fruit. A portion is around 80–100g. Always serve fruit with protein, fats and healthy carbohydrates.

Lunches and dinners

I like to treat lunch and dinner as similarly sized meals. I want a lunch that is going to take me easily through until suppertime, helping me avoid that mid-afternoon slump and any need for snacking before dinner.

When I'm putting together lunch or dinner at home, I tend to follow the 1, 2, 3, 4, 5 approach, choosing one item from each category in the chart opposite.

Suggesting exact serving amounts is tricky, as requirements will differ depending on your build, as well as many other lifestyle factors, although I do give some guidelines here, and some more advice on pages 31–36 and 304. Choose amounts to suit your frame and activity levels.

For plant-based meals, where beans or lentils may be a commonly used protein source, remember to use healthy wholegrains, nuts, seeds, tempeh and tofu to top up your protein.

Fridge-raid meals

There will inevitably be times – possibly multiple times a week – when we find that the day has run away with us, or we only have twenty minutes to make and eat lunch. In these moments, it's tempting to just make a sandwich and carry on... but is there a better way of approaching this and stilling hitting your balanced plate goal? This is where the perfect plate fridge-raid comes in!

Using the 1, 2, 3, 4, 5 approach, it becomes simple to put a quick plate of food together that you will enjoy and that will serve you – using whatever you have in your fridge and cupboards. See over the page for more on step 5 – the Bells and Whistles!

THE 1, 2, 3, 4, 5 APPROACH

STEP 1: CHOOSE YOUR PROTEIN

Start by building your plate around your protein. Proteins should take up around ¼ of your plate. Below are approximate serving sizes, but these would depend on your personal requirements, and whether you are combining your proteins – also remember protein is found in other foods on your plate, e.g. healthy carbohydrates. I like to mix-and-match a variety of proteins to make up my ¼ plate, e.g. lentils and tofu, halloumi and chickpeas, chicken and beans, which can optimise protein and also top up the fibre!

- 150g cooked beans or lentils, tofu, tempeh or seitan
- 110–150g oily fish, white fish, shellfish, poultry or meat
- 60–90g cheese, e.g. feta, halloumi, goat's cheese or mozzarella
- 2–3 eggs
- 50–75g unsalted, raw nuts or seeds

STEP 2: ADD YOUR VEGETABLES

Add half a plate of vegetables (around 200–250g). Choose at least three different types and mix up the colours. These can be cooked, chopped into a salad, grated, cut into crudités, stir-fried, roasted, in a soup, threaded on to kebabs – be creative!

STEP 3: ADD A HEALTHY CARBOHYDRATE (AS A SIDE)

These should be around ¼ of your plate, which is 1–3 tablespoons of pasta or grains (30–50g dry weight); 50g–75g of heavier seeded breads. This may not work for every meal, so don't worry if you miss this part out now and then. Also, remember that beans and lentils can also be used as a healthy carb – aim for 2–3 tablespoons, which is around 65–110g.

STEP 4: THINK ABOUT HEALTHY FATS

Have you used healthy fats to cook with? Or as a dressing? Around 1 tablespoon per meal is about right. Or are there healthy fats as part of your food – e.g. in fatty fish or avocado? If not, think about how you can add some. Maybe make a quick mustard or tahini dressing in a jam jar (page 171 or 176), or add some olives, nuts or seeds to your plate.

STEP 5: ADD THREE THINGS

Up the nutrients and diversity by adding three ingredients. For example, walnuts, olives, fermented veggies such as sauerkraut or kimchi, fresh herbs, shards of Parmesan, pumpkin seeds, microgreens, sesame seeds, a spoonful of hummus or even a bowl of miso soup. (See page 94 for more ideas.)

BONUS: ADD A FRUIT

Enjoy a piece of fruit at your meals if you like! It could be part of your meal, e.g. apple in your salad, or try the Halloumi Salad with Pomegranate Salsa (page 198). Preferably, opt for lower glycaemic fruits, such as berries, apples, pears or kiwis (see page 36 for more lower-glycaemic options).

NOW ADD THREE THINGS TO YOUR PLATE – THE BELLS AND WHISTLES

I love to ADD IN rather than take away. Adding a few foods to your plate can make your meals more sustaining and even more nutrient-dense, meaning that we are more likely to hit our nutrient targets for the day – and up our plant points, too. It also makes our meals more interesting and enjoyable to eat! A few extras such as those listed below, stashed in your fridge or store cupboard, can instantly transform a simple meal into something really special.

Some of my favourites include:

- Fermented foods, such as sauerkraut, live yoghurt, kefir, miso or kimchi. These foods are a rich source of live probiotic bacteria (page 21).
- Seaweed flakes, which are a good source of iodine, iron, calcium and magnesium.
- A spoon of hummus or guacamole for extra fibre and healthy fats. Avocado is also good source of vitamin E, B6 and folate. See my recipes on page 269–271.
- Shards of Parmesan or a sprinkling of feta cheese. Parmesan is fantastic for topping up calcium, with around 1,000mg per 100g, while feta adds great flavour and also protein.
- Crispy baked chickpeas (page 186) make a great protein and fibre top-up, and add texture too.
- Green pesto or tomato salsa (page 205 or 242) give a punch of flavour and can top up our plant points. Making your own pesto means you can pack in more basil, garlic, olive oil and nuts, while tomatoes are rich in the antioxidant lycopene.
- Microgreens, which are sprouted seeds, are a concentrated source of nutrients as well as beneficial plant compounds.
- Nuts and seeds, for their beneficial fats, fibre and minerals, such as magnesium and zinc.

NUTRITIONAL INFORMATION

At the top of each of my recipes, I've shown the total amount of protein and fibre (in grams) and the maximum number of plant points per serving. (Your actual plant points total will depend on whether you have consumed any of the ingredients already that week; see page 70 for more information.) These totals are for the complete balanced plate recipe, including the 'to serve' instructions, but not for any variations I have suggested. On pages 296–303, you'll also find the calories for my recipes.

On pages 296–303 I've also provided the nutritional information for some of the separate components of my recipes. For example, I've given the breakdown for the beans in my Any Bean Shakshuka (page 138) on their own, in case you wish to serve them without bread – or with an alternative bread – and the seeded wraps from page 183, so you can use them with alternative fillings.

I don't encourage keeping a tally of everything you are eating, though. If you are following my six principles, you will be consuming sufficient protein and fibre at your mealtimes, and more than meeting your 30 plant points per week.

Please remember that nutritional information is only ever an estimation too, as values may vary depending on the ingredients you use. My main wish is to provide you with a toolkit to better health and a positive approach to eating for now and the long term.

Key to symbols

G   Gluten-Free

D   Dairy-Free

V   Vegetarian

Vg   Vegan

    Make-One-Take-One

MEAL PLANNER WEEK 1

	Breakfast	Lunch	Dinner
Monday	Jewelled granola breakfast bowl (page 108)	Sweet potato and feta frittata (page 135) (Make-One-Take-One)	Lentil, pea and crispy aubergine dhal (page 212) (Make-One-Take-One)
Tuesday	Sweet potato and feta frittata (page 135) (Make-One-Take-One)	Lentil, pea and crispy aubergine dhal (page 212) (Make-One-Take-One)	Firecracker chicken (page 208)
Wednesday	Carrot cake overnight oats (page 115)	Burrata and peach salad (page 190)	Prawn fishcakes with soba noodle salad and wasabi dipping sauce (page 206)
Thursday	Harissa beans on toast (page 126)	Wasabi super green soup (page 164)	Beef chilli with lentils and chocolate (with black rice) (page 219) (Make-One-Take-One)
Friday	Creamy chocolate chia pudding (page 125)	Beef chilli with lentils and chocolate (with avocado and sour cream) (page 219) (Make-One-Take-One)	Pesto and walnut crust salmon (page 205)
Saturday	Turkish eggs brunch (page 131) OR Tofu scramble (page 122)	Sticky peanut tofu poke bowl (page 180) (Make-One-Take-One)	Dijon chicken with tarragon (page 217)
Sunday	Any bean shakshuka (page 138)	Chicken Caesar salad with Parmesan chickpea croutons (page 186)	Thai fish curry with sesame zoodles (page 235)

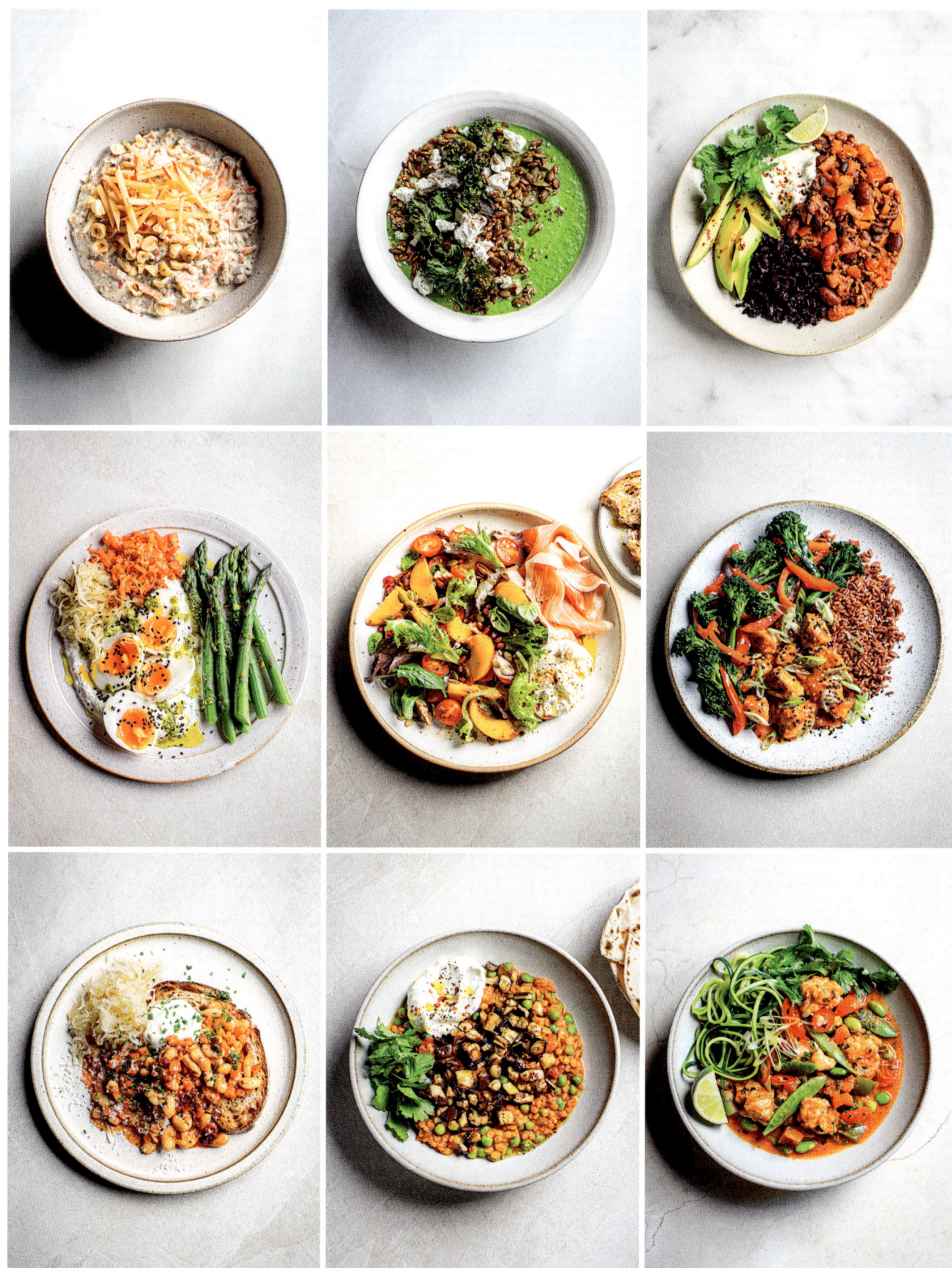

MEAL PLANNER WEEK 2

	Breakfast	**Lunch**	**Dinner**
Monday	Sunrise sprinkles with yoghurt and berries (page 112)	Sticky peanut tofu poke bowl (page 180) (Make-One-Take-One)	Shepherdess pie with cheesy bean and parsnip mash (page 221) (Make-One-Take-One)
Tuesday	Cherry bakewell baked oats (page 132)	Shepherdess pie with cheesy bean and parsnip mash (page 221) (Make-One-Take-One)	Sticky trout with salad (page 231) (Make-One-Take-One)
Wednesday	Super green bread with mozzarella, tomato and pesto (page 254)	Sticky trout with salad (page 231) (Make-One-Take-One)	Tandoori chicken salad with raita (page 232)
Thursday	Gut-boosting breakfast bowl (page 118)	Mozzarella and vegetable seeded wraps with tuna salad (page 183)	Crispy gochujang with stir-fried vegetables (page 246)
Friday	Berry pancake stack (page 140)	Halloumi salad with pomegranate salsa (page 198)	Pork loin with smoky beans (page 240)
Saturday	Chocolate cherry breakfast bowl (page 120)	Asparagus and goat's cheese flan (page 169) (Make-One-Take-One)	Mackerel fishcakes with watercress cream (page 244)
Sunday	New York-style smoked salmon bagel (page 128)	Asparagus and goat's cheese flan (page 169) (Make-One-Take-One)	Chicken and kale burgers with tomato salsa salad (page 242)

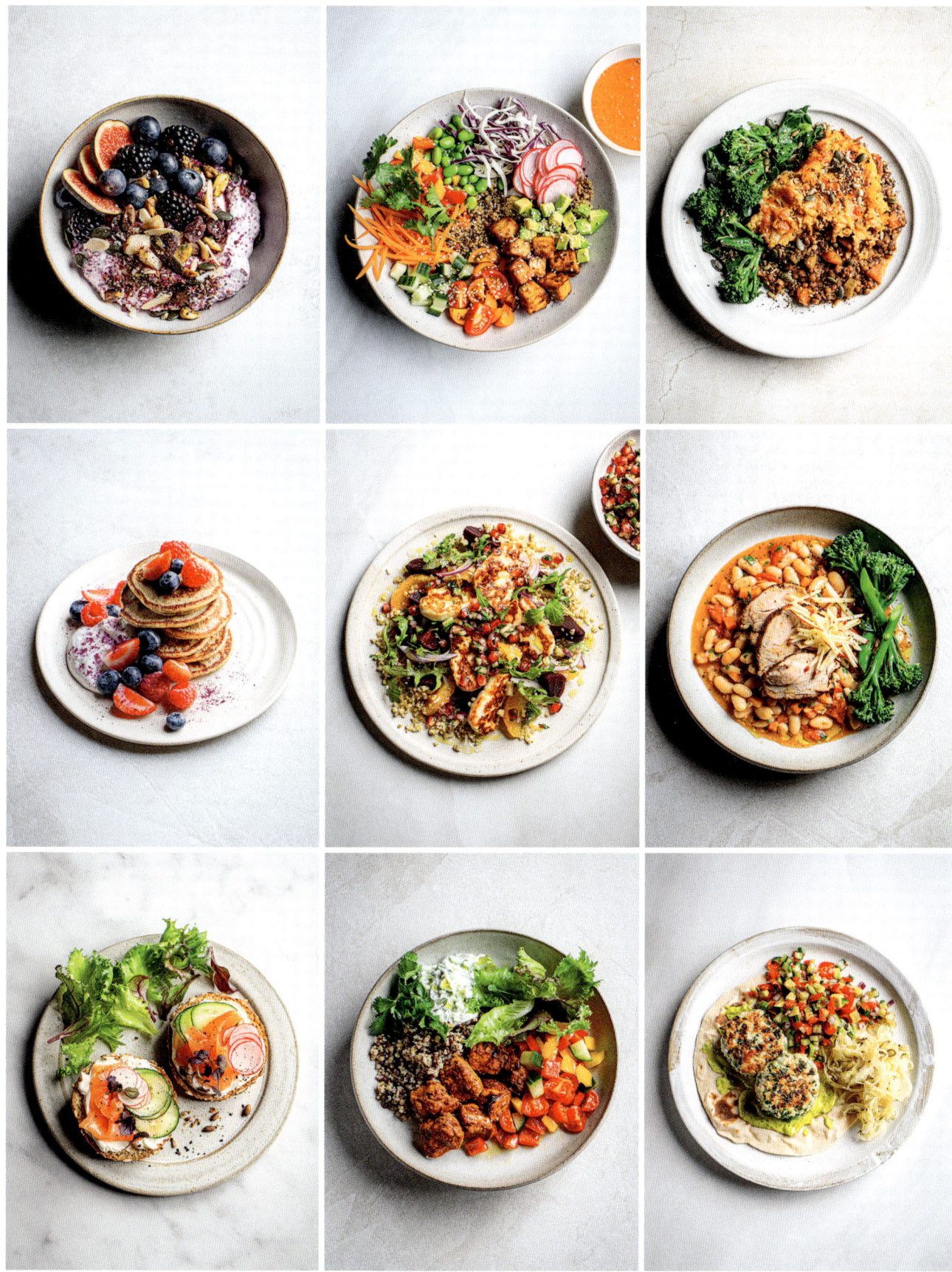

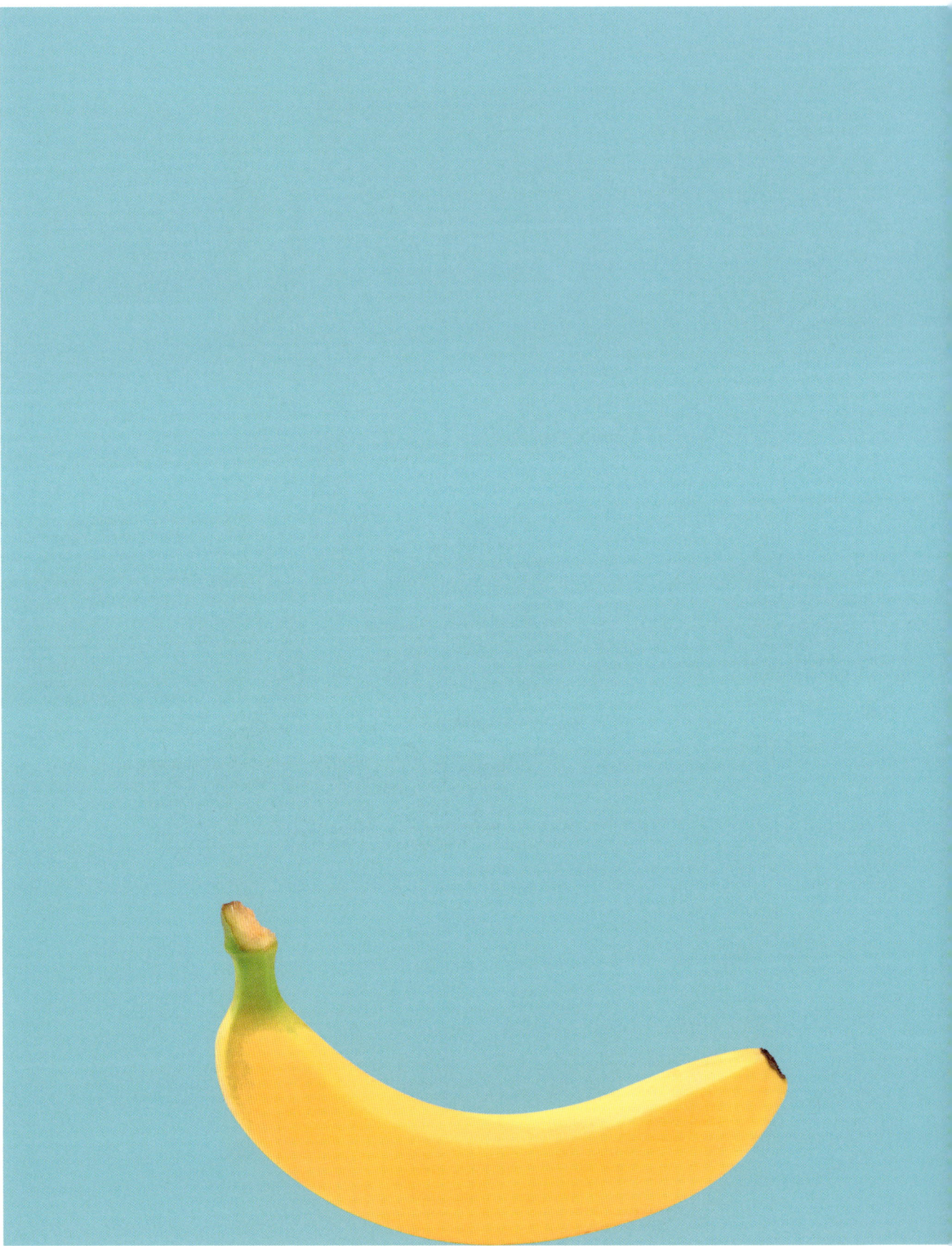

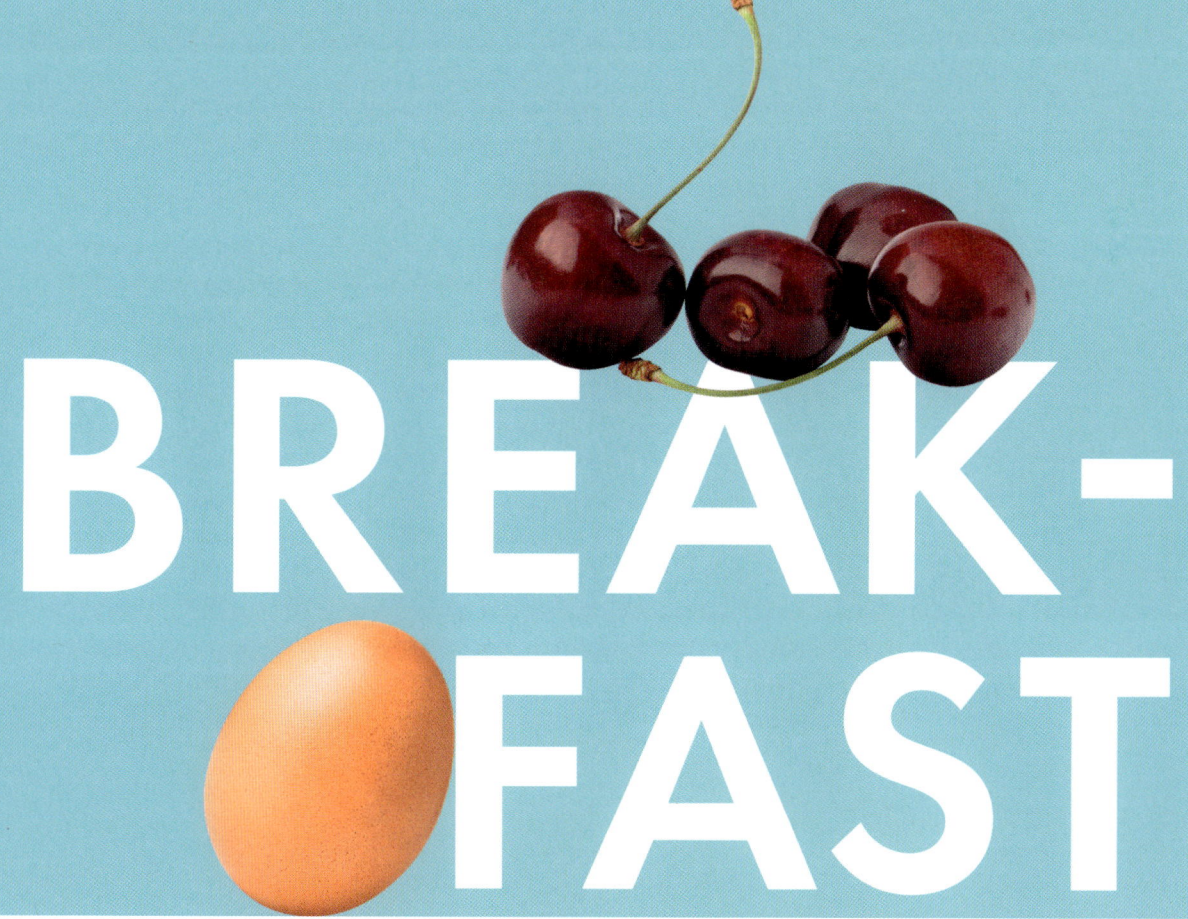

The choices we make at breakfast lay the foundation for our energy and focus, and influence our food choices for the rest of the day. Breakfast, at its core, is about 'breaking the fast'. After 12–14 hours without food, our body needs nourishment to refuel.

If our breakfast is balanced and contains sufficient nutrition, we are less likely to start the vicious cycle of snacking and more likely to make healthier choices.

The recipes in this chapter are designed to fit into your lifestyle throughout the week, whatever your morning demands from you. You'll find recipes you can prepare in advance, portable 'jam jar' breakfasts (see my lists on page 104), and relaxed brunch ideas like Turkish Eggs (page 131) for when you have a bit more time. From speaking to my clients, I've found that we tend to be creatures of habit when it comes to our breakfast choices, so to start with I suggest you choose three or four recipes from this chapter and make them part of your regular breakfast rotation. Varying your breakfast choice throughout the week means you'll benefit from a wider range of nutritients – and more plant points!

Sweet or savoury – or somewhere in between?

You'll see that some recipes lean towards savoury, while others are a little sweeter, but you'll notice a common theme: I rarely include any added sugars. Instead, natural sweetness comes from whole fruits, or I allow the savoury flavours of my chosen ingredients to take centre stage. Veggies for breakfast? Yes! I use plenty of vegetables at breakfast! Remember that vegetables and whole fruits not only supply us with nutrients and fibre, but also slow down our digestion, keeping our energy and appetite on an even keel.

We are often advised to start the day with a savoury breakfast, but what does that really mean and where does fruit fit in?

When we think of sweet breakfasts, we're likely to picture foods like toast with jam or marmalade, almond croissants, pastries, pancakes drizzled with syrup, or smoothies made from bananas or with apple juice. Most supermarket breakfast cereals also fall into this category. Although breakfast cereals are often marketed as healthy choices with impressive health promises, they are often low in protein and healthy fats while being high in fast-digesting carbohydrates and added sugars. The suggested serving size is also very small – usually only around 30g.

This might deliver as little as 100–150 kcals, which is not going to lead to an energised and productive morning! In addition, since in reality we are likely to be pouring ourselves a much larger portion than recommended, the sugar levels shown on the packet are far lower than what we are actually eating. Healthier options, such as porridge, can also shift into 'sweet' territory when topped with honey or maple syrup, but even without these obviously sweet extras, porridge still lacks adequate protein and healthy fats. While these breakfasts may be comforting and enjoyable, they often provide a rapid spike in blood sugar that can leave you feeling tired or hungry again by mid-morning.

When it comes to savoury options, great go-to choices are cooked egg-based breakfasts, like omelettes and scrambled or poached eggs. I love eggs in the morning, as they are quick to prepare and a great source of nutrition. You can also add fillings to omelettes to up their nutritional value, like cooked spinach or courgette or grated cheese – or see my Turmeric and Coriander Folded Omelette recipe on page 153, which I have served on a slice of my Super Green Bread. Beans, such as my Harissa Beans on Toast (page 126) or Any Bean Shakshuka (page 138), will also set you up well for the day. Or, we can follow the lead of many European countries by topping nutritionally dense rye bread with cheeses, fish and vegetables (see pages 148–153 for my quick topping ideas). Protein-rich savoury breakfasts like these are great choices for stabilising blood sugar levels.

Then there are the breakfasts that are neither sweet in the traditional sense but are also not savoury, sitting somewhere in the middle. It's perfectly possible to have a sweeter-sounding breakfast, such as the Berry Pancake Stack (page 140), and still hit all your goals nutritionally. Just because you have had some fruit in the morning, it doesn't mean you've had a 'sweet' breakfast.

Many of the breakfasts I make for myself at home are based around yoghurt, and in particular naturally thicker Greek yoghurts, which are higher in protein. Together with nuts and seeds, which are rich in fibre and healthy fats, and topped with lower-glycaemic whole fruits (see page 36), you can still enjoy a well-balanced breakfast that is a bit sweeter to start the day if that's what you prefer. When you eat your fruit whole, the sugars are still contained within the plant's cell walls, meaning they will take longer to break down and hit your bloodstream. Try it for yourself in my Sunrise Sprinkles with Yoghurt and Berries (page 112) – the perfect quick-assembly breakfast.

Portable breakfasts

Perfectly balanced and full of goodness, prep these grab-and-go breakfasts the night before and pack them into a jam jar (or other container) to take with you.

- Jewelled Granola Breakfast Bowl (page 108)
- Sunrise Sprinkles with Yoghurt and Berries (page 112)
- Carrot Cake Overnight Oats (pages 115 and 116)
- Gut-Boosting Breakfast Bowl (page 118)
- Creamy Chocolate Chia Pudding (page 125)
- Harissa baked beans (page 126) (take in a hot food flask)
- 2 boiled eggs on a bed of chopped veggies with cottage cheese
- An apple with some cheese cubes, walnuts and pumpkin seeds
- Cottage cheese, grated carrot and oatcakes or crackers (page 261) (pack the oatcakes or crackers separately so they don't go soggy)
- Greek yoghurt with a good palmful of any mixed nuts and seeds, with berries

Make-ahead breakfasts

If you haven't got long in the morning, prepare these in advance to quickly warm up or assemble for breakfast in minutes.

- Cherry Bakewell Baked Oats (page 132)
- Sweet Potato and Feta Frittata (page 135)
- Harissa baked beans (page 126)
- Any Bean Shakshuka (page 138)
- Egg Muffins (page 272) with watercress
- Granola jars: Chocolate Cherry Granola (page 119) or Jewelled Granola Breakfast Bowl (page 108)
- Red Lentil Bagels (page 267) with toppings
- Whisk up eggs and chopped veg the night before, ready to make a quick omelette
- Mix cooked chicken, avocado, cottage cheese, chopped peppers, onion, tomatoes and mustard together for a quick toast topper

HUNGRY AFTER OATS?
A NEW WAY TO EAT YOUR OATS

Rolled oats can be a healthy addition to our diet, as they contain a type of soluble fibre called beta-glucan, which has been shown to play a role in lowering cholesterol. Oats also contain some protein, but you will need to top this up for a completely balanced breakfast. Ways to do this include adding a spoonful of nut butter to your oats, topping them with nuts and seeds, and/or stirring through chia seeds or flaxseeds – you can even stir an egg into your porridge while it cooks, you won't taste it at all! I've also mixed ground almonds into the Cherry Bakewell Baked Oats (page 132) for extra protein and fibre – and to add to the Bakewell flavour. Chia seeds, nuts and seeds provide good amounts of protein and fibre to both my granola recipes (pages 107 and 119), but the Jewelled Granola Breakfast Bowl (page 108) has an incredible 30g of protein because I've served it alongside a generous amount of Greek yoghurt, and the Chocolate Cherry Breakfast Bowl (page 120), served with quark, has 31g of protein, so also consider what you are serving your oats with.

Interestingly, while some people feel full all morning after their bowl of porridge, others can find themselves hungry a couple of hours later. This can be explained by blood sugar fluctuations that occur in many people after eating oats. If our blood sugars increase too fast, they are likely to drop quickly again mid-morning. This is the exact time when we may start to feel tired and hungry. Mild fluctuations in our blood sugars are perfectly normal and nothing to be concerned about; however, a series of glucose spikes and dips during the day can sometimes leave us feeling worse and can affect the quality of our day (see pages 18–19 for more on blood sugars).

For this reason, I have created my Carrot Cake Overnight Oats in two ways (pages 115 and 116). Both contain extra protein, but one has less energy coming from the oats, and more from seeds. Try both to see which one suits you best by assessing how you feel mid-morning, noticing when you first feel hungry again after eating.

Unrolling your oats: why the type of oat matters

The type of oats we use can also make a difference to how quickly we digest them and how full they make us feel.

- **Steel-cut oats** These are often sold as pinhead oats in the UK. They are roughly chopped oat grains. Because the grain is mostly intact, it is harder for our body to break down, meaning that these oats have a gentler effect on our blood sugars. As they are 'chunkier', they also usually require a longer cooking time.

- **Rolled oats** Traditional rolled oats can be thick or thin. It is best to choose thicker oats if you can, as these are likely to break down more slowly. These have been lightly steamed and passed between large rollers to flatten. They are perfect for soaked oats and porridge.

- **Quick oats** These oats are steamed for longer, which partially cooks the oats. They are mostly cut into smaller pieces before being rolled into thinner flakes and dried. They are often sold as 'quick oats' that generally cook in a few minutes. Because they have a larger surface area and are pre-cooked, they break down the quickest in our digestive tract and are much more likely to cause blood sugar spikes. Avoid oats labelled 'quick-cook' or those that can be prepared in the microwave.

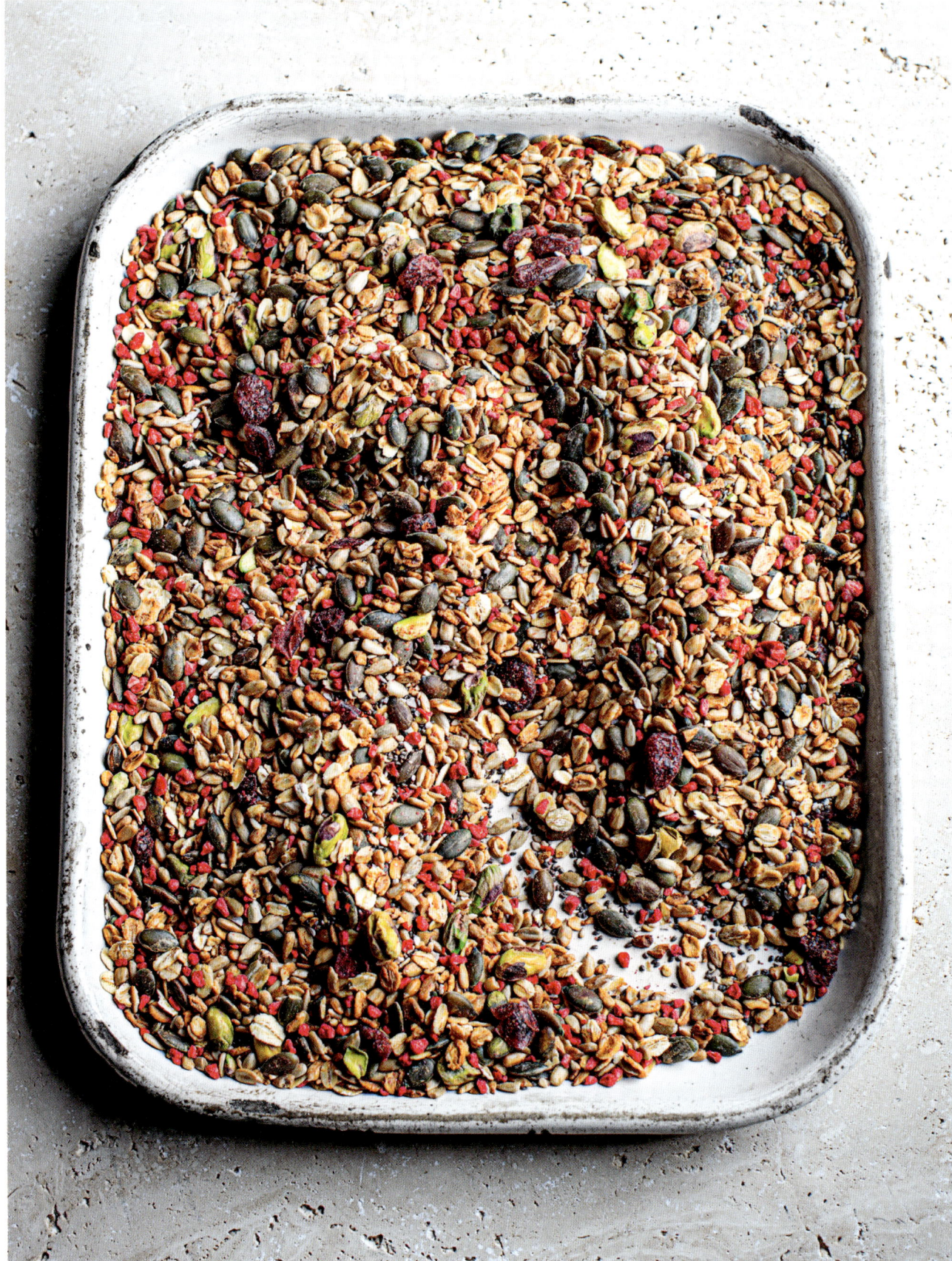

PER SERVING
PROTEIN: 6G
FIBRE: 4G
PLANT POINTS: 8.5

**MAKES 28 SERVINGS
(40G PER SERVING)**

300g gluten-free (or regular) rolled oats
200g sunflower seeds
200g pumpkin seeds
100g sesame seeds
zest and juice of 1 orange
25ml extra virgin olive oil
a little maple syrup (optional)

'Jewels' – to add after cooking
100g pistachio nuts
50g chia seeds
100g dried cranberries
a sprinkling of freeze-dried raspberries (optional)

JEWELLED GRANOLA

Joy in a jar! This granola is nutritious, delicious and visually striking due to the cranberries, freeze-dried raspberries and pistachio nuts. The trick with granola is to balance the oats with slow-release seeds and to combine them with protein-rich foods, like yoghurt, to keep your energy on an even keel and your cravings at bay. Using the granola as a topping, rather than the main component, helps keep things balanced (see the example on page 32). It's colourful, enjoyable to eat and is always stocked in my cupboard. The freeze-dried raspberries are an optional extra that add colour and can be swapped for extra cranberries if you prefer.

---

1. Preheat the oven to 180°C fan. In a ceramic dish or roasting tray, mix together the oats, sunflower seeds, pumpkin seeds, sesame seeds, orange zest and juice, and the extra virgin olive oil. If you like, you can add a little maple syrup before it goes into the oven, although I don't think it needs it as the cranberries will add extra sweetness at the end. Bake for 25 minutes, or until lightly golden.

2. Turn the oven off and leave the tray inside to cool completely. This allows it to crisp up without overcooking the seeds.

3. Once completely cool, stir in the pistachio nuts, chia seeds, dried cranberries and a sprinkling of dried raspberries, if using. Transfer to an airtight container.

Storage: Store in an airtight container for up to 2 weeks.

PER SERVING
PROTEIN: 30G
FIBRE: 10G
PLANT POINTS: 11.5

SERVES 1
200g Greek yoghurt
10g milled flaxseeds
a splash of milk
40g Jewelled Granola (page 107)
a handful of fresh fruit
50g pomegranate seeds

JEWELLED GRANOLA BREAKFAST BOWL

We eat with our eyes, and this breakfast bowl brings a burst of colour to your morning routine and works well with a variety of fruits. I like to use raspberries, blueberries, strawberries, oranges or even kiwi, so you can adapt your bowl to what's in season. It's a quick and easy option that you can throw together in the morning and take with you in a pot, making it a great portable breakfast that delivers on taste, nutrition and convenience. I use well-strained Greek yoghurt or other thick varieties with around 10g of protein per 100g to ensure optimal protein. I've also added flaxseeds for extra protein and fibre, but if you don't have any, you can leave them out – it will still be a delicious, well-balanced start to the day.

---

1. Spoon the Greek yoghurt into a bowl. If using the flaxseeds, mix them in first, using a little milk to loosen. Top with the granola and the fruit.

Storage: Best served immediately, but can be prepared and stored in the fridge for up to 12 hours in an airtight container.

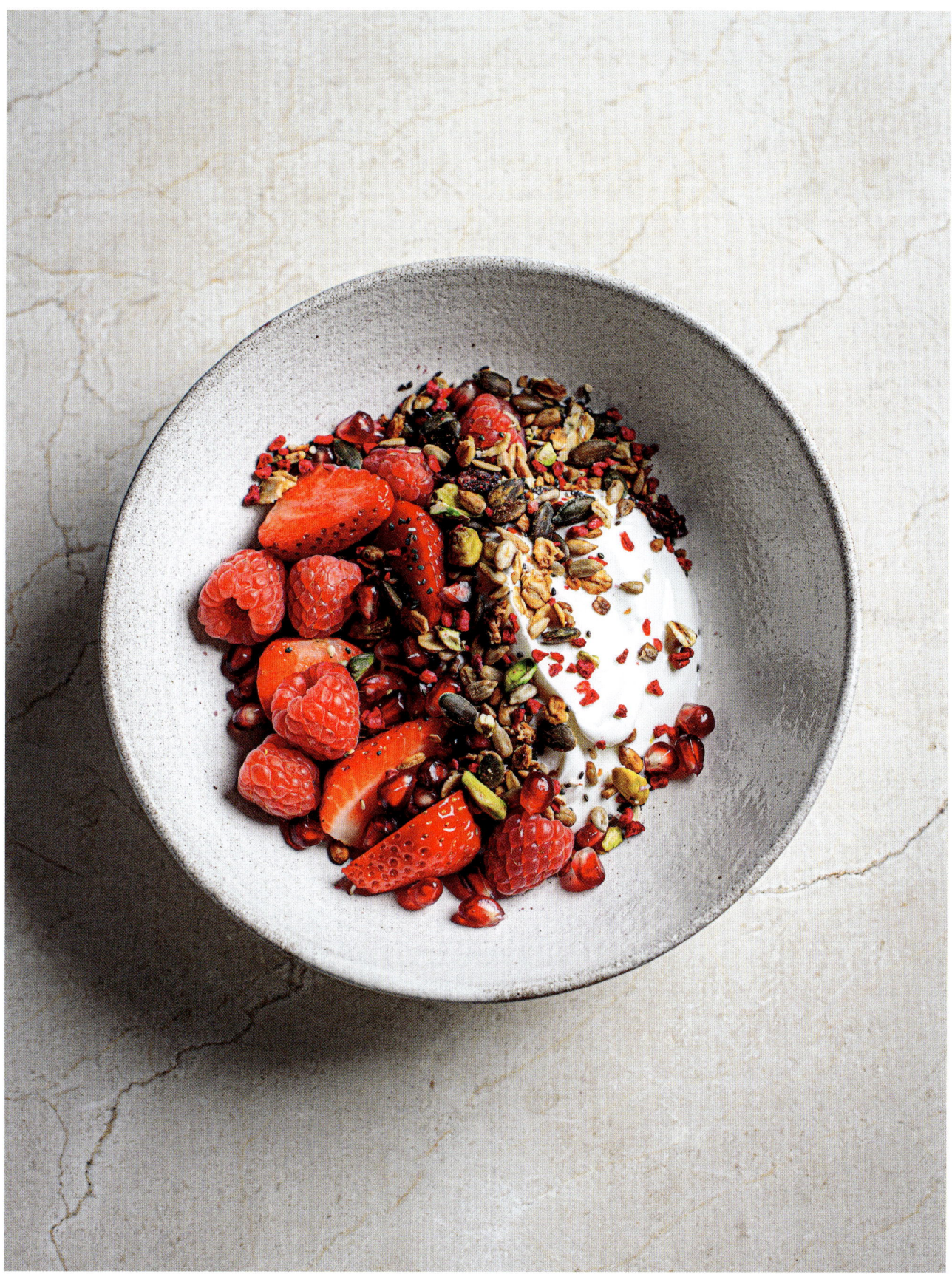

PER SERVING
PROTEIN: 8G
FIBRE: 8G
PLANT POINTS: 12

**SERVES 6
(50G PER SERVING)**

25g sunflower seeds
25g pumpkin seeds
25g almonds,
    chopped or flaked
25g milled flaxseeds
25g pistachio nuts
25g milled hemp seeds
25g chia seeds
25g Brazil nuts,
    roughly chopped
25g walnuts,
    roughly chopped
25g dried cranberries
25g coconut flakes
25g one of the following:
    dried pitaya powder,
    acai, cranberry or
    blueberry powder

SUNRISE SPRINKLES

This is a very simple and delicious way of eating more plant points and is a true gut-boosting breakfast. This sunrise mix looks stunning in the jar and even better in your breakfast bowl (page 112). The addition of dried berry powders brings both a burst of colour and natural sweetness. I used pitaya powder, which is made from dried pink dragon fruit and can be sourced from lots of online retailers. The vibrant pink colour comes from betacyanins, which are polyphenols and antioxidants. You can easily swap this for dried cranberry, blueberry or acai powder, all of which work brilliantly. If you're missing any seeds on this list, use what you have to make your own unique version. This also makes a fantastic gift when kept layered in the jar.

1. Put all the ingredients into a large jar. You can layer them one at a time to create a striking visual effect and then shake the jar before using.

Storage: Store in an airtight jar in a cool, dry place and use within 3 weeks.

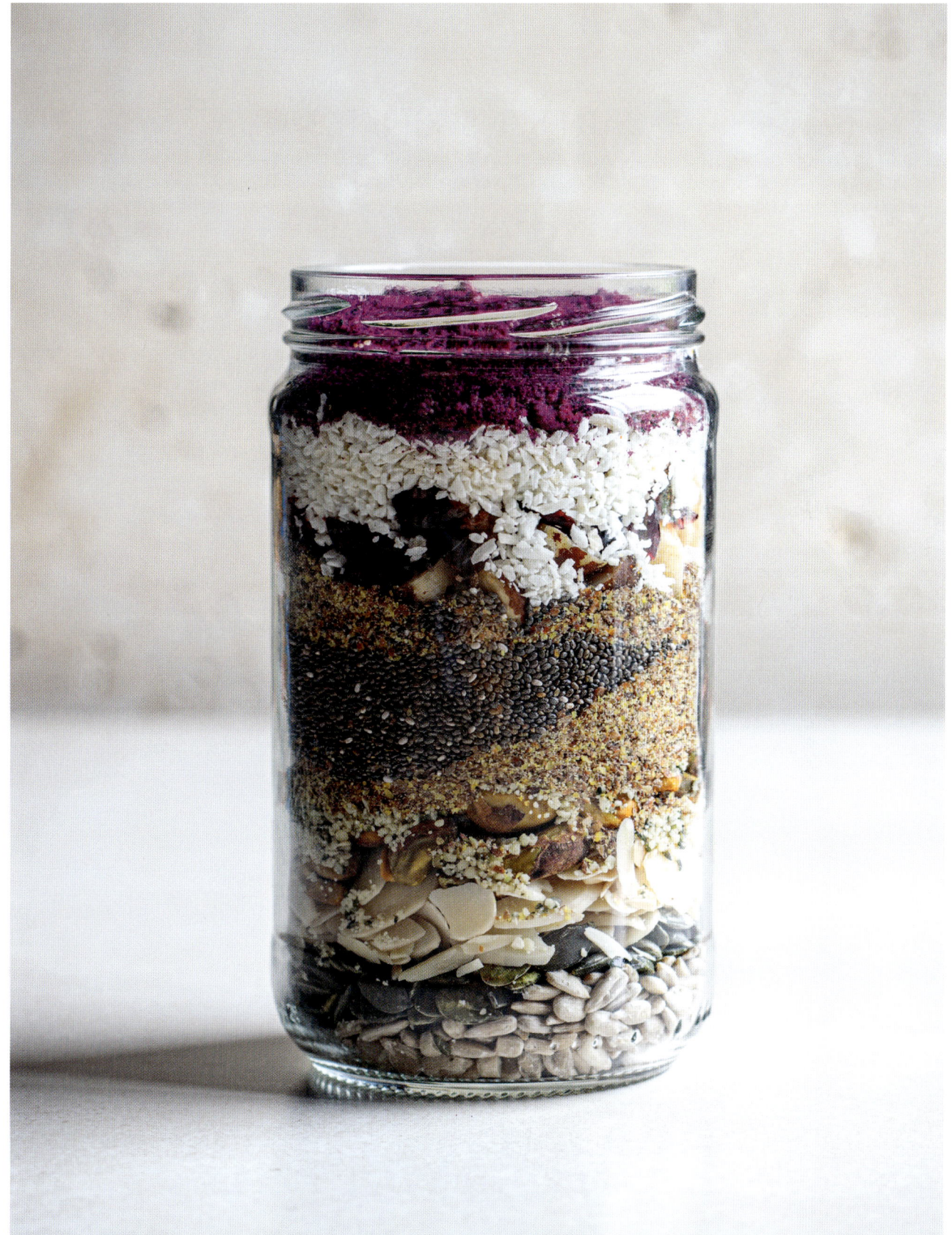

PER SERVING
PROTEIN: 30G
FIBRE: 10G
PLANT POINTS: 15

SERVES 1

200g Greek yoghurt
50g Sunrise Sprinkles (page 110)
80g mixed berries or chopped fruit (e.g. blackberries, strawberries, raspberries, blueberries, figs)

SUNRISE SPRINKLES WITH YOGHURT AND BERRIES

This bright and nourishing way to start your day is guaranteed to put a smile on your face in the morning. Adding your Sunrise Sprinkles (page 110) to yoghurt is one of the most delicious and cheerful ways to enjoy them, as they turn your yoghurt a vibrant pink. Berry powders, especially bright pink pitaya powder or dried berry powders, add a subtle sweetness as well as rich colour. This bowl offers the perfect nutritional balance at breakfast, delivering 30g of protein and 10g of fibre per serving. It also transports well, so you can take it with you.

---

1. Stir most of the Sunrise Sprinkles into the yoghurt until well combined. Top with the berries or chopped fruit, then scatter over the rest of the sprinkles.

Storage: Best served immediately, but can be prepared and stored in the fridge for up to 12 hours in an airtight container.

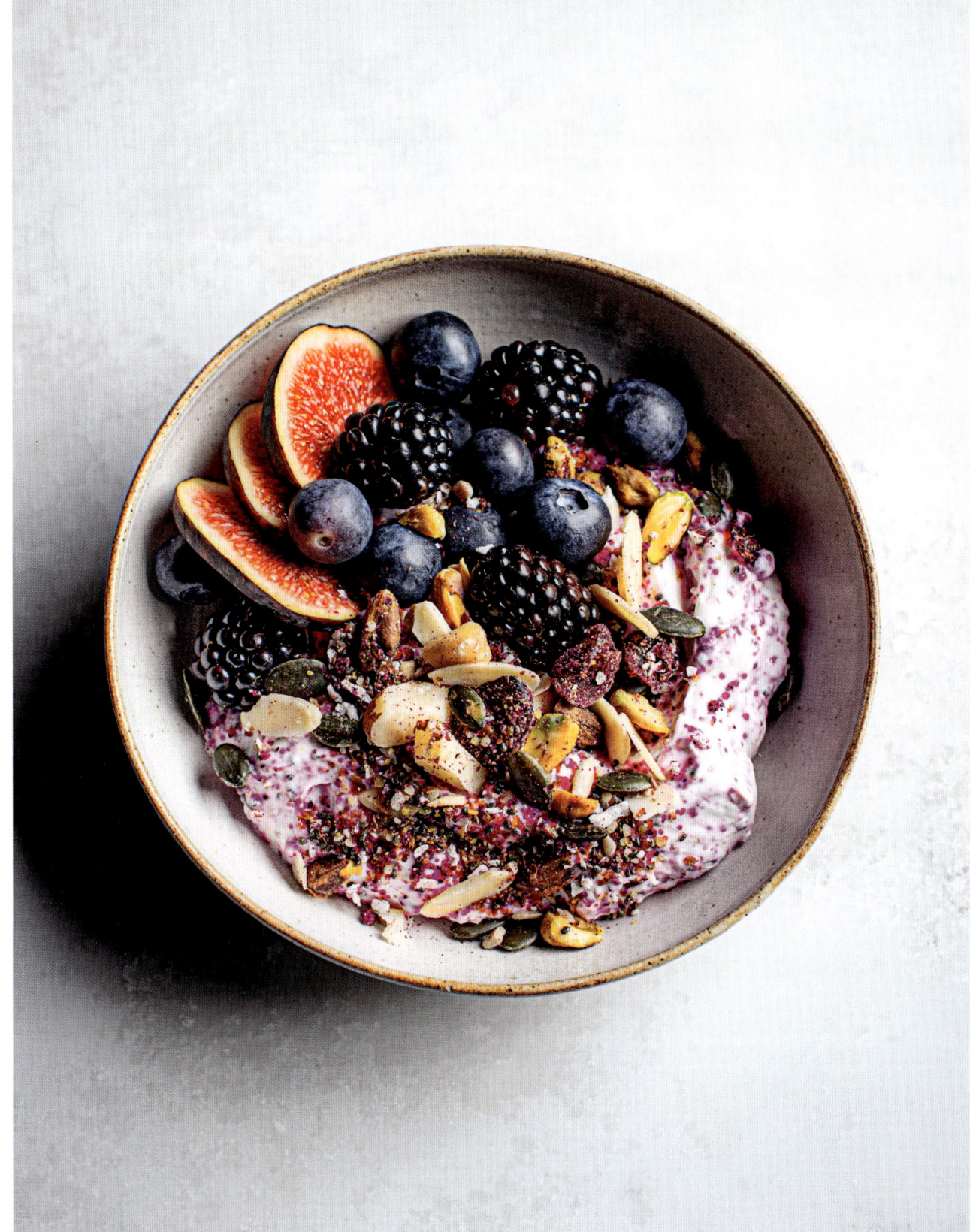

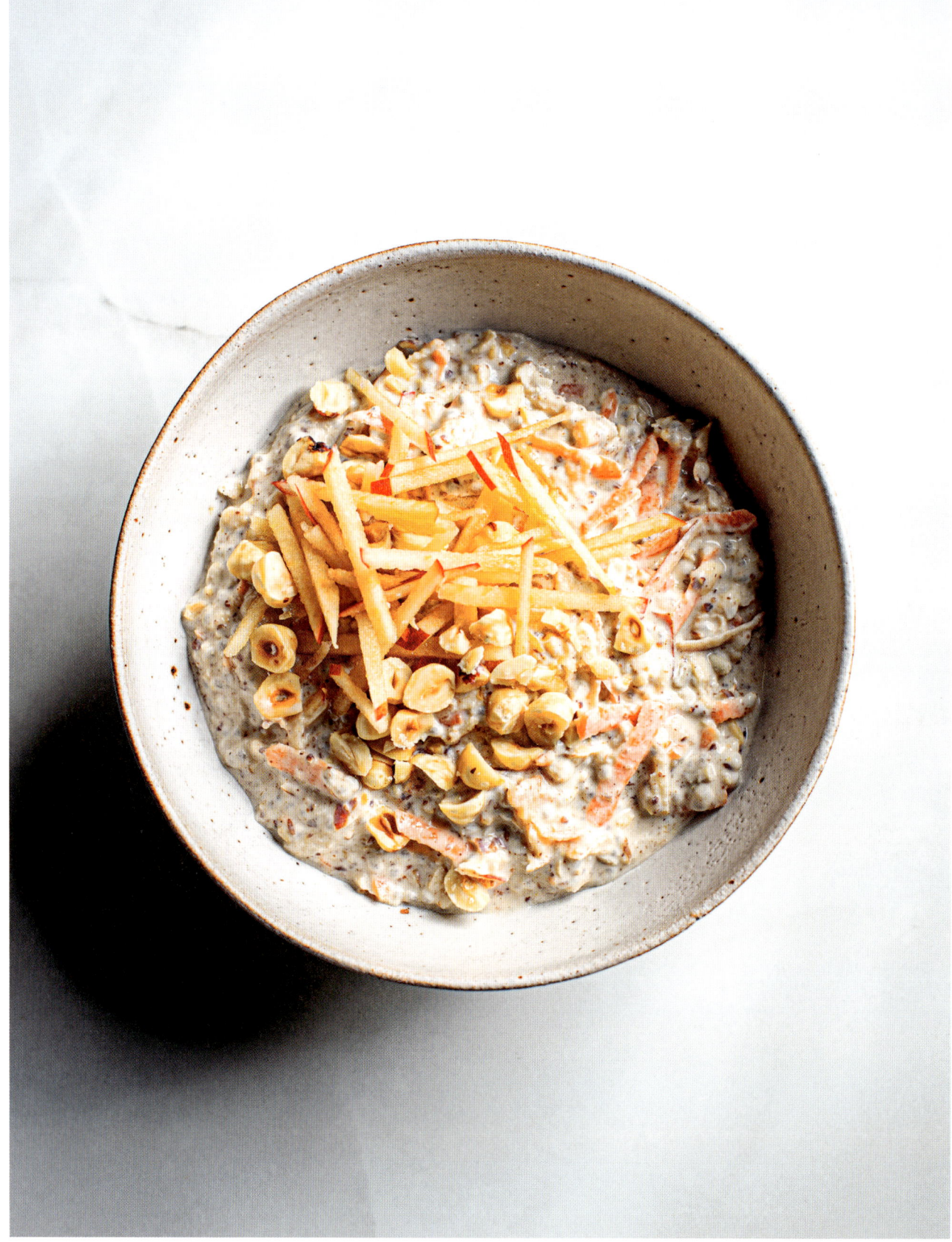

PER SERVING
PROTEIN: 30G
FIBRE: 10G
PLANT POINTS: 5.5

SERVES 1

40g gluten-free (or regular) rolled oats
10g chia seeds
150g Greek yoghurt
½ carrot, grated
½ apple, grated
150–200ml milk of choice (I used soya milk, which is the closest nutritionally to semi-skimmed cow's milk)
a pinch of ground cinnamon
a pinch of ground ginger
10g chopped hazelnuts
1 teaspoon honey or maple syrup (if required)

To serve (optional)
extra apple, grated
a few chopped hazelnuts

CARROT CAKE OVERNIGHT OATS 1

Balancing the carbohydrates in oats with protein helps slow digestion and support energy levels. Here, Greek yoghurt provides that protein boost, with extra soluble fibre from chia seeds. The oats soften in around 2 hours, chia seeds in 20 minutes, so this can be made in the morning if you're not eating right away, or soaked overnight. This recipe has 40g of oats per portion, which is an average serving and is likely to work better for some people than others (see page 105). You can replace the Greek yoghurt with Greek soya yoghurt if you prefer. See also my other version of these overnight oats on page 116, made with fewer oats and more seeds.

1. Mix all the ingredients together in a jam jar or bowl. Stir through the honey or maple syrup if you would prefer it to be a little sweeter. Cover and refrigerate overnight.

2. Stir in a little more milk to loosen the consistency before serving, if needed, as it may thicken overnight. Top with a little more grated apple and chopped hazelnuts if you like.

Storage: Store in the fridge; best eaten within 24 hours.

PER SERVING
PROTEIN: 30G
FIBRE: 11G
PLANT POINTS: 7.5

SERVES 1
10g chia seeds
10g milled flaxseeds
10g sunflower seeds
10g gluten-free (or regular) rolled oats
150g Greek yoghurt
150ml milk (or 75ml milk of choice and 75ml kefir)
½ carrot, grated
½ apple, grated
a pinch each of ground cinnamon and ground ginger
10g chopped hazelnuts or almonds
1 teaspoon honey or maple syrup (if required)

To serve (optional)
extra apple, grated
a few chopped hazelnuts

CARROT CAKE OVERNIGHT OATS 2

This version includes fewer oats and more fibre-rich seeds than the version on page 115, to create a slower energy release alternative. The yoghurt and other ingredients remain unchanged, making it easy to compare how you feel after you have eaten it. I've used soya milk, which contains slightly more protein than almond milk, but cow's milk or any plant milk works well. I also replaced half the milk with kefir to boost the probiotic bacteria for extra gut support. I like my oats without extra sweetening, but you have the option to choose. (See opposite for my recipe for a large batch of oat mix.)

---

1. Mix all the ingredients in a jar or bowl, stirring through the honey or maple syrup if you prefer it to be a little sweeter. Cover and refrigerate overnight.

2. In the morning, stir in a little more milk to loosen the consistency.

Storage: Store in the fridge; best eaten within 24 hours.

PER SERVING
PROTEIN: 7G
FIBRE: 8G
PLANT POINTS: 4

**SERVES 10
(40G PER SERVING)**

100g gluten-free (or regular) rolled oats
100g chia seeds
100g milled flaxseeds
100g sunflower seeds

LARGE JAR OF OAT MIX

If you enjoyed the second recipe for Carrot Cake Overnight Oats (opposite) and found it worked best for you, save time by preparing a larger jar of the oat mix in advance. This versatile oat mix can be used as a base for any overnight oats or can be gently heated with 150ml milk for a hot porridge – add 150g of Greek yoghurt after cooking to boost the protein, and top with fruit for extra fibre.

---

1. Combine all the ingredients in an airtight jar.

Storage: Store in an airtight container in the fridge or a cool, dry cupboard for up to 2 weeks.

PER SERVING
PROTEIN: 30G
FIBRE: 12G
PLANT POINTS: 5

SERVES 1

1 tablespoon milled flaxseeds (about 15g)
1 tablespoon milled chia seeds (about 15g) (or you can use an extra 1 tablespoon milled flaxseeds instead)
100–150ml kefir (or milk of choice)
150g Greek yoghurt
100g fresh berries (e.g. blueberries, blackberries, strawberries, raspberries)
a drizzle of almond butter or 1 tablespoon of nuts (e.g. pistachios, almonds or hazelnuts)

Tip: You can mill your seeds in a coffee grinder or a small blender, or use pre-milled seeds. I use around 30g combined weight of milled chia and flaxseeds.

GUT-BOOSTING BREAKFAST BOWL

This is one of my go-to breakfasts that I make multiple times a week. It's filling, delicious, your gut bugs will love it and you can take it with you! This breakfast bowl contains the three Ps for optimum gut health: prebiotics, probiotics and polyphenols (see page 68 for more on these). The prebiotics are the soluble fibre, found in the flaxseeds, chia seeds and berries; the probiotics are the live bacteria, such as strains of Lactobacillus, found in the yoghurt and kefir, which can have a positive effect on our health as they pass through the gut; and the polyphenols in the vibrantly coloured berries are not only incredible antioxidants, but also get metabolised by the gut bacteria to make other healthy substances that further support our health. This well-balanced, gut-nourishing bowl provides around 30g of protein and up to 12g of fibre, making it a brilliant start to the day.

---

1. Mix the seeds with the kefir (or milk) and stir through the yoghurt. Add more kefir (or milk) if necessary to reach the right consistency. The mixture should be loose and not stiff, as the seeds can absorb a lot of liquid.

2. Top with berries and drizzle with almond butter or top with nuts of your choice.

Variation: This is also gorgeous made with grated frozen peaches and pistachios – like eating a sorbet for breakfast! Or with chopped kiwis – keep the skin on for even more fibre.

PER SERVING
PROTEIN: 6G
FIBRE: 5G
PLANT POINTS: 6.25

**MAKES 15 SERVINGS
(40G PER SERVING)**

120g gluten-free (or regular) rolled oats
120g sunflower seeds
120g pumpkin seeds
25g maple syrup
2 tablespoons extra virgin olive oil
1 teaspoon vanilla paste
a pinch of sea salt
75g cacao nibs
50g dried cherries
75g chia seeds

CHOCOLATE CHERRY GRANOLA

Chocolate and cherry, for me, are the perfect combination, especially when served with creamy yoghurt and fresh cherries. This breakfast takes me back to my time living in Germany and captures all the indulgence of a Black Forest gâteau (Schwarzwälder Kirschtorte). Unlike most shop-bought granolas, this version is more nutrient-dense, thanks to the addition of twice as many nuts and seeds as oats. The cacao nibs give it an intense chocolatey flavour, while also delivering on polyphenols, magnesium and iron. Adding the cherries at the end keeps them sweet and juicy and prevents them from overcooking and becoming bitter in the oven. I have purposely kept the added sugars low in this recipe, but you can use a little more maple syrup if you like.

1. Preheat the oven to 180°C fan. In a large bowl, combine the rolled oats, sunflower seeds, pumpkin seeds, maple syrup, extra virgin olive oil, vanilla paste and sea salt. Mix well, then spread in a thin layer on a baking sheet or in a ceramic baking dish lined with baking paper.

2. Bake for 25 minutes, stirring halfway through, until lightly golden. Remove from the oven and allow to cool fully – the granola will become crunchy as it cools.

3. Meanwhile, grind the cacao nibs in a small blender or a coffee grinder until they have the texture of a coarse flour.

4. Once the granola has cooled, stir in the ground cacao nibs, dried cherries and chia seeds.

Storage: Store in an airtight jar at room temperature for up to 2 weeks.

PER SERVING
PROTEIN: 31 G
FIBRE: 7G
PLANT POINTS: 7.25

SERVES 1
200g quark
40g Chocolate Cherry Granola (page 119)
80g fresh cherries or other berries

CHOCOLATE CHERRY BREAKFAST BOWL

Quark is a thick dairy product that is similar to a thick yoghurt and also has some resemblance to a soft cheese, but with a creamy, indulgent texture. It is higher in protein than Greek yoghurt and is usually low in fat, so the two can be used interchangeably in many of my recipes. If you like granola, but want to enjoy a perfectly balanced breakfast, this is a great choice. This recipe is ideal for a quick morning meal and also travels well, making it perfect for a jam-jar breakfast on the go.

1. Spoon the quark into a bowl or jar and top with the granola and fresh cherries or berries. Alternatively, layer the ingredients in a tall glass, finishing with the cherries or other berries on top.

Storage: Refrigerate if preparing in advance. Best enjoyed within 24 hours.

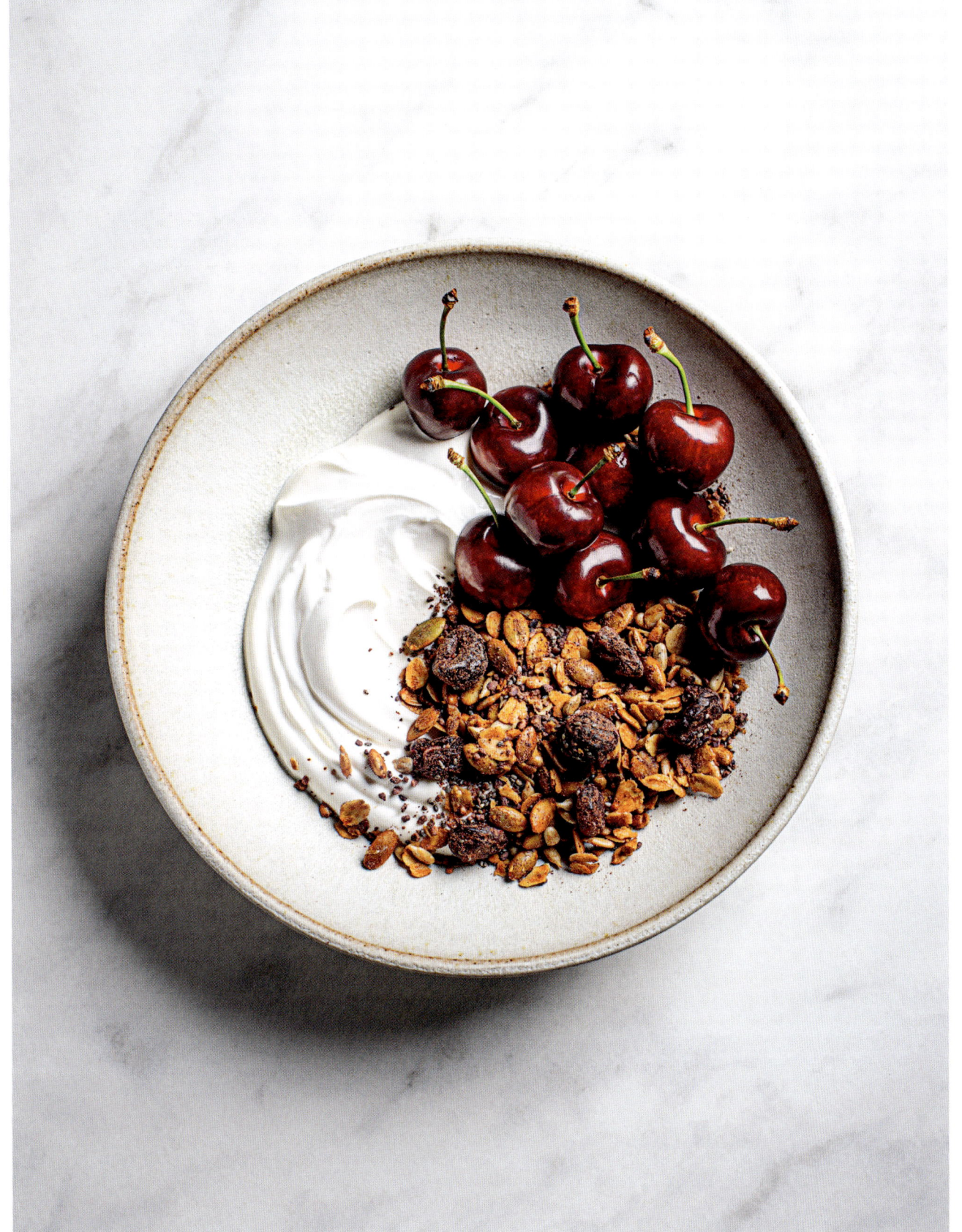

PER SERVING
PROTEIN: 33G
FIBRE: 13G
PLANT POINTS: 14.5

SERVES 2

½ teaspoon ground turmeric
½ teaspoon sweet paprika
2 tablespoons nutritional yeast (with added B12 if possible) (see Tip)
200g firm, plain tofu, drained and patted dry
1 tablespoon extra virgin olive oil
1 garlic clove, crushed, or 1 teaspoon garlic powder
30–80ml vegetable stock
1 red pepper, diced
200g vine tomatoes, chopped
50g kale or baby spinach
¼ teaspoon sea salt, or black salt (kala namak) for an eggy flavour

To serve

2 slices of Seed and Nut Loaf (page 253) or Carrot and Courgette Yoghurt Loaf (page 256) (Note, the Carrot and Yoghurt Loaf isn't vegan or dairy-free)
a small handful of fresh coriander and parsley, chopped
2 spring onions, chopped
a pinch of chilli flakes (optional)

Tip: You can use Parmesan instead of nutritional yeast, although this will, of course, make it unsuitable for vegans and vegetarians and it won't be dairy-free.

TOFU SCRAMBLE

This breakfast offers a delicious way to enjoy a plant-based meal with a convincing scrambled egg taste. Black salt (kala namak), a volcanic rock salt, gives the scramble an unmistakably 'eggy' flavour. Nutritional yeast is rich in protein and fibre and is often fortified with vitamin B12, which can be a great addition to vegetarian and plant-based diets. I use it here to give a gentle 'cheesy' taste. To add a healthy carbohydrate, I've served the tofu scramble with a slice of my Carrot and Courgette Yoghurt Loaf (page 256), which isn't vegan, so for a fully plant-based breakfast, choose the Seed and Nut Loaf (page 253), or a wholegrain bread. Alternatively, serve the scramble on a grilled portobello mushroom.

1. Measure the turmeric, paprika and nutritional yeast into a small bowl. Crumble the tofu into another bowl by hand or using a fork.

2. Heat the extra virgin olive oil in a frying pan over a medium heat, add the tofu and garlic or garlic powder, and stir until warmed through. Slowly add the vegetable stock, just enough to moisten the tofu mixture. The quantity of stock needed may vary depending on the tofu used.

3. Stir in the red pepper, vine tomatoes, kale or spinach, and the mixed spices and nutritional yeast, with your choice of salt. Cook for 2–3 minutes, until the vegetables soften slightly.

4. Serve with a slice of my carrot and yoghurt loaf, and garnish with chopped coriander, parsley, spring onions and a pinch of chilli flakes if using.

Storage: Store in an airtight container in the fridge for up to 2 days. Reheat in a frying pan over a low heat with a splash of water or extra virgin olive oil.

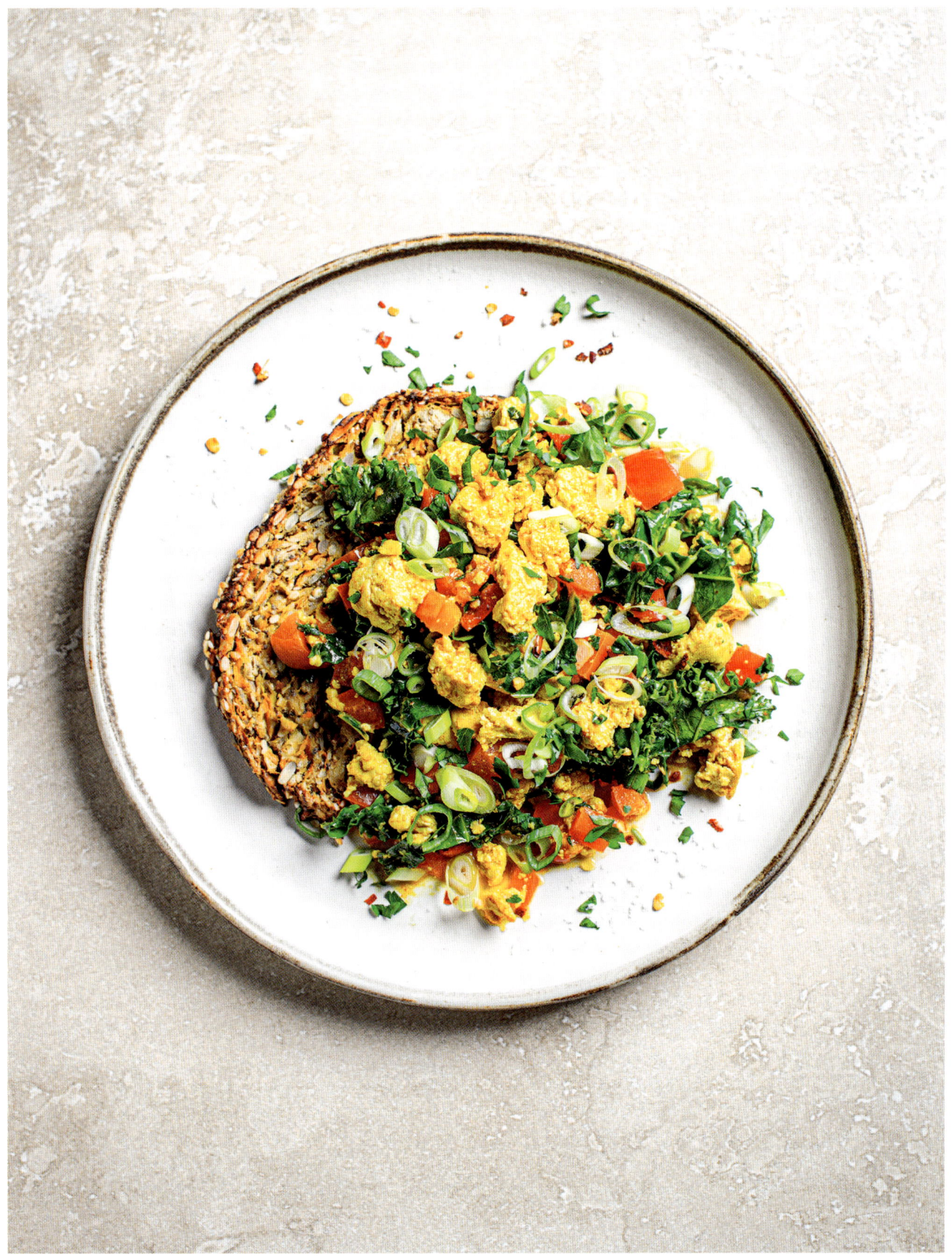

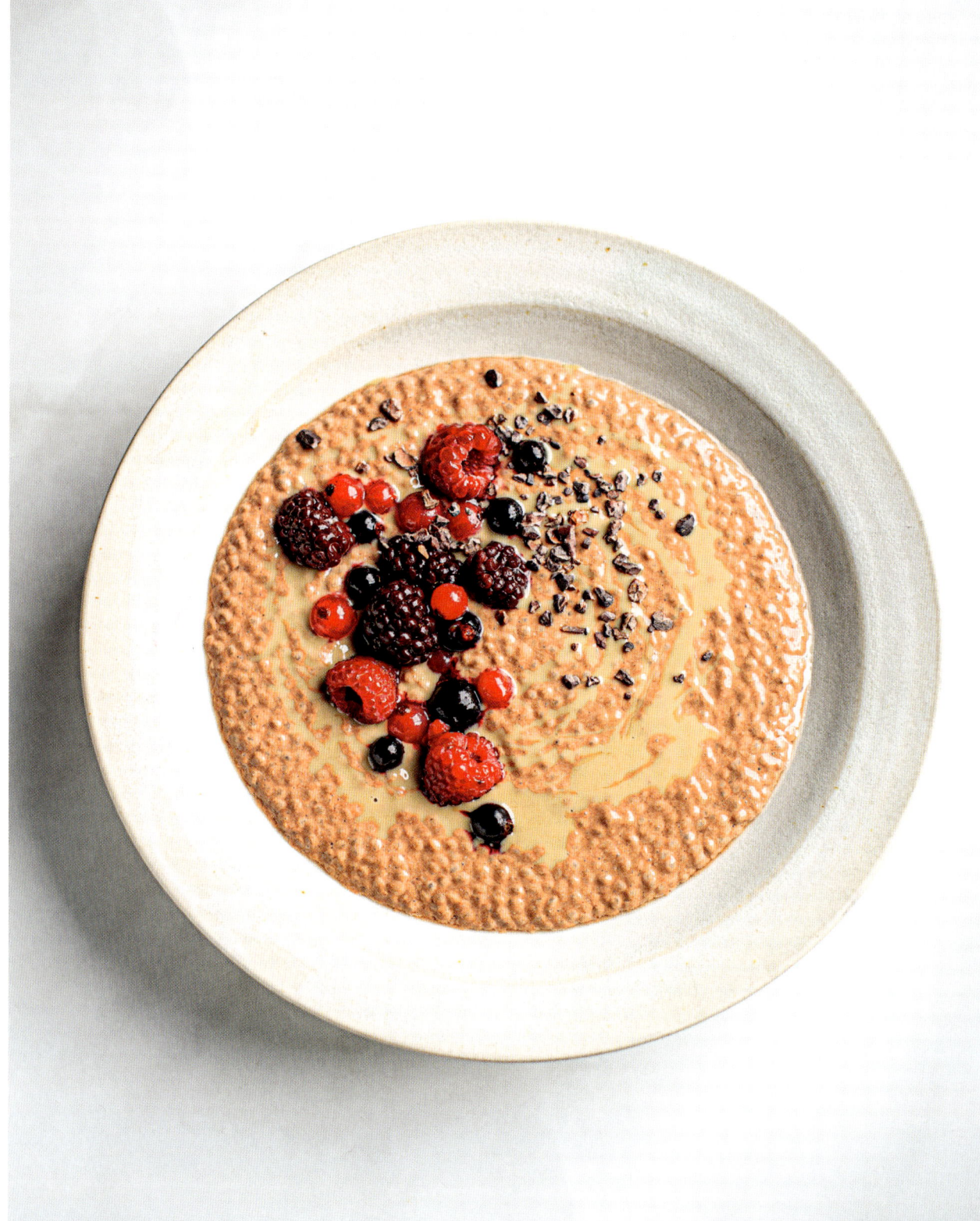

PER SERVING
PROTEIN: 27G
FIBRE: 13G
PLANT POINTS: 5.75

SERVES 1
2 tablespoons chia seeds
   (about 20g)
150g Greek yoghurt
100ml almond milk
   (or other plant milk)
1 teaspoon maple syrup
5–10g raw cacao powder,
   to taste

To serve
80g mixed berries
   (e.g. redcurrants, blackcurrants,
   blackberries and raspberries)
1 teaspoon tahini
a pinch of cacao nibs
a little maple syrup, if desired

CREAMY CHOCOLATE CHIA PUDDING

This is a great breakfast for anyone who is new to chia seeds, or if you find their texture a little 'gloopy'! You can enjoy this pudding as it is, but for a smoother consistency, you can blend the soaked mixture before serving to create a smooth, rich, mousse-like texture which many people prefer. Cacao powder has hidden benefits and is a surprisingly rich source of fibre. Just 10g contains around 3g of fibre, so it is great to sneak into your recipes. This breakfast also travels well, making it an excellent option for busy mornings. You can buy your berries frozen for convenience. I've also given you the option of sweetening it with extra maple syrup on serving, to suit your taste buds.

---

1. In a bowl, combine the chia seeds, Greek yoghurt, almond milk, maple syrup and cacao powder, to taste. Stir well and leave to soak for 30 minutes, allowing the chia seeds to swell and absorb the liquid. If the mixture becomes too thick, add a little more milk to reach the consistency you like.

2. For a smoother pudding, blend the mixture in a food processor until creamy.

3. Taste and adjust the sweetness if needed, then spoon into a bowl. Top with mixed berries, a drizzle of tahini, and a sprinkle of cacao nibs for crunch. Drizzle with a little extra maple syrup, if desired.

Storage: Keep refrigerated and consume within 24 hours.

PER SERVING
PROTEIN: 22G
FIBRE: 15G
PLANT POINTS: 7.5

SERVES 2

1 medium red onion, finely chopped
1 garlic clove, crushed
1 tablespoon extra virgin olive oil
1 medium carrot, scrubbed and finely diced
1 red pepper, diced
1 x 400g tin or jar of flageolet beans (or other white beans) (240g drained weight)
1 teaspoon harissa paste
1 tablespoon lemon juice
1 tablespoon chopped fresh herbs (e.g. parsley or chives), plus extra to serve
sea salt and freshly ground black pepper

To serve
2 tablespoons Greek yoghurt (around 50g)
2 slices of sourdough bread or Super Green Bread (page 254) or Carrot and Courgette Yoghurt Loaf (page 256)
30g Parmesan (or vegetarian hard cheese), grated
50g sauerkraut or kimchi

HARISSA BEANS ON TOAST

Creamy beans are comfort food on a plate, but making your own is simple and takes less than twenty minutes. Beans are incredibly versatile and are also gentle on our blood sugars, due to their high fibre content. I have boosted the protein in this dish with some yoghurt and cheese, which softens the heat of the harissa and gives a rich, creamy texture. The quality of your bread really matters – a traditional sourdough bread is fermented, which makes it easier for us to digest. Using bean liquid adds creaminess, but you can replace it with water if you prefer, particularly if you are sensitive to the gassy effects of beans. (This is because bean water contains some of the carbohydrates that cause gas.) There is no need to peel the carrots – a good scrub is enough, as many of the nutrients are found just beneath the skin. I've served my harissa beans with a slice of seeded sourdough but they're also great with the Super Green Bread (page 254) or Carrot and Courgette Yoghurt Loaf (page 256) – both of these will make it gluten-free.

1. Sauté the onion and garlic in a frying pan with the extra virgin olive oil over a medium heat for around 5 minutes, until softened and translucent. Add the diced carrot and red pepper and cook for a further 3 minutes, until just tender.

2. Add the beans with their liquid (if using), the harissa paste, lemon juice and chopped herbs and season with salt and pepper. Simmer gently for 5–8 minutes, until the mixture thickens and becomes creamy.

3. Remove from the heat and stir through the Greek yoghurt, or spoon the beans over the toasted sourdough and serve with the yoghurt on the side. Top with grated Parmesan, a little extra fresh herbs and a spoonful of sauerkraut.

Storage: Store the cooked bean mixture in an airtight container in the fridge for up to 3 days.

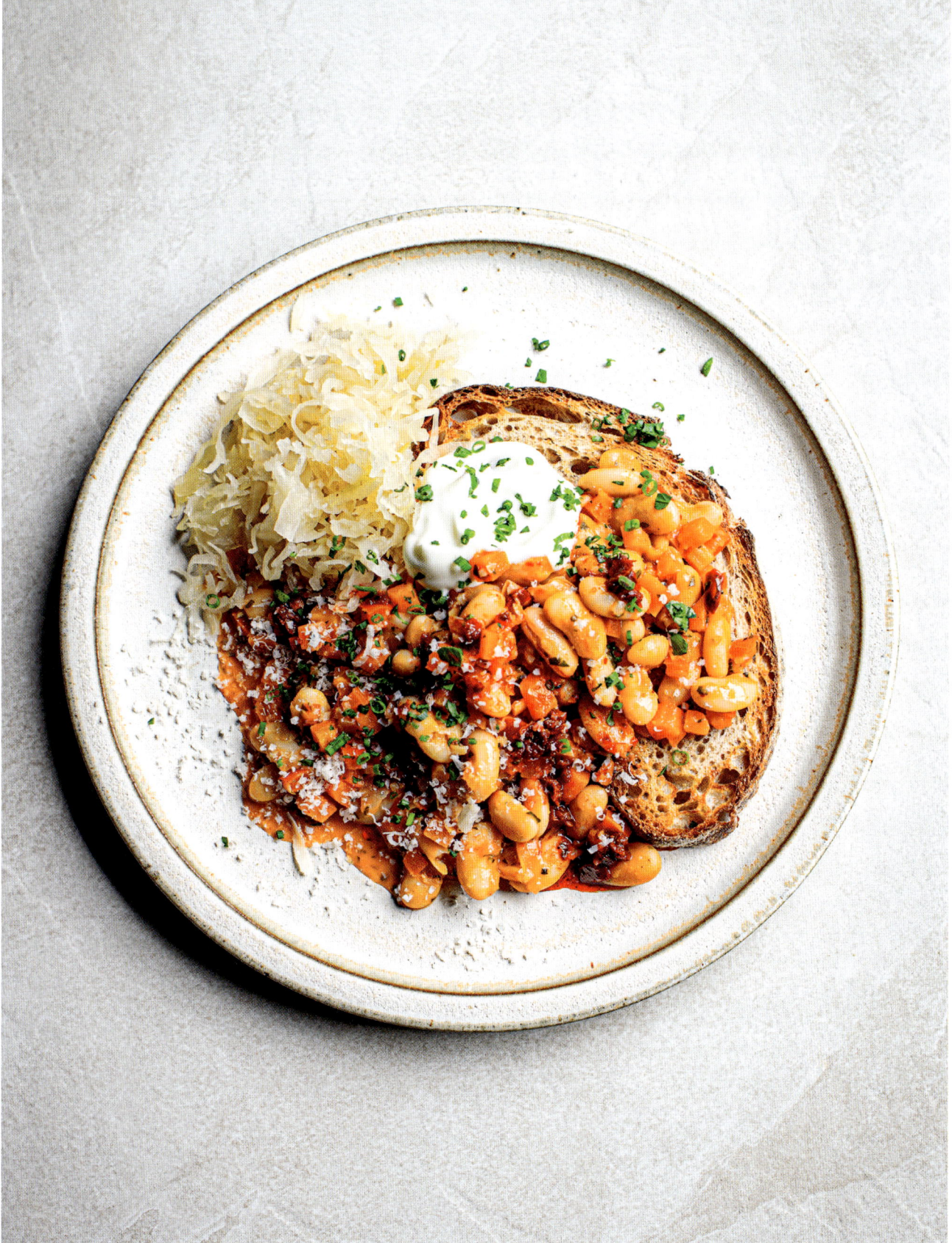

PER SERVING
PROTEIN: 25G
FIBRE: 9G
PLANT POINTS: 4.5

SERVES 1

1 Red Lentil Bagel (page 267)
25g quark or soft cream cheese
50g smoked salmon or trout
100–150g salad
  (e.g. cucumber, radish, tomato, red onion, salad leaves or microgreens)
freshly ground black pepper

NEW YORK-STYLE SMOKED SALMON BAGEL

Who doesn't love a New York bagel! My Red Lentil Bagel recipe (page 267) is completely gluten-free and perfectly balanced, and because they are higher in protein and fibre they keep you feeling full up for longer. Whenever I make these, no one can quite believe that they are made from lentils! I have paired mine with quark to boost the protein and give an extra creamy texture, but you can swap this for a cream cheese if you prefer.

---

1. Slice your bagel in half. Toast if desired, then spread the quark or cream cheese evenly over the base.

2. Top with slices of smoked salmon or trout, then add the sliced vegetables on top and on the side of the plate. Sprinkle with freshly ground pepper and serve immediately.

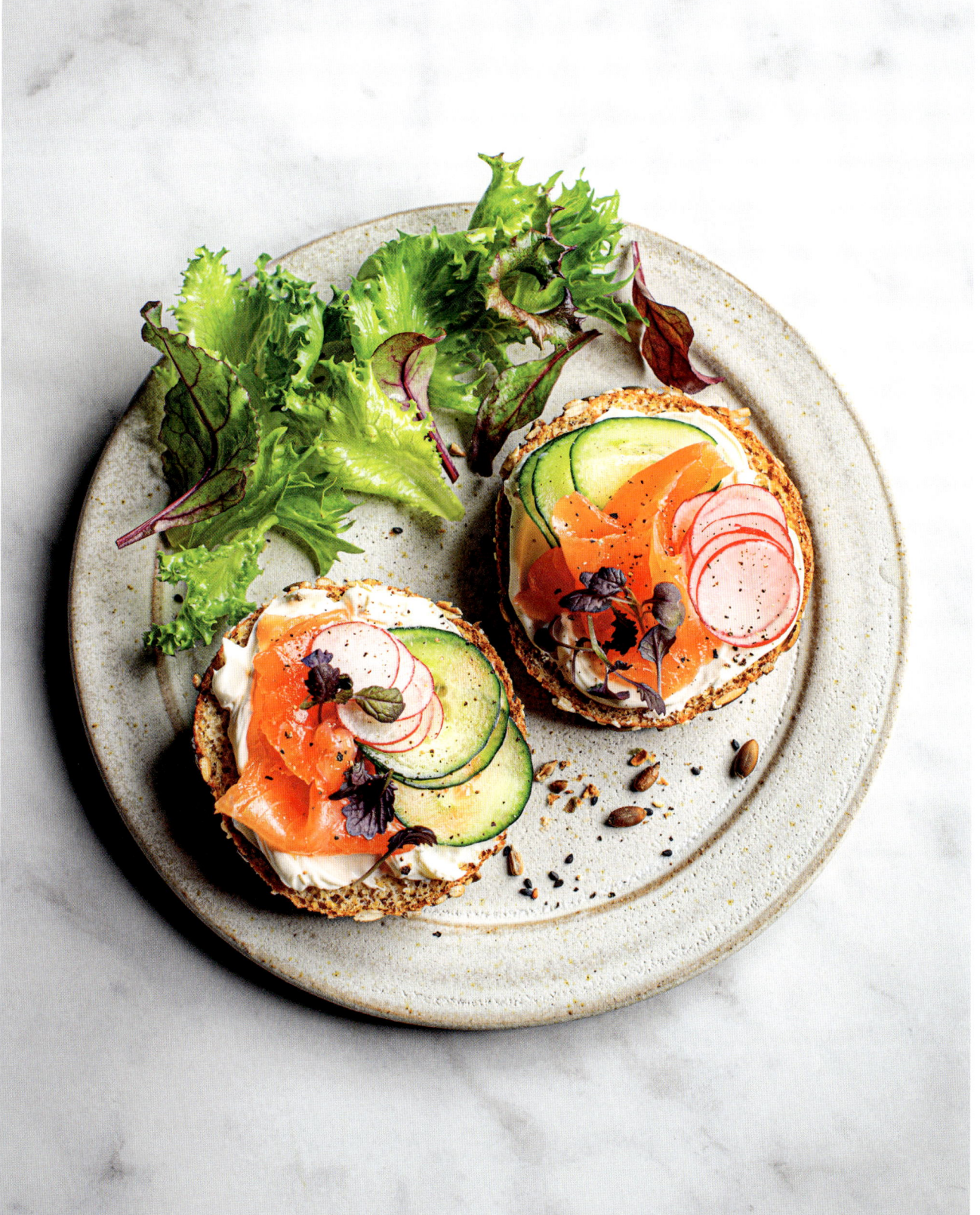

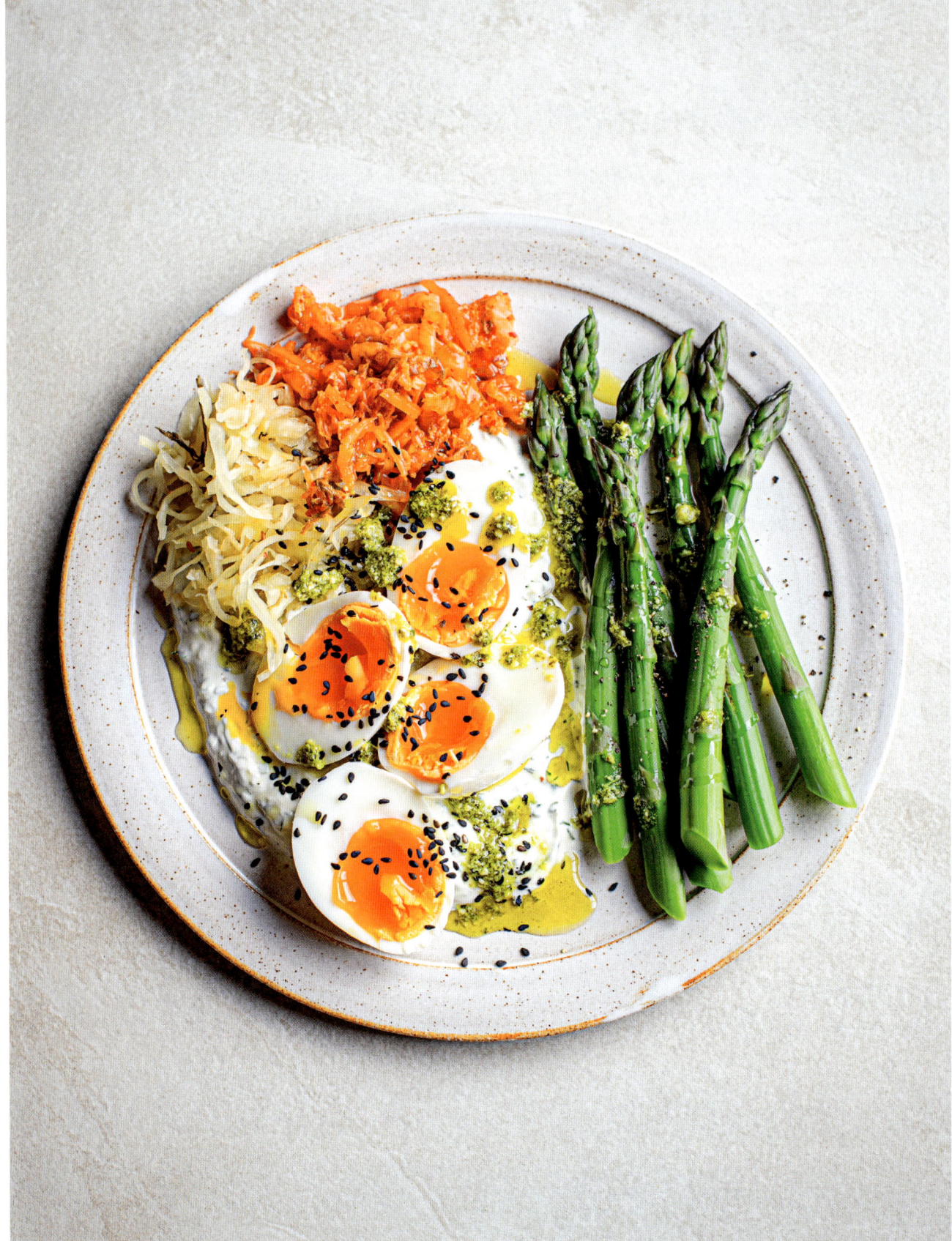

PER SERVING
PROTEIN: 29G
FIBRE: 6G
PLANT POINTS: 6.25

SERVES 2
200g Greek yoghurt
1 tablespoon extra virgin olive oil
2 garlic cloves, crushed
1 tablespoon lemon juice
a small handful of mixed chopped herbs (e.g. parsley, chives, dill)
sea salt and freshly ground black pepper
4 eggs
300g asparagus, ends trimmed

To serve
1 spoonful of kimchi (around 50g per serving)
1 spoonful of sauerkraut (around 50g per serving)
a swirl of Green Pesto (page 205) (or vegetarian pesto)
a pinch of black sesame seeds

TURKISH EGGS BRUNCH

This is one of my favourite brunch recipes for a lazy Sunday. It is a lovely way of serving eggs with a creamy garlic yoghurt sauce. The dish is packed with probiotic bacteria to support our gut health, with a combination of fermented vegetables and live yoghurt. I love to top the eggs with a swirl of homemade Green Pesto (page 205), which I always keep on hand, for extra protein and fibre, rather than the more traditional harissa butter. I have served it without bread but, if you like, you can use a slice of sourdough or my Super Green Bread (page 254) to scoop up the last of the sauce.

1. In a bowl, combine the yoghurt, extra virgin olive oil, garlic, lemon juice and chopped herbs and season with salt and pepper. Spread the yoghurt mixture across two plates or shallow bowls.

2. Pierce your eggs and cook them in simmering water with the lid on for 6 minutes, along with the trimmed asparagus, which will cook in around the same time.

3. Remove the eggs from the pan and plunge them into ice-cold water to stop the cooking process, and to keep the egg yolks soft. Drain the asparagus and place it on the serving plates with the yoghurt. Add the kimchi and sauerkraut.

4. Peel the eggs, place them on top of the yoghurt, and cut them in half to show their deliciously gooey centres. Top with a swirl of pesto and sprinkle with black sesame seeds.

PER SERVING
PROTEIN: 25G
FIBRE: 10G
PLANT POINTS: 4

SERVES 2
1 ripe banana, mashed
80g gluten-free (or regular) rolled oats
40g ground almonds
200g destoned frozen (and defrosted) or fresh cherries
½ teaspoon vanilla paste
200ml milk of choice (I used almond milk)
10g flaked almonds

To serve
200g quark or Greek yoghurt

CHERRY BAKEWELL BAKED OATS

I have a secret love of Bakewell tart and all things almond, and I wanted to bring this into a breakfast that could be both delicious and healthy. Adding ground almonds helps lower the glycaemic response of the oats, while a mashed banana provides natural sweetness along with fibre, some resistant starch and potassium. Cherries bring in more sweetness and give an antioxidant boost, and the generous spoonful of quark or Greek yoghurt adds creaminess and helps balance the dish with enough protein to support energy levels through the morning. For a dairy-free option, swap the yoghurt for Greek-style soya yoghurt and use a plant-based milk. This breakfast can be made in advance and reheated before serving.

1. Preheat the oven to 180°C fan and lightly grease a small ceramic dish, about 10cm x 15cm in size.

2. In a mixing bowl, combine the mashed banana, oats, ground almonds, cherries, vanilla paste and milk. Stir until well mixed, then pour the mixture into the prepared dish.

3. Sprinkle the flaked almonds over the top and bake in the oven for 30–35 minutes, until golden and set in the centre. Serve warm, with a generous helping of quark or Greek yoghurt.

Storage: Allow to cool completely before storing. Keep in an airtight container in the fridge for up to 3 days. Reheat gently in the oven or enjoy it cold. Suitable for freezing for up to 1 month; defrost overnight in the fridge before serving.

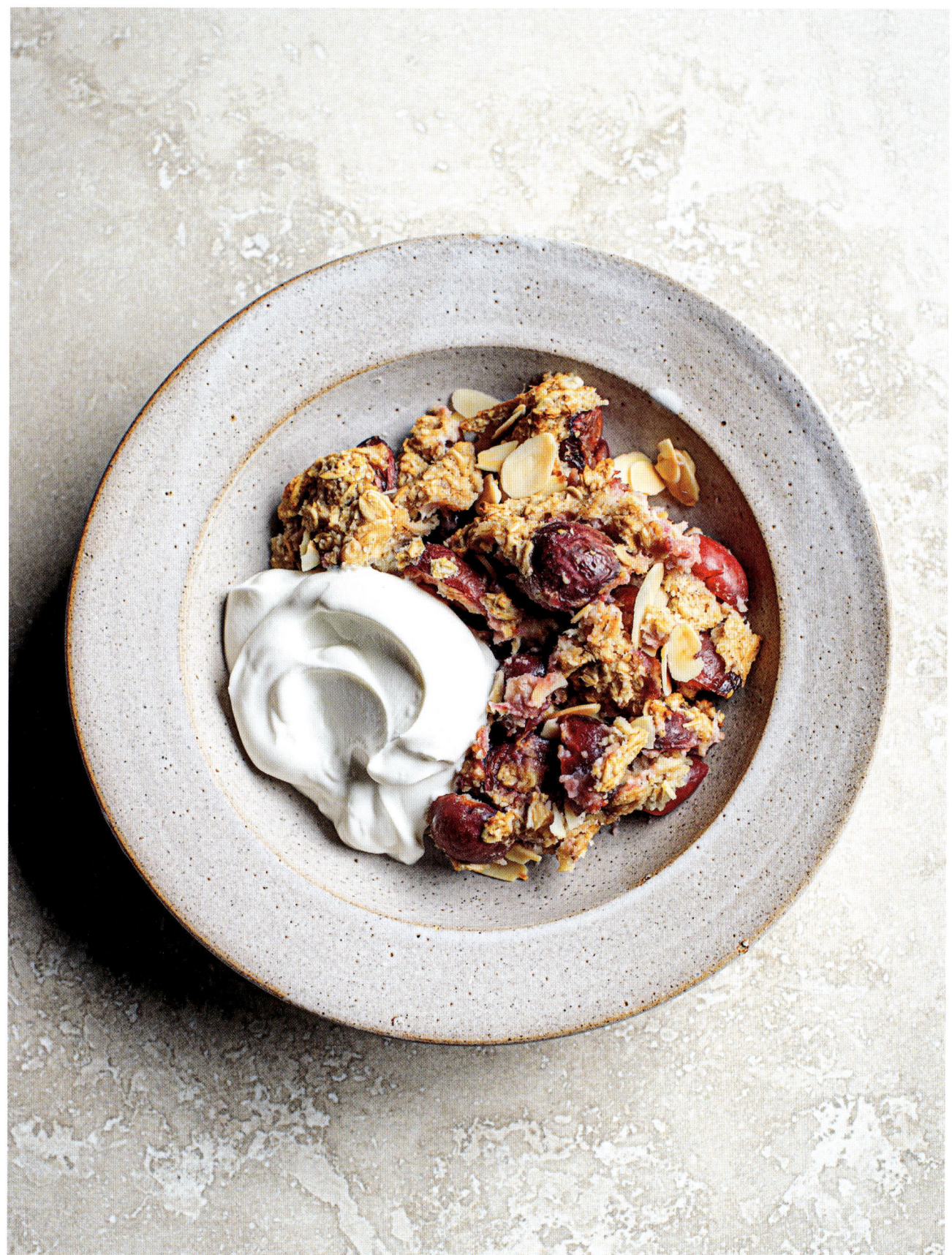

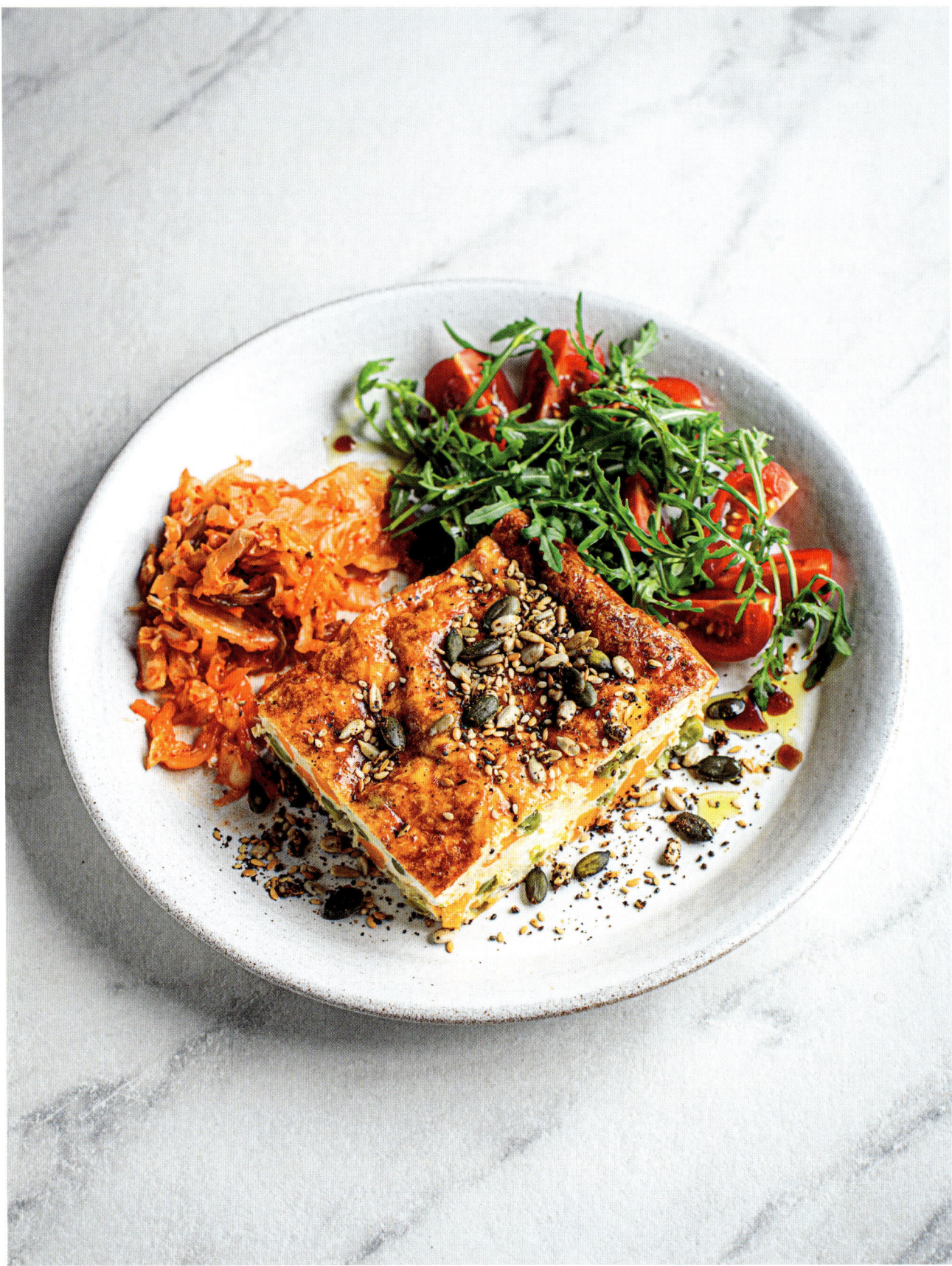

PER SERVING
PROTEIN: 28G
FIBRE: 11G
PLANT POINTS: 9.5

SERVES 6

1 red onion, finely diced
1 tablespoon extra virgin olive oil
250g sweet potato, peeled and diced
250g frozen peas
8 eggs
200g Greek yoghurt
sea salt and freshly ground black pepper
200g feta
30g Parmesan (or vegetarian hard cheese), grated

To serve (per serving)
1 tablespoon (15 g) Savoury Seed Mix (page 136)
50g kimchi
mixed salad, with 30ml French dressing

SWEET POTATO AND FETA FRITTATA

I love yoga and attend a least one in-person class each week. Afterwards, we visit a local café where sweet potato frittata is my favourite go-to brunch. I wanted to make a version that aligns with my Triple 30 principles and contains sufficient protein to start the day. This version is ideal to make in advance and is easy to transport – it also makes a perfect lunch to take with you on the go! I cut larger portions for lunch, so the frittata serves 6 for breakfast and 4 at lunch. At lunchtime, serve it with a large mixed salad (about 250g) comprising at least three different vegetables. Peas are often the unsung hero in a recipe, yet most people have some in their freezer. With around 5g of protein and 5g of fibre per 100g, peas can really boost the nutrition in your meals. I have also added my Savoury Seed Mix (page 136) to increase the fibre and the plant diversity, and kimchi for an extra boost of probiotic bacteria.

1. Preheat the oven to 180°C fan. In a frying pan, gently sauté the red onion in the extra virgin olive oil over a low heat for 7–10 minutes, until soft and caramelised.

2. Bring a small pan of water to the boil and add the diced sweet potato. Cover and cook for 4 minutes, then add the frozen peas and cook for 2 more minutes. Drain and allow the steam to evaporate so the vegetables are dry. The sweet potato should still be slightly undercooked.

3. In a large bowl, whisk the eggs and Greek yoghurt together. Season with salt and pepper, then crumble in the feta and mix gently. Fold through the cooked onion, sweet potato and peas.

4. Line a ceramic dish (about 25cm x 15cm) with non-stick baking paper. Pour in the egg mixture and sprinkle the grated Parmesan over the top. Bake for about 1 hour, or until golden brown and puffed up in the centre.

5. Allow to cool slightly before slicing. Serve with the savoury seed mix, kimchi and a mixed salad.

Storage: Keep in an airtight container in the fridge for up to 3 days. Reheat in the oven or air fryer at 180°C for 5 minutes, until hot all the way through.

PER 15G SERVING
PROTEIN: 3G
FIBRE: 3G
PLANT POINTS: 6.75

MAKES 425G

75g sunflower seeds
75g pumpkin seeds
100g whole flaxseeds
75g sesame seeds
50g hemp seeds
50g chia seeds
a pinch of chilli flakes or cayenne pepper
1 teaspoon tamari or soy sauce (Note, soy sauce isn't gluten-free)
1 teaspoon extra virgin olive oil

SAVOURY SEED MIX

This versatile seed mix is an easy way to increase your plant points while adding flavour, protein and fibre to your meals. Sprinkle a spoonful over soups, salads or any meal to enhance both nutrition and texture. A tablespoon delivers 3g of protein and 3g of fibre to your plate, which can really help you reach your target of 10g of fibre per meal. The jar contains 425g of seeds, so make up the weight with any seeds or nuts if you are missing any ingredients.

1. Preheat the oven to 160°C fan. In a large bowl, mix together all the ingredients.

2. Spread the mixture evenly on a baking tray and bake for 12 minutes, stirring once halfway through, until the seeds are slightly golden. Allow to cool completely, then transfer to an airtight jar.

Storage: Store in an airtight jar and use within 3 weeks.

PER SERVING
PROTEIN: 26G
FIBRE: 13G
PLANT POINTS: 3

SERVES 2

4 tablespoons chia seeds (around 50g)
200ml milk of choice (I have used unsweetened soya)
50ml coconut milk (from a tin)
30g coconut flakes
300g Greek yoghurt

To serve
around 100g fruit of choice (I like chopped kiwi or berries)

Tip: You can freeze any extra tinned coconut milk in an ice cube tray so that you can easily add a cube or two to soups, stews or porridge.

HOT COCONUT CHIA PORRIDGE

In this porridge I have combined chia seeds with milk, tinned coconut milk, coconut flakes, Greek yoghurt and berries for a warming, fibre-rich breakfast. Chia seeds are mini powerhouses when it comes to nutrition. They contain high levels of soluble fibre to help support gut health, and they are also surprisingly rich in micronutrients, such as calcium, iron, zinc and magnesium. Chia seeds swell up and can absorb many times their own weight in liquid, so we need to make sure that we soak or cook them before consuming them. Drinking sufficient water throughout the day helps to keep these little seeds 'puffed up', which can also help to keep our gut moving.

---

1. Put the chia seeds, milk, coconut milk and coconut flakes into a saucepan and heat gently, stirring well. Cover with a lid and simmer over a very low heat for around 25 minutes, stirring occasionally. Check the consistency and add a splash more milk if needed.

2. Once the porridge has thickened and the chia seeds have softened, stir in the Greek yoghurt.

3. Serve topped with fresh fruit.

PER SERVING
PROTEIN: 28G
FIBRE: 13G
PLANT POINTS: 6.75

SERVES 2
1 tablespoon extra virgin olive oil
1 red onion, thinly sliced
1 large garlic clove, crushed
1 teaspoon ground cumin
½ teaspoon ground coriander
a pinch of chilli flakes
1 x 400g tin or jar of black beans, rinsed and drained (240g drained weight)
1 x 400g tin of chopped or cherry tomatoes
2 eggs

Toppings
1 small avocado, sliced
a handful of rocket and/or coriander leaves
2 spring onions, thinly sliced
50g feta
a pinch of chilli flakes (optional)
50g Greek yoghurt
sea salt and freshly ground black pepper

ANY BEAN SHAKSHUKA

This is a fun take on the traditional shakshuka. It's packed with fibre and protein, so will fill you up and you'll be less likely to think about food between meals. The tomato and bean base is deep and rich, ideal for scooping up with your favourite bread – I suggest a slice of sourdough or my Seed and Nut Loaf, Super Green Bread or Carrot and Courgette Yoghurt Loaf (pages 253, 254 or 256). The recipe can easily be doubled for a family meal and can even work well as a quick lunch.

---

1. Heat the extra virgin olive oil in a large frying pan over a medium heat. Add the red onion and garlic and cook for around 5 minutes until softened. Stir in the ground cumin, ground coriander and chilli flakes, and cook for 1 minute. Add the black beans and tinned tomatoes, stirring to combine. Simmer gently for about 8 minutes, until the mixture thickens and the flavours develop, adding a splash of water if needed.

2. Meanwhile, cook the eggs in a separate pan. Fried, poached or soft-boiled eggs work well. (I like to cook the eggs separately to avoid the beans sticking to the bottom of the pan, as stirring is tricky once the eggs are cooking.) For soft-boiled eggs, cook for 6½ minutes and plunge into ice-cold water to stop the cooking process, before peeling. To poach, heat a pan of simmering water, crack each egg into an oiled ladle, gently lower into the water and release once the white starts to set. Cook for 2–3 minutes, until the whites are set and the yolks are runny. Remove with a slotted spoon and keep warm.

3. Divide the tomato and bean base between two plates. Top each with an egg, sliced avocado, rocket and/or coriander leaves, spring onions, a sprinkle of crumbled feta, chilli flakes (if using) and the Greek yoghurt. Season with salt and pepper. Enjoy on its own, or with your choice of bread.

Storage: Best served immediately. The tomato base can be stored in an airtight container in the fridge for up to 3 days, without any of the toppings.

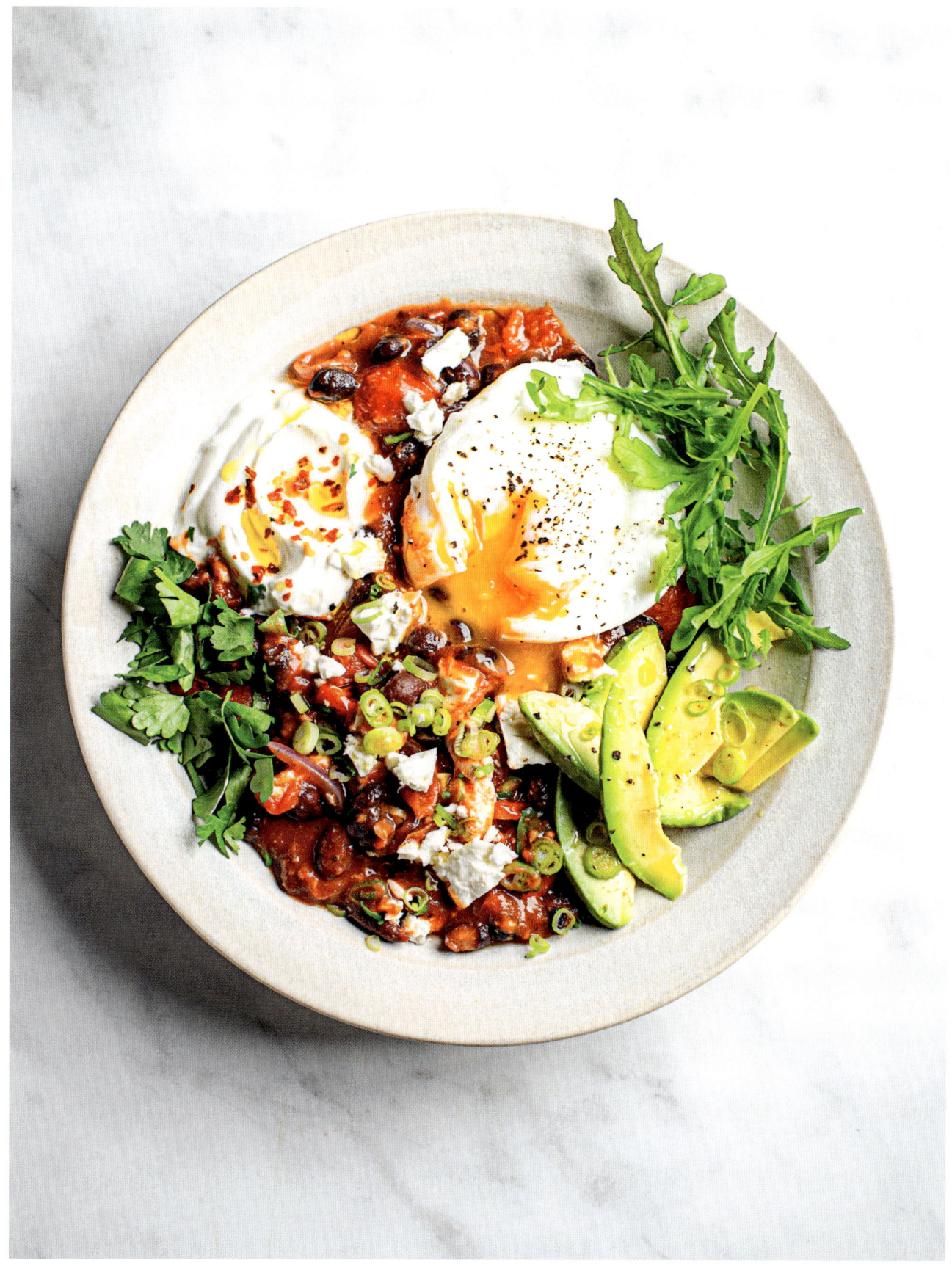

PER SERVING
PROTEIN: 27G
FIBRE: 11G
PLANT POINTS: 6.25

SERVES 2
MAKES 12 MINI PANCAKES

80g gluten-free (or regular) rolled oats or oat flour
1 ripe banana
2 eggs
75g Greek yoghurt
25g milled flaxseeds (or ground almonds)
½ level teaspoon baking powder
¼ teaspoon vanilla paste or extract
25ml milk of choice (I used soya milk)
a little extra virgin olive oil (or avocado oil if you prefer a milder taste), for frying

To serve
a generous spoonful of Greek yoghurt (around 75g per serving)
150g fresh berries (e.g. raspberries, blueberries, blackberries, strawberries)
a pinch of dried blueberry, acai or pitaya powder (optional)

BERRY PANCAKE STACK

Who doesn't enjoy a stack of pancakes? This version is less stodgy than your usual pancake stack and lighter in texture, and can be more than just a weekend treat. These pancakes can help to sustain your energy and are healthy too. I like to make them with milled flaxseeds for an extra fibre boost, but you can swap these for ground almonds if you prefer. Some berries, such as raspberries and blackberries, are made up of clusters of 'mini' fruits called drupelets. This structure means that they can contain nearly twice the fibre content of single berries, such as blueberries.

---

1. If using rolled oats, blend them first into a flour in a food processor. This should take around 10 seconds at high speed.

2. Add the banana, eggs, yoghurt, flaxseeds (or ground almonds), baking powder and vanilla, and blend until smooth. (If you are using oat flour, you can mix all the ingredients together in a bowl, but remember to mash the banana first with a fork.)

3. Slowly add the milk to reach a thick but pourable consistency. Note: if using flaxseeds, you may need slightly more milk; with ground almonds, slightly less.

4. Heat a little oil in a frying pan over a medium heat and drop in spoonfuls of the pancake mixture to form small circles. Allow the surface to set and bubbles to form, then flip and cook the other side. Each side should take around 1–2 minutes.

5. Stack the pancakes on plates and top with Greek yoghurt, fresh or defrosted berries, and a sprinkling of dried berry powder, if using.

Storage: Leftovers can be stored in an airtight container in the fridge for up to 3 days. These pancakes also freeze well for up to 2 months. Reheat in an oven or air fryer for 3–4 minutes at 160°C.

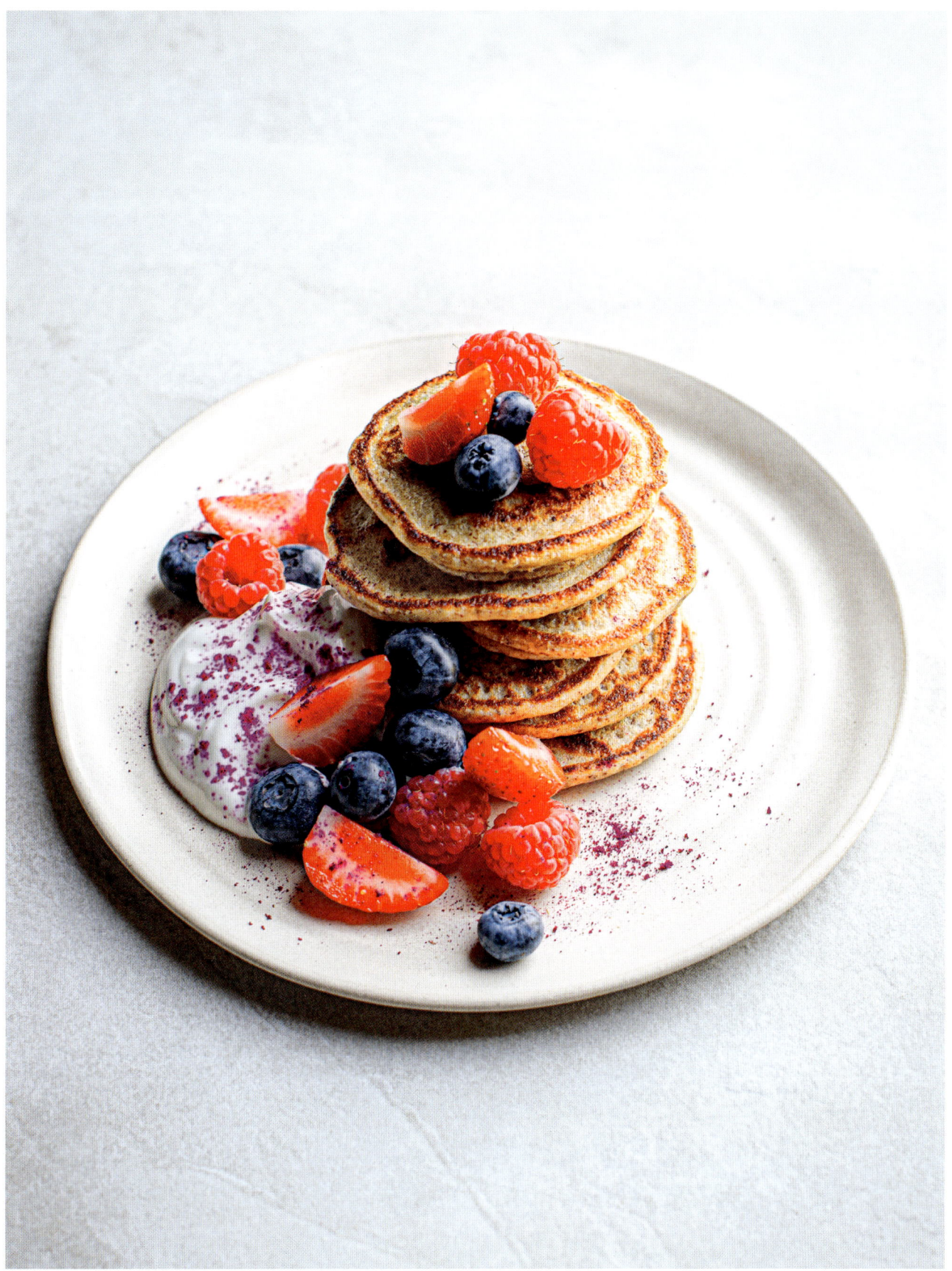

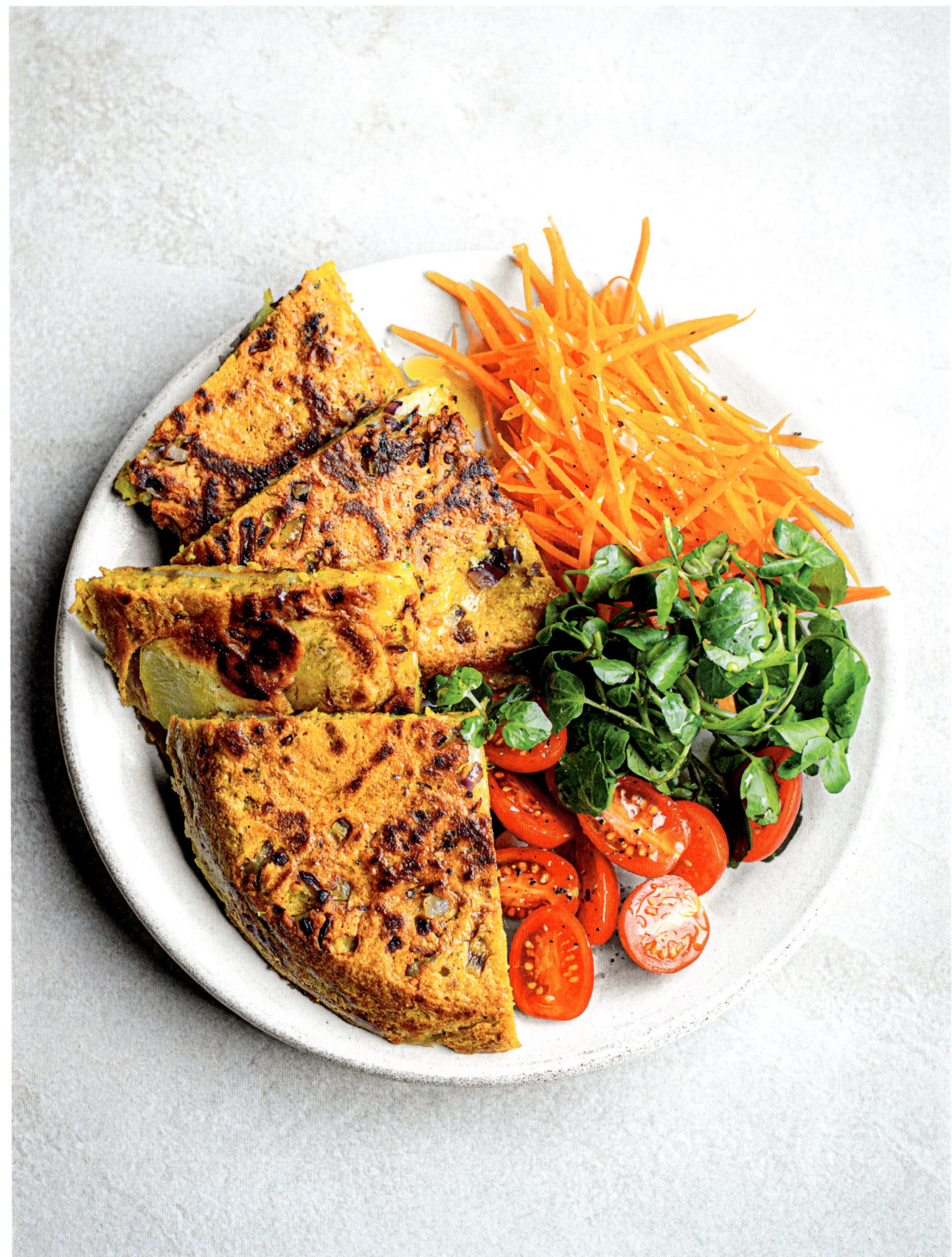

PER SERVING
PROTEIN: 28G
FIBRE: 15G
PLANT POINTS: 7.5

SERVES 2

200g chickpea (gram) flour
350ml filtered water
¼ teaspoon sea salt, or black salt (kala namak) for an eggy flavour
1 teaspoon ground cumin
1 teaspoon ground coriander
1 teaspoon ground turmeric
¼ teaspoon chilli flakes
1 medium courgette, grated
15g nutritional yeast
1 tablespoon extra virgin olive oil
1 medium red onion, finely diced
150g peeled potato, very thinly sliced (use a mandoline if possible)

To serve
For breakfast: Serve with vegetables (e.g. watercress, tomatoes or grated carrot).
For lunch: Serve with a generous portion of mixed salad (half a plate!)

BREAKFAST CHICKPEA TORTILLA

I am often asked about savoury breakfast options that are plant-based or egg-free yet still provide plenty of protein and fibre. This can be a challenge without resorting to protein powders as a top-up, but chickpeas are naturally rich in both protein and fibre and make a great alternative to eggs in this egg-free tortilla. I have used plenty of warming spices to create a rich and satisfying tortilla. The nutritional yeast adds flavour and protein, but you can leave it out if you prefer. Ideal for make-ahead breakfasts, this also works well as a filling lunch with a generous salad.

---

1. Whisk the chickpea flour, water, salt and spices together in a mixing bowl or food processor until smooth. Stir in the grated courgette, and nutritional yeast, if using. For best results, set the mixture aside for around 30–60 minutes to thicken.

2. Heat the extra virgin olive oil in a small frying pan over a medium heat. Add the red onion and sauté for 2 minutes. Add the sliced potato and cook, stirring regularly, for 4–5 minutes until the potato begins to soften and turn lightly golden. Remove half the onion and potato and set aside for the second tortilla.

3. Pour in half the batter, spreading it evenly over the vegetables. Do not stir at this stage. Reduce the heat to medium-low to avoid it catching on the base, and cover the pan with a lid to create steam. Cook for around 10 minutes, or until the mixture is fully set on top.

4. Carefully flip the tortilla using a fish slice or spatula. Cook for 5–8 minutes on the other side until golden and cooked through.

5. Repeat with the remaining onion, potatoes and batter.

6. Arrange on plates with vegetables or salad of your choice, e.g. watercress, tomatoes and red onion.

Storage: Store in an airtight container in the fridge for up to 3 days. Can be reheated easily in the oven or in an air fryer for 6 minutes at 160°C.

PER SERVING
PROTEIN: 33G
FIBRE: 7G
PLANT POINTS: 4.25

SERVES 2
1 teaspoon extra virgin olive oil, plus more for oiling
125g asparagus spears, ends trimmed
200g vine tomatoes
2 eggs
2 kipper fillets (around 120g each)

To serve
1 slice of rye pumpernickel bread (½ a slice per serving)
1 heaped tablespoon sauerkraut per serving
a pinch of chilli flakes (optional)

KIPPERS AND EGGS

Kippers are smoked herrings. They have fallen slightly out of favour, but they still remain an excellent source of omega-3 fats and protein. While their flavour is quite strong, they can be a delicious and nutrient-rich addition to your breakfast rotation. Because kippers are naturally salty, they are best enjoyed occasionally rather than as an everyday breakfast. Cooking them gently by poaching in hot water helps to reduce any strong kitchen smells (which is probably one of the main reasons people avoid cooking them!) and keeps preparation quick and simple. This dish is a great example of a balanced savoury breakfast.

---

1. Heat the extra virgin olive oil in a deep-sided frying pan over a medium-high heat and cook the asparagus spears and whole tomatoes for around 5–6 minutes, until softened and lightly charred. Add a splash of water if needed to prevent sticking and to gently create some steam. Transfer to a plate and keep warm.

2. Using the same frying pan, fill it halfway with hot water. Once it is gently simmering, carefully lower the whole eggs into the water and cook for 6½ minutes. Remove and plunge into ice-cold water to stop them cooking, then peel. Alternatively, to poach your eggs, bring the water to a gentle simmer. Crack each egg into an oiled ladle, gently lower into the water and release once the white starts to set. Cook for 2–3 minutes, until the whites are set but the yolks are still runny. Remove with a slotted spoon and keep warm.

3. Keeping the hot water in the pan, add the kipper fillets, turn off the heat, and cover with a lid. Allow the kippers to poach for around 5 minutes, until fully cooked.

4. Assemble all the ingredients on 2 plates and serve with a spoonful of sauerkraut on the side and a sprinkle of chilli flakes, if you like.

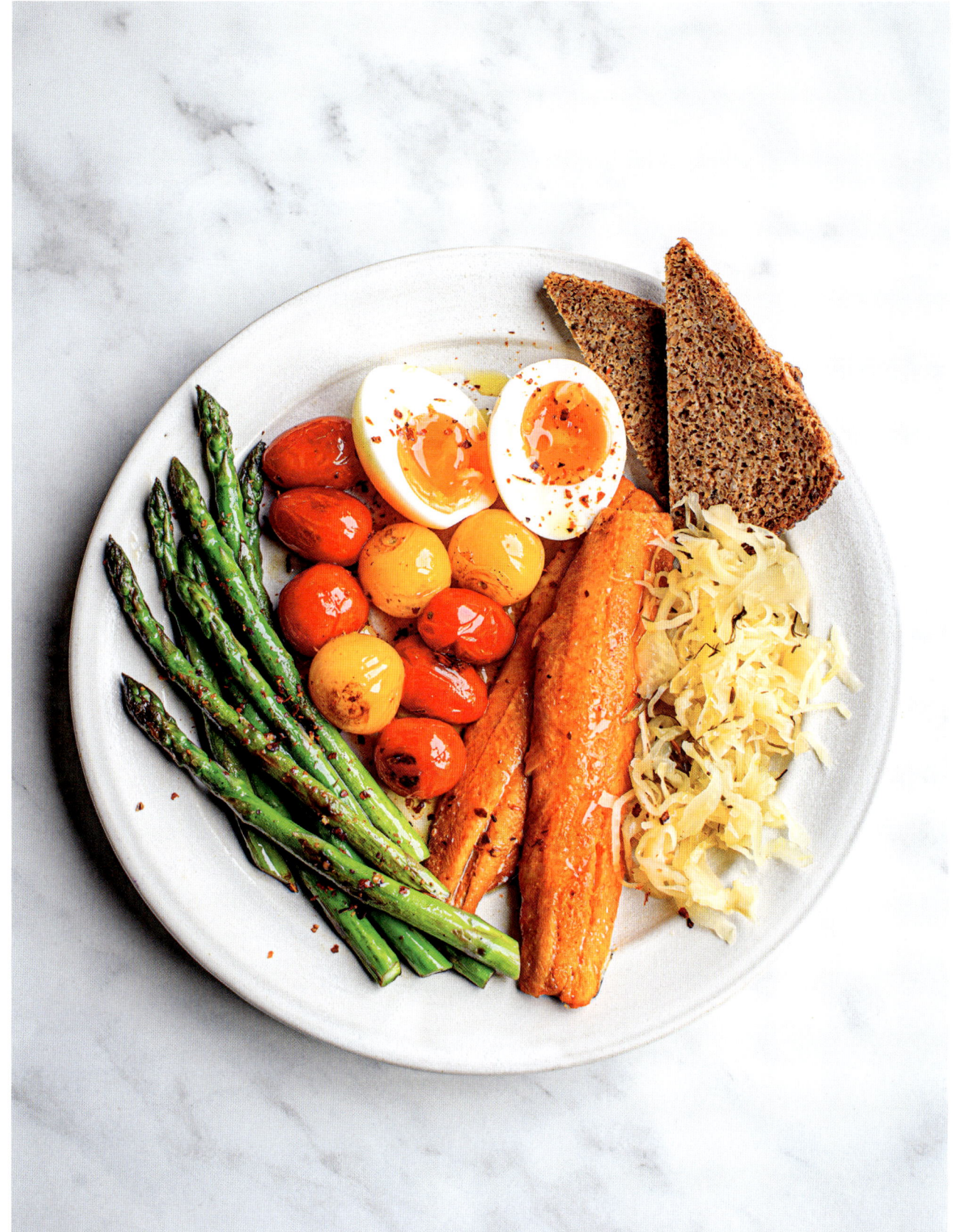

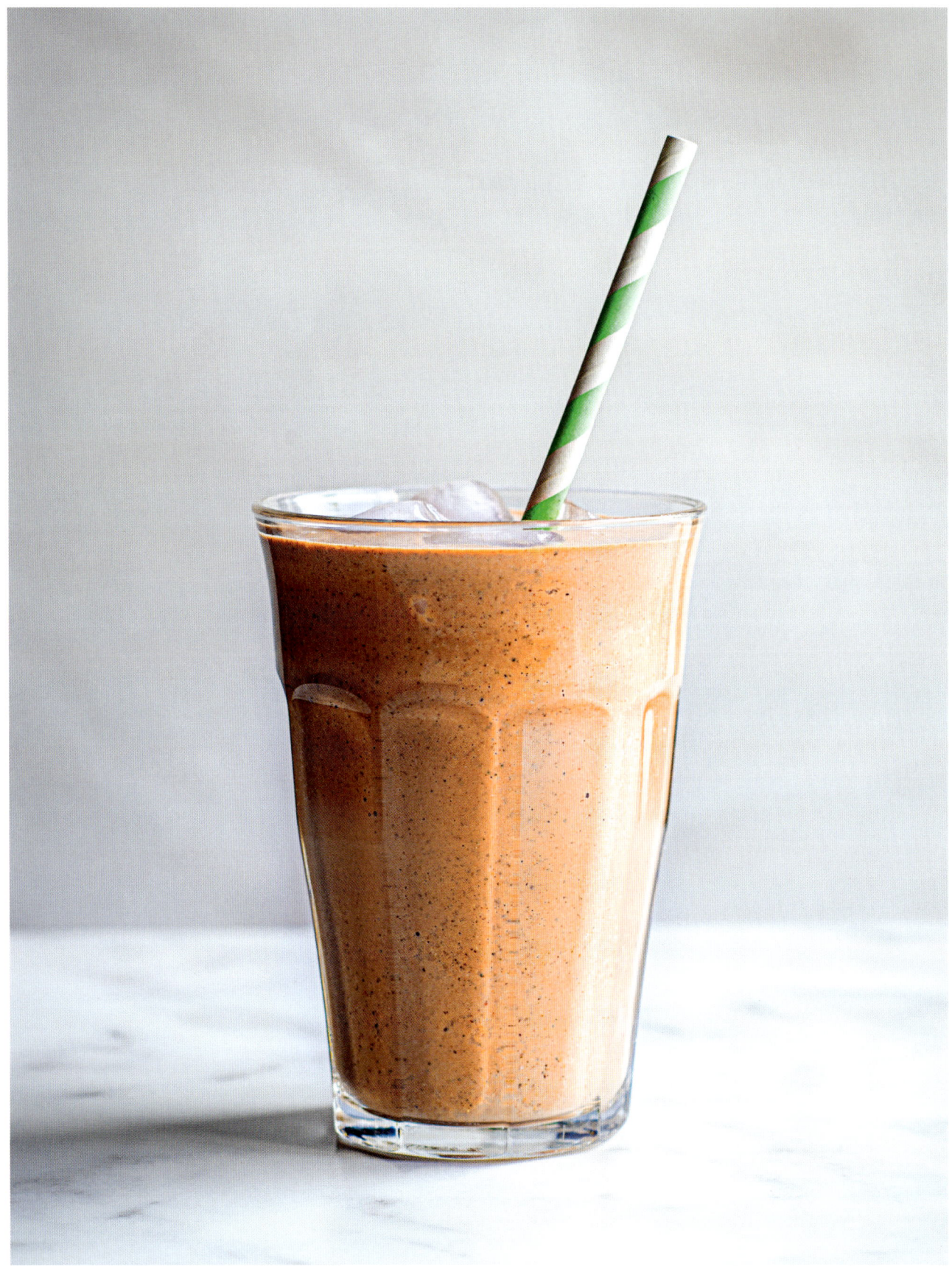

PER 100ML
PROTEIN: 3G
FIBRE: 0.4G
PLANT POINTS: 1.25

MAKES 500ML

50g shelled hemp seeds
   (or flaked almonds
   or cashew nuts)
500ml filtered water
½ teaspoon ground cinnamon

QUICK HEMP MILK

Shelled hemp seeds contain around 33g of protein per 100g, making them an ideal for plant-based milk. As they are already soft, they don't need soaking first. A powerful bullet blender works well, but you can also use a stick blender. I don't strain my nut milk, but simply give it a good shake before using. Most nut milks contain on average only 2–4 per cent nuts, but this version contains 10 per cent seeds, and as it is a 'no-strain' recipe, you get to enjoy even more of the natural protein, fibre and healthy fats. Use it in any of the recipes in this book – it's great in shakes (see below), porridge and even dairy-free lattes! Other nuts that work well for no-soak milk are flaked almonds and cashew nuts.

1. Blend the hemp seeds, water and cinnamon together in a high-speed blender until smooth and creamy.

Storage: Store for up to 3 days in an airtight glass bottle or jam jar in the fridge. Shake well before use.

PER SERVING
PROTEIN: 22G
FIBRE: 10G
PLANT POINTS: 4.25

SERVES 1

50g shelled hemp seeds
10g chia seeds
10g cacao powder
   or cacao nibs
1 banana
¼ teaspoon ground cinnamon
250ml filtered water

To serve
3 ice cubes

HEMP AND CHOCOLATE SHAKE

This shake provides an impressive 10g fibre and can be used as a fibre top-up or a lighter breakfast. Cacao powder blends easily into the smoothie and is a great source of magnesium and antioxidants, whereas cacao nibs will give a little 'crunch'. I have increased the hemp seeds from the hemp milk recipe (above) to make a creamier, shake. If you would like it sweeter, add 1 teaspoon of maple syrup.

1. Blitz the hemp seeds, chia seeds, cacao powder or nibs, banana, cinnamon and water together in small, high-speed blender until smooth and creamy. Pour over ice cubes into a glass and serve.

Storage: Best served fresh, but can be stored in a food flask or in the fridge for a few hours. Shake well before use.

HEALTHY BREAD TOPPERS

If time is short, you can use a slice of one of my breads, such as my Seed and Nut Loaf (page 253), Super Green Bread (page 254), Carrot and Courgette Yoghurt Loaf (page 256), Naked Loaf (page 258) or a Red Lentil Bagel (page 267), and pile on one of these quick and easy fillings to create a completely balanced breakfast or light meal. The bread topper recipes really need a good quality bread to balance them properly and ensure you meet your fibre goals. If you are not going to use one of the breads in this book, opt for a heavier rye bread, a seeded bread, a pumpernickel-style bread or a wholegrain sourdough as an alternative. To top up the fibre further, add some crunchy vegetable sticks, such as carrot, celery or red pepper on the side.

PER SERVING
PROTEIN: 25G
FIBRE: 7G
PLANT POINTS: 12.25

SERVES 1

1 slice of Super Green Bread (page 254)
30g cream cheese
1–2 tomatoes or ½ beef tomato
60g tinned sardines (in brine or extra virgin olive oil), drained weight
microherbs, to serve (optional)

SARDINES ON TOAST

Sardines are a superfood in my opinion! For extra calcium, buy the sardines with bones – one tin can have more calcium than a glass of milk. The bones are very soft, and the calcium is in a form that is easily absorbed by the body.

1. Toast your bread and spread with the cream cheese. Slice your tomato and arrange on the bread, then top with the sardines and a few microherbs, if using.

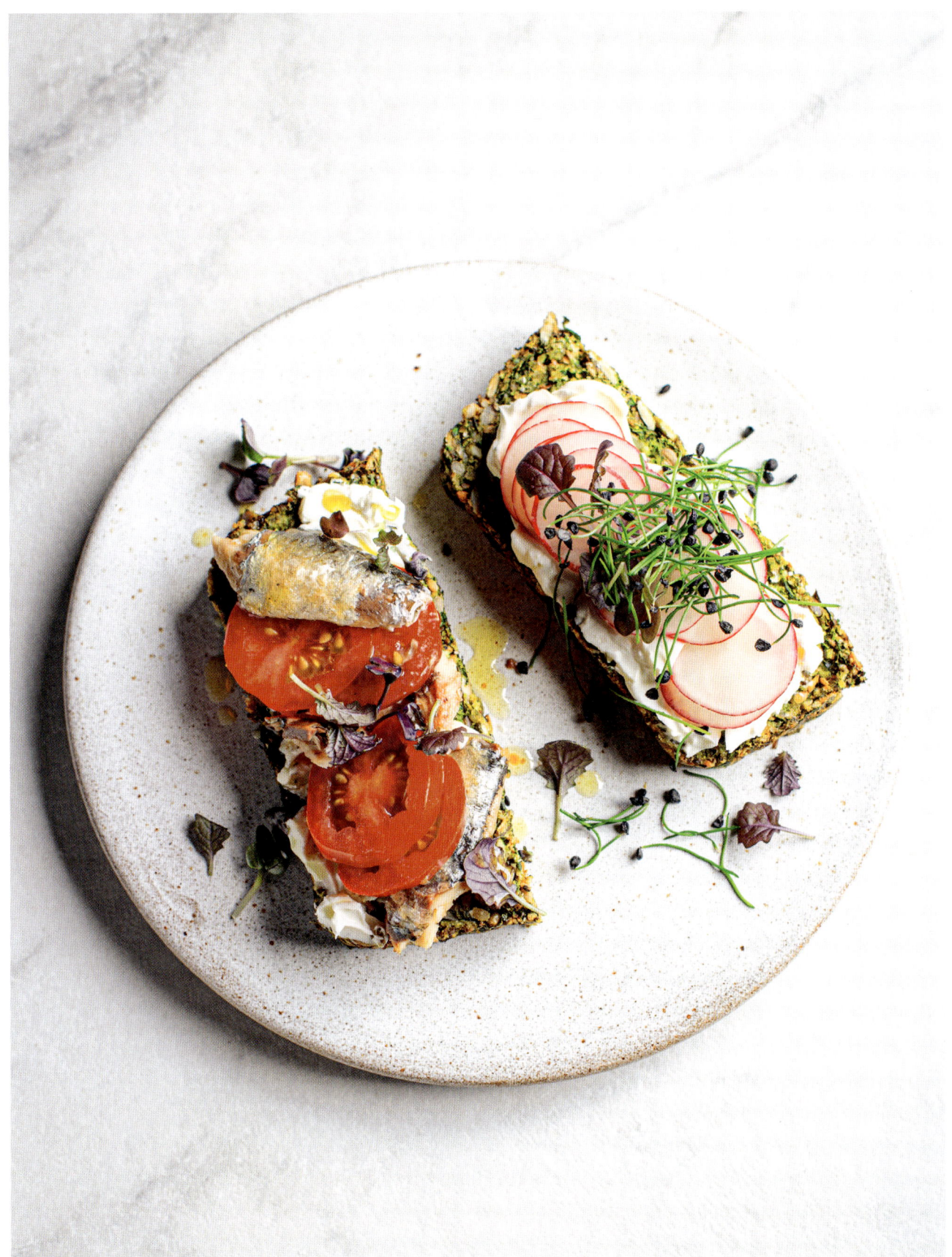

PER SERVING
PROTEIN: 24G
FIBRE: 11G
PLANT POINTS: 14.5

SERVES 1
100g quark
1 tablespoon Sunrise Sprinkles (page 110)
1 slice of Naked Loaf (page 258)
100g strawberries, sliced, or a mixture of sliced strawberries and blueberries

QUARK WITH STRAWBERRIES AND SUNRISE SPRINKLES

This is a fun way of having a sweeter topping on your bread that still packs in the fibre and plant points. I like to use quark as it is thicker and creamier than yoghurt and is less likely to slide off your bread! Use 2 slices of bread if you are hungry!

1. Mix the quark with the sprinkles and spread over your bread. Serve with sliced strawberries on top.

PER SERVING
PROTEIN: 22G
FIBRE: 14G
PLANT POINTS: 11.25

SERVES 1
1 egg
½ avocado
sea salt and freshly ground black pepper
a splash of lemon juice
1 slice of Carrot and Courgette Yoghurt Loaf (page 256)
25g Savoury Seed Mix (page 136)

AVOCADO AND SEEDS

Avocado on toast, while delicious, can be low in protein which we need to keep us well fuelled and energised. Adding the savoury seeds increases the protein, but adding a boiled, fried or poached egg really balances this meal.

1. Fill a pan halfway with hot water. Once it is gently simmering, carefully lower the whole egg into the water and cook for 6½ minutes. Remove and plunge into ice-cold water to stop it cooking, then peel. Alternatively, to poach your egg, bring the water to a gentle simmer. Crack the egg into an oiled ladle, gently lower into the water and release once the white starts to set. Cook for 2–3 minutes, until the white is set but the yolk is still runny.

2. Meanwhile, smash the avocado with some salt and pepper and a splash of lemon juice. Spread on the bread and sprinkle over the savoury seeds. Top with the egg (halved if soft-boiled).

PER SERVING
PROTEIN: 24G
FIBRE: 9G
PLANT POINTS: 11.75

SERVES 1

1 slice of Seed and Nut Loaf (page 253)
1 tablespoon Green Pesto (page 205) (or vegetarian pesto)
80g mozzarella, sliced
100g tomatoes, sliced

MOZZARELLA WITH TOMATO AND PESTO

This is a classic combination of flavours that is simple to prepare and doubles up beautifully as a quick mid-morning brunch or lunch.

1. Toast your bread and spread it with the pesto. Top with slices of mozzarella and sliced tomato.

PER SERVING
PROTEIN: 29G
FIBRE: 9G
PLANT POINTS: 13.75

SERVES 1

1 slice of Super Green Bread (page 254)
75g halloumi, cut into 2 or 3 slices
2 teaspoons Green Pesto (page 205) (or vegetarian pesto)
¼ avocado, sliced
1 large tomato, sliced
chilli flakes (optional)

QUICK FRIED HALLOUMI

Halloumi is the perfect cheese to fry or grill. Crispy on the outside and soft in the centre, I use it a lot as it is so versatile.

1. Toast your bread. Fry the halloumi slices in a dry pan over a medium-high heat for 1–2 minutes on each side, until golden on the outside and soft in the centre.

2. Spread the toast with the pesto and layer on the avocado and tomato slices, then top with the halloumi. Add a few chilli flakes if you like a little spice.

BREAKFAST 151

PER SERVING
PROTEIN: 33G
FIBRE: 7G
PLANT POINTS: 10.75

SERVES 1

2 eggs, boiled for 6 minutes and cooled
100g cottage cheese (I like to use full-fat)
1 tablespoon finely chopped pickled gherkins
a few chives, chopped
sea salt and freshly ground black pepper
1 slice of Super Green Bread (page 254)
a bed of watercress

SMASHED EGGS

Eggs are packed with essential nutrients and can be a convenient and healthy breakfast choice. To top up the protein and keep you going until lunchtime, I have teamed mine with cottage cheese and added some pickled gherkins for extra flavour.

1. Peel the cooled boiled eggs and mash them in a bowl with the cottage cheese, using a fork.

2. Stir in the gherkins and chives, and season with salt and pepper. Top the bread with watercress and spoon over the topping.

PER SERVING
PROTEIN: 27G
FIBRE: 10G
PLANT POINTS: 15

SERVES 1

100g quark (or 50g cream cheese)
6 radishes, grated or sliced
a little chopped cress
1 slice of Super Green Bread (page 254)
1 tablespoon Savoury Seed Mix (page 136)
¼ cucumber, sliced
microherbs (optional)

QUARK AND RADISH

Using quark instead of cream cheese helps to boost the protein; however, you can swap it for 50g of cream cheese if you prefer.

1. Mix the quark with the grated radish and chopped cress.

2. Spread over the bread. Top with the savoury seed mix, cucumber slices and microherbs, if you like, and you are good to go!

PER SERVING
PROTEIN: 24 G
FIBRE: 11 G
PLANT POINTS: 13.75

SERVES 1

1 tablespoon extra virgin olive oil
1 tablespoon Green Pesto (page 205) (or vegetarian pesto)
2 eggs
1 slice of Super Green Bread (page 254)
¼ ripe avocado
a few cherry tomatoes, roughly chopped

PESTO FRIED EGGS

Everyone needs to try pesto fried eggs. In my opinion, it's the only way to eat fried eggs! Once you have tried it, there will be no going back.

1. Swirl the extra virgin olive oil into a frying pan over a medium heat and stir through the pesto. Fry your eggs for 2–5 minutes, depending on how soft you like them, allowing the pesto to become lightly golden around them. Feel free to flip your egg if you would like the top cooked.

2. Spread your bread with the avocado and top with tomatoes and your delicious pesto eggs.

PER SERVING
PROTEIN: 21 G
FIBRE: 9 G
PLANT POINTS: 11.25

SERVES 1

2 eggs
½ teaspoon ground turmeric
sea salt and freshly ground black pepper
1 teaspoon olive oil
1 slice of Seed and Nut Loaf (page 253)

To serve
50g sliced tomato
50g sliced cucumber
a sprinkle of chopped fresh coriander

TURMERIC AND CORIANDER FOLDED OMELETTE

Surprisingly, I haven't manage to squeeze an omelette recipe into this book yet, so here is one now! You can omit the turmeric and coriander if you prefer, though the light spices and eggs work perfectly together.

1. Beat the eggs in a small bowl with the turmeric and some salt and pepper.

2. Heat the oil gently in a frying pan over a medium heat and add the beaten eggs. Pull the omelette away from the sides of the pan, swirl in more of the egg mixture and allow to cook and set.

3. Fold the omelette in half and then into quarters and place on your bread. Add some sliced tomato and cucumber on the side and sprinkle with fresh coriander to serve.

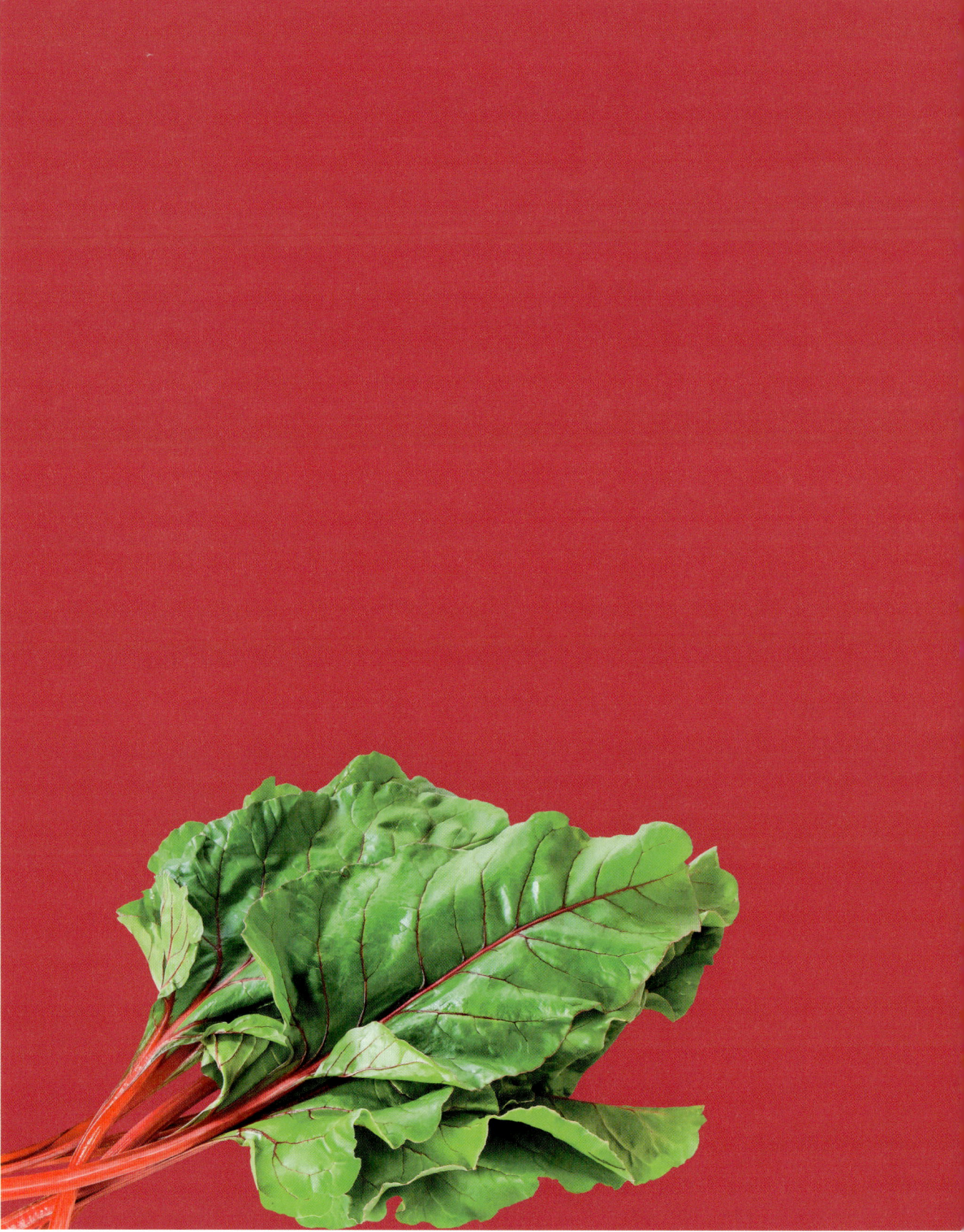

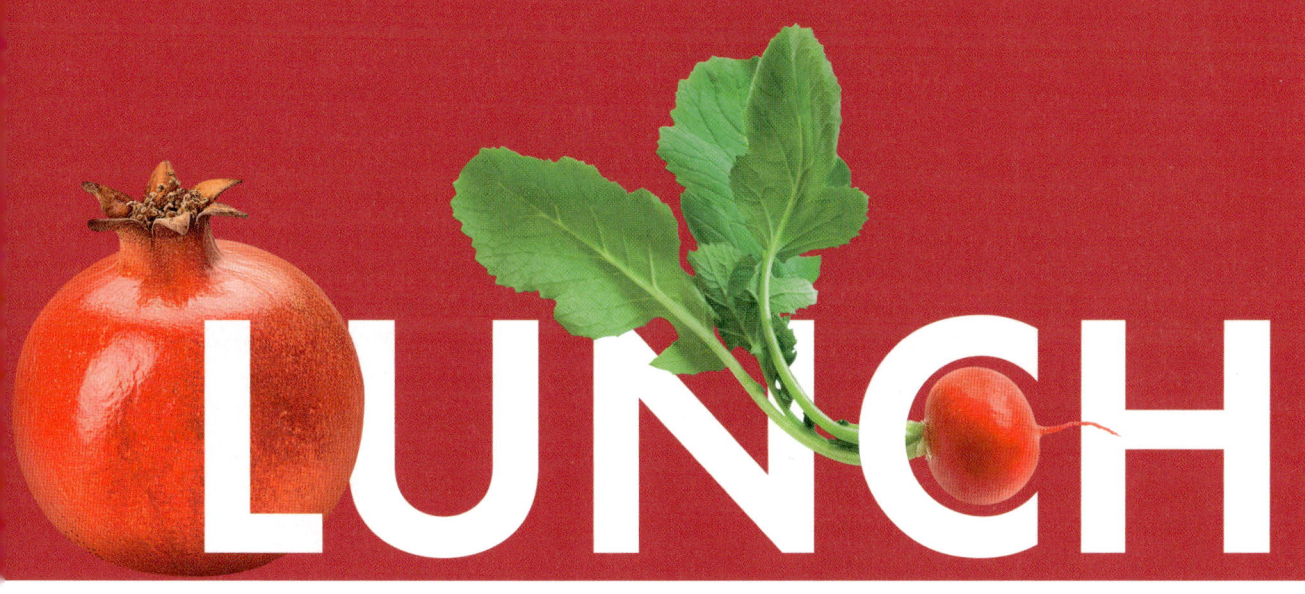

Many people go for lighter options at lunchtime, but I encourage my clients to focus on providing similar amounts of energy, balanced across protein, fibre, plant points and nutrients, at both lunch and dinner to satisfy them throughout the afternoon and into the evening. Skimping on lunch can often backfire, leading to eating more or snacking later in the day. Even if your goal is weight loss, I still recommend proportioning these meals equally. The advantage of this is that you can also swap your lunch or dinner interchangeably – and you can have leftovers from your evening meal for lunch the next day.

For most people, lunch needs to be quick to assemble or something you can take in a lunchbox. You'll see I've included plenty of soup and salad recipes in this lunch chapter, such as my Sunshine Soup (page 174) and Citrus Mackerel Salad (page 160). Soups are perfect to prep ahead, salads are speedy to make, and both can be taken with you to work. One gadget that makes salads even easier – and that I would literally not be without – is my vegetable dicer. They are inexpensive and mean that you can create a salad in just a few minutes.

I also often use my Make-One-Take-One approach, making an extra portion of my evening meal or cooking an extra element to turn into a quick lunch the next day. You'll see this in my Roasted Vegetable, Feta and Puy Lentil Salad (page 163) and Sticky Peanut Tofu Poke Bowl (page 180). I've highlighted the recipes I suggest for Make-One-Take-One at the top of each page, but also see the Make-One-Take-One recipes in the Dinner chapter for meals that make great lunch leftovers.

On some days, lunch may need to be more of a fridge-raid affair, but it's still important to make it balanced, with optimum proportions of protein, fibre and healthy fats – that's why keeping a well-stocked pantry is always a good idea! Once you know the secret to putting together a perfect plate (see pages 92–95), you'll be able to effortlessly put together a fridge-raid meal to leave you feeling your best all afternoon.

Don't be afraid to change my recipes to suit your tastes and to fit the ingredients you have in your kitchen. It's fine to swap broccoli for kale, for example in my Wasabi Super Green Soup (page 164), interchange chicken and prawns, or tofu and halloumi, or to add some seitan or tempeh to increase the plant proteins in your diet. Sometimes you may just look at the photo and find it is enough inspiration to create a recipe of your own. You may want to dial down – or up! – the spices according to your tastes, or include your own favourite ingredients. In short, don't be limited by what my recipes say. You'll be surprised how most recipes are quite flexible, so if you have some extra ingredients and want to include them, go for it!

Super soups

Soups are a great lunch option, especially in cooler weather. They can be batch-cooked and stored in the fridge or frozen, and they are easy to transport. Stored in an airtight container, soups will stay fresh in the fridge for up to 2–3 days, or you can freeze them in individual portions for up to 3 months.

Soups are also a great way of eating more vegetables, but because they usually have a high water ratio and can be low in protein, the classic soup and bread combination doesn't always fill us up all afternoon. The way to turn your soup into a balanced meal is to add even more fibre and protein so that you feel properly satiated and energised. You can still have some of your favourite bread or crackers (especially if you choose one of mine on pages 253–261, which are high in protein and fibre), but adding extra protein to your soup can be a gamechanger for your appetite.

When making a soup for four people, I use around 1kg of vegetables, so each portion has around 250g. Then I think about how to up the protein. Below are some of my favourite ways. Remember, seeds, nuts, beans, lentils, breads or crackers give you a healthy fibre top-up too!

- Fried halloumi squares or spicy fried tofu pieces (page 180)

- Toasted sunflower and pumpkin seeds

- Cooked white beans or chickpeas (to thicken a soup or left whole)

- Crispy fried spicy chickpeas with halloumi (page 184)

- Cooked red or green lentils or red lentil pasta

- Crumbled feta

- 2 poached eggs

- Whipped Feta and Bean Dip (page 175) with Seeded Crackers (page 261) or one of my homemade breads (pages 253–258)

- Hummus (pages 269–271) and Seeded Crackers (page 261) or one of my homemade breads (pages 253–258)

- Mackerel Pâté with Seeded Crackers (pages 194 and 261)

- Red Lentil Polpette (page 176)

- My Red Lentil Bagel (page 267)

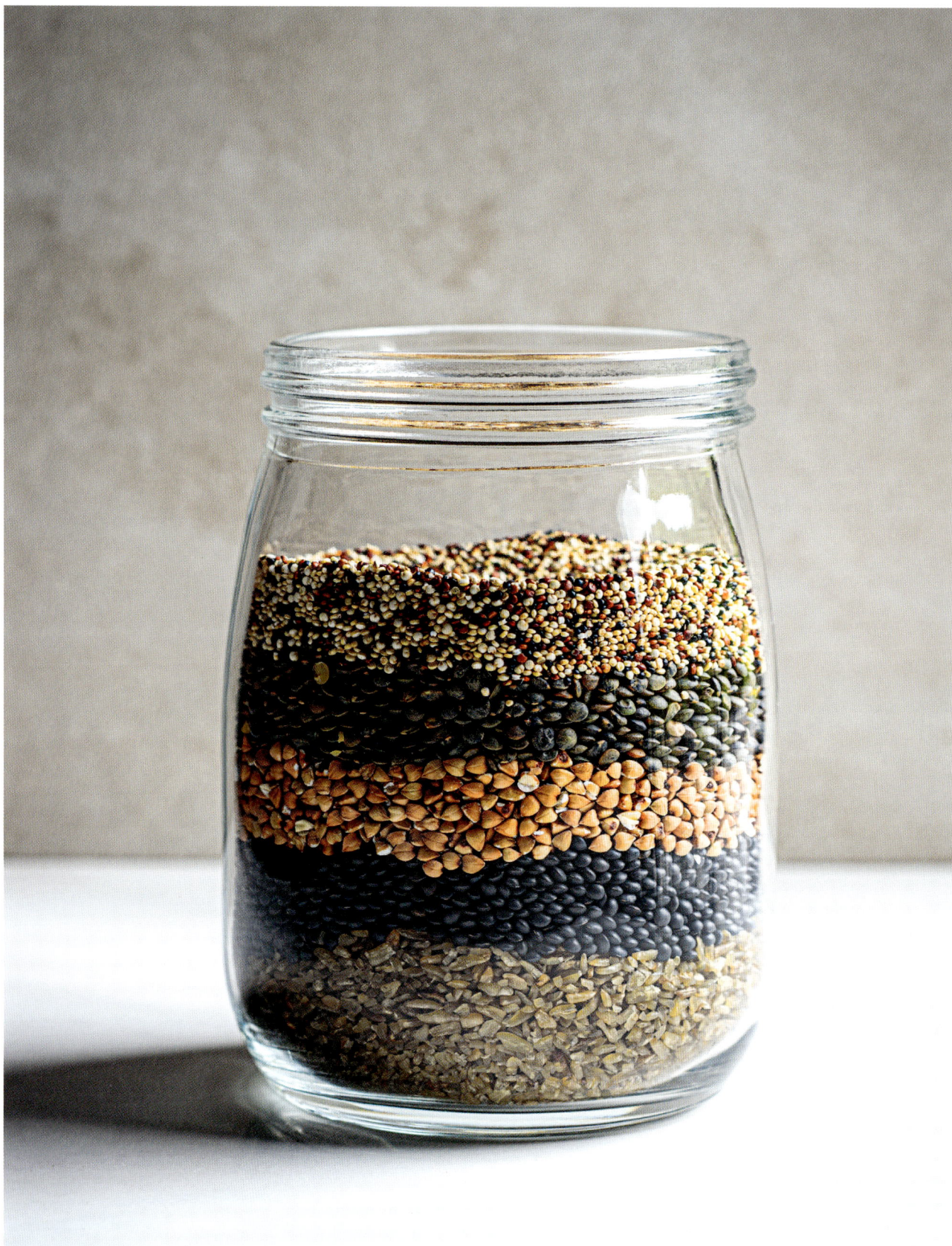

PER SERVING
PROTEIN: 8G
FIBRE: 6G
PLANT POINTS: 5

SERVES 10
50G (DRY WEIGHT) PER PORTION

100g whole buckwheat groats (or cracked bulgur wheat)
100g freekeh
100g quinoa
100g black beluga lentils
100g Puy lentils

To cook
sea salt or vegetable stock powder or bouillon

GRAIN AND LENTIL HEALTHY CARB MIX

I came up with this idea while trying to think up ways to increase plant points at our meals with blood-sugar-friendly grains. Having some of this mix cooked up in the fridge and ready to go means you can add it to salads and soups, or enjoy it as a side dish. The simplicity comes from the fact that all these grains and legumes cook in around 25 minutes, meaning that it is possible to cook them all in the same pan. This is a fantastic way to bring healthy carbohydrates into your meal, to sustain you for longer. Black beluga lentils contain high levels of polyphenols, which give them a darker appearance, and since different types of lentils count as separate plant points, this mix makes it an easy way to boost yours! At 6g of fibre per serving, it's also a genius way of topping up your fibre. To make this gluten-free, use buckwheat groats, quinoa, black lentils, Puy lentils, millet or amaranth.

1. Mix all the grains together in a large jar and give it a good shake!

2. Put 50g of the grain and lentil mix per person into a large saucepan and cover with twice as much water to grains and lentils. Season with sea salt or vegetable stock powder. Bring to a gentle simmer and cook for 20–25 minutes with the lid on, or until all the components are tender. Drain thoroughly, rinse in hot water and fluff with a fork.

3. Serve warm as a side, stir into soups, allow to cool and mix through salads with herbs and dressing.

Storage: The grains store well uncooked in an airtight jar for a few weeks. Once cooked, store in an airtight container in the fridge for up to 3 days.

PER SERVING
PROTEIN: 30G
FIBRE: 18G
PLANT POINTS: 9.5

SERVES 2

1 orange, sliced
1 small fennel bulb, finely sliced
80g watercress
½ red onion, finely sliced
150g cooked baby beetroot, quartered
1 x 400g tin or jar of chickpeas, rinsed and drained (240g drained weight)
2 fresh mackerel fillets
1 tablespoon extra virgin olive oil
30g olives
1 tablespoon pumpkin seeds
1 tablespoon sauerkraut

Dressing
2 tablespoons lemon juice
2 tablespoons extra virgin olive oil
sea salt and freshly ground black pepper

CITRUS MACKEREL SALAD

Oily fish is a reliable source of omega-3 fatty acids. The advantage of eating some of our omega-3 from fish is that they are present in a form called EPA and DHA, which is easy for the body to take up and use; we call these the 'active' forms. Plant omega-3 (called ALA) requires a series of conversions via enzymes to create active forms, which are far less efficient (see page 62). Omega-3 fats are important for cell membranes, cell signalling and cardiovascular and brain health, so eating oily fish a few times a week is a great way of meeting our requirements. Mackerel is also a good source of selenium and contains some iodine, both of which are necessary for a healthy thyroid. If you are short of time, you can swap fresh mackerel for smoked mackerel fillets.

---

1. To make the dressing, whisk the lemon juice and extra virgin olive oil together in a small bowl. Season with salt and pepper to taste. Set aside.

2. Arrange the orange slices, fennel slices, watercress, red onion, beetroot and chickpeas on serving plates.

3. Pan-fry the mackerel fillets, skin side down, in extra virgin olive oil in a heavy-based frying pan over a medium-high heat. Cook for around 3–4 minutes on each side until cooked through. Ensure that the pan is not too hot and press the fish gently with a fish slice while cooking to help prevent the skin from buckling.

4. Place the cooked mackerel fillets on top of the vegetables and orange slices. Scatter over the olives and pumpkin seeds. Drizzle with the lemon dressing and serve with some gut-loving sauerkraut on the side.

Storage: Best enjoyed fresh. Store any leftovers in an airtight container in the fridge for up to 24 hours.

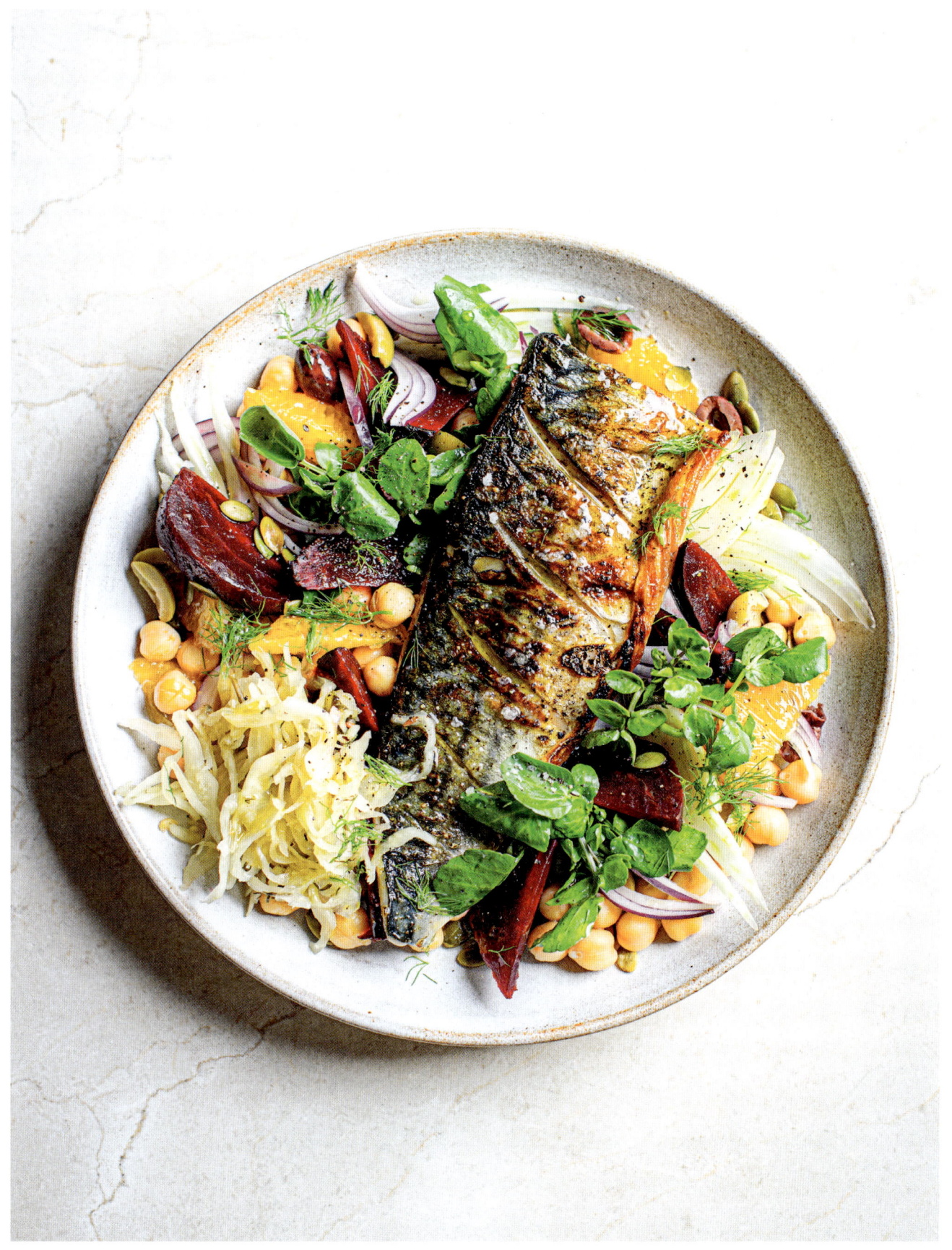

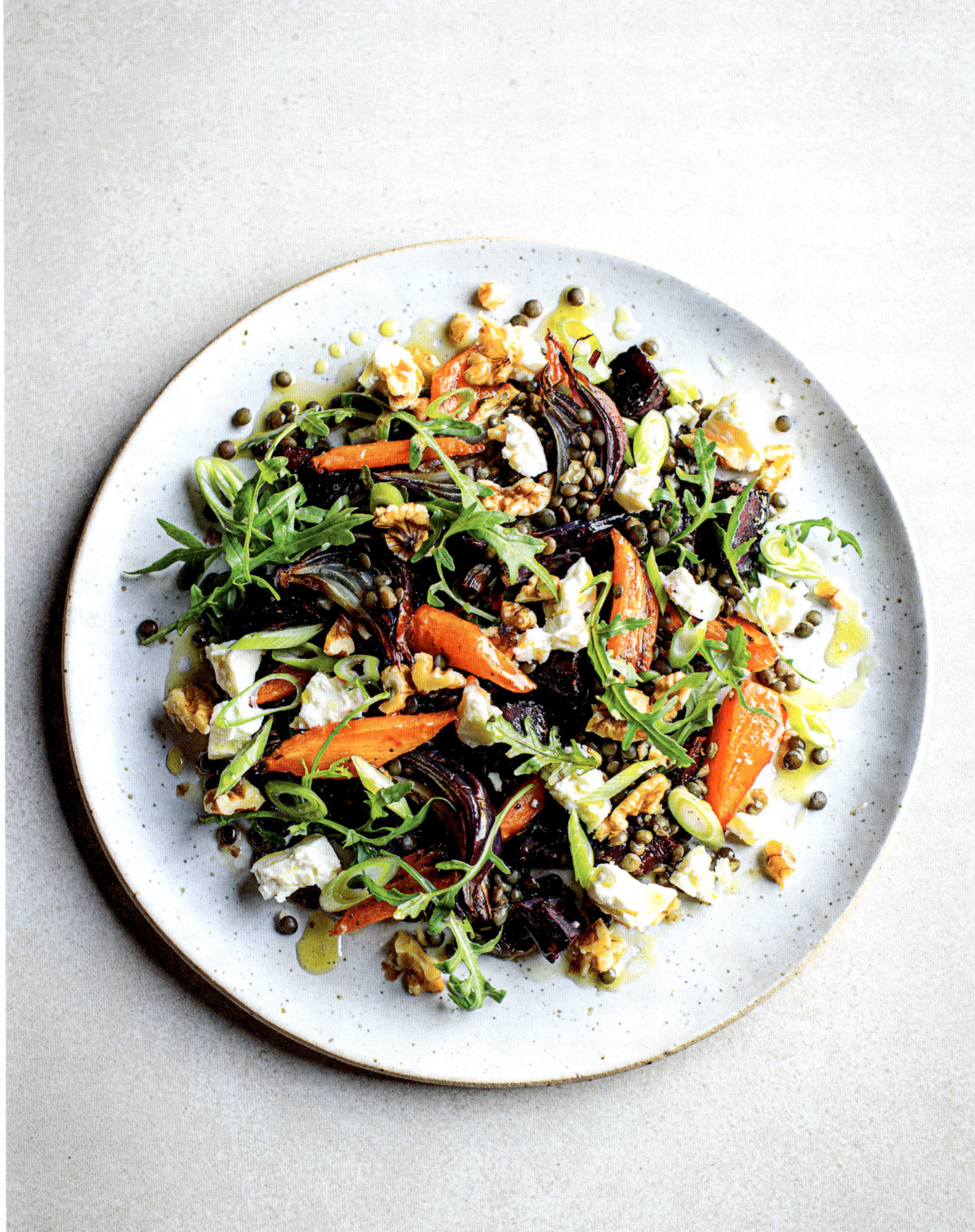

PER SERVING
PROTEIN: 26G
FIBRE: 14G
PLANT POINTS: 8.25

SERVES 4

200g dried Puy lentils (or around 400g ready-cooked lentils)
a little sea salt or vegetable stock powder or bouillon
250g fresh beetroot, peeled
1 red onion
250g carrots
2 tablespoons extra virgin olive oil
1 teaspoon dried herbs (e.g. thyme, sage, rosemary, oregano)
200g feta, crumbled
120g rocket or mixed salad leaves
4 spring onions, finely sliced
100g walnut halves, roughly chopped

Dressing

2 tablespoons extra virgin olive oil
2 tablespoons lemon juice
sea salt and freshly ground black pepper

ROASTED VEGETABLE, FETA AND PUY LENTIL SALAD

You don't need lots of fancy ingredients to make a balanced plate; often you can make a great meal out of leftovers or foods you already have in your fridge. Whenever the oven is on, I love to roast a tray of vegetables – anything from pumpkin to carrots, onions, beetroot, fennel or swede. Roasted vegetables make a perfect base for a salad or a side dish. This salad was one that my son Alex, who is a great cook, made for me one day, using the roasted vegetables he found in the fridge – the perfect fridge-raid lunch. It's also a good example of topping up your protein with extra plant proteins, in this case the Puy lentils. Lentils are a great addition to salads, keeping you full for longer and stopping you feeling hungry mid-afternoon. You can buy lentils ready-cooked for convenience.

---

1. If using dried lentils, put them into a pan with at least twice as much water to lentils, and a little sea salt or vegetable stock. Cook with the lid on over a medium heat for around 25 minutes, until just al dente. They should still hold their shape. Drain and allow to cool. If using ready-cooked lentils, cook for just a few minutes to soften and warm through.

2. Preheat the oven to 200°C fan. Chop the beetroot, onion and carrot into even-sized pieces. The smaller the pieces, the faster they will roast, so try to keep them uniform. Place in a ceramic baking dish. I like to keep the colours separate, otherwise the beetroot has a habit of turning the carrots purple. Drizzle over the extra virgin olive oil and sprinkle with dried herbs. Roast for around 40 minutes, until tender and golden at the edges. Allow to cool.

3. In a large bowl, combine the cooled roasted vegetables with the crumbled feta, cooked Puy lentils, rocket or salad leaves, chopped spring onions and walnuts.

4. Whisk the dressing ingredients together, or shake together in a jar, and pour over the salad. Fold together gently before serving.

Make-One-Take-One: Store the salad without dressing in an airtight container in the fridge for up to 2 days. Mix in the dressing just before serving.

PER SERVING
PROTEIN: 27G
FIBRE: 15G
PLANT POINTS: 9.25

SERVES 4

Soup
1 tablespoon extra virgin olive oil
1 large onion, finely diced
2 garlic cloves, crushed
500–600ml vegetable stock (or chicken bone broth)
1 large head of broccoli, cut into florets
300g frozen petits pois or peas
200g baby spinach
1 teaspoon wasabi paste
sea salt and freshly ground black pepper
pinch of sumac (optional)

Toppings
200g mixed sunflower, pumpkin and sesame seeds
1 tablespoon tamari or soy sauce (Note, soy sauce isn't gluten-free)
1 rounded teaspoon wasabi paste
100g kale or cavolo nero, stalks removed and roughly cut
1 tablespoon extra virgin olive oil

To serve
100g feta, crumbled

Tip: Avoid overcooking the soup, which will dull its vibrant green colour.

WASABI SUPER GREEN SOUP

This soup is quite a showstopper due to its vibrant green colour, which practically shouts 'healthy'! Green vegetables contain the pigment chlorophyll, and at the heart of each chlorophyll molecule is an ion of magnesium, which is why green leafy vegetables are rich in this important mineral. This soup can be made and served in around 20 minutes. Sumac is a deep red spice made from dried, ground sumac berries and adds a slightly zesty, fruity flavour. It is a higher-fibre soup, so have a smaller portion if you are still getting used to more fibre. If you are feeling especially hungry, serve with the Rosemary and Sea Salt Seeded Crackers on page 261.

---

1. Preheat the oven to 200°C fan and line a baking tray with baking parchment. To make the toppings, mix the seeds with the tamari and wasabi. Spread on one half of a baking tray lined with baking parchment. Rub the kale or cavolo nero with 1 tablespoon of extra virgin olive oil and spread on the other half of the tray. Roast for 6–8 minutes until crisp and fragrant, taking care not to burn them.

2. Meanwhile, for the soup, heat 1 tablespoon of extra virgin olive oil in a large saucepan over a medium heat. Gently sauté the onion for around 5 minutes until softened, then add the garlic and cook for another 2 minutes.

3. Pour in 500ml of the stock and add the broccoli florets, holding the rest of the stock back to adjust the consistency at the end. Simmer for 3–4 minutes, then add the frozen peas and spinach and cook for a further 2 minutes, just until tender.

4. Remove from the heat and stir in the wasabi paste, then season with salt, pepper and the sumac, if using. Allow to cool slightly.

5. Blend the soup using a stick blender, until smooth. Add a little of the remaining stock if you would like it a little looser.

6. Ladle into bowls and top with the roasted seeds, kale or cavolo nero and crumbled feta.

Storage: Store in an airtight container in the fridge for up to 3 days. The soup can also be frozen for up to 2 months. Store the toppings separately and add when serving.

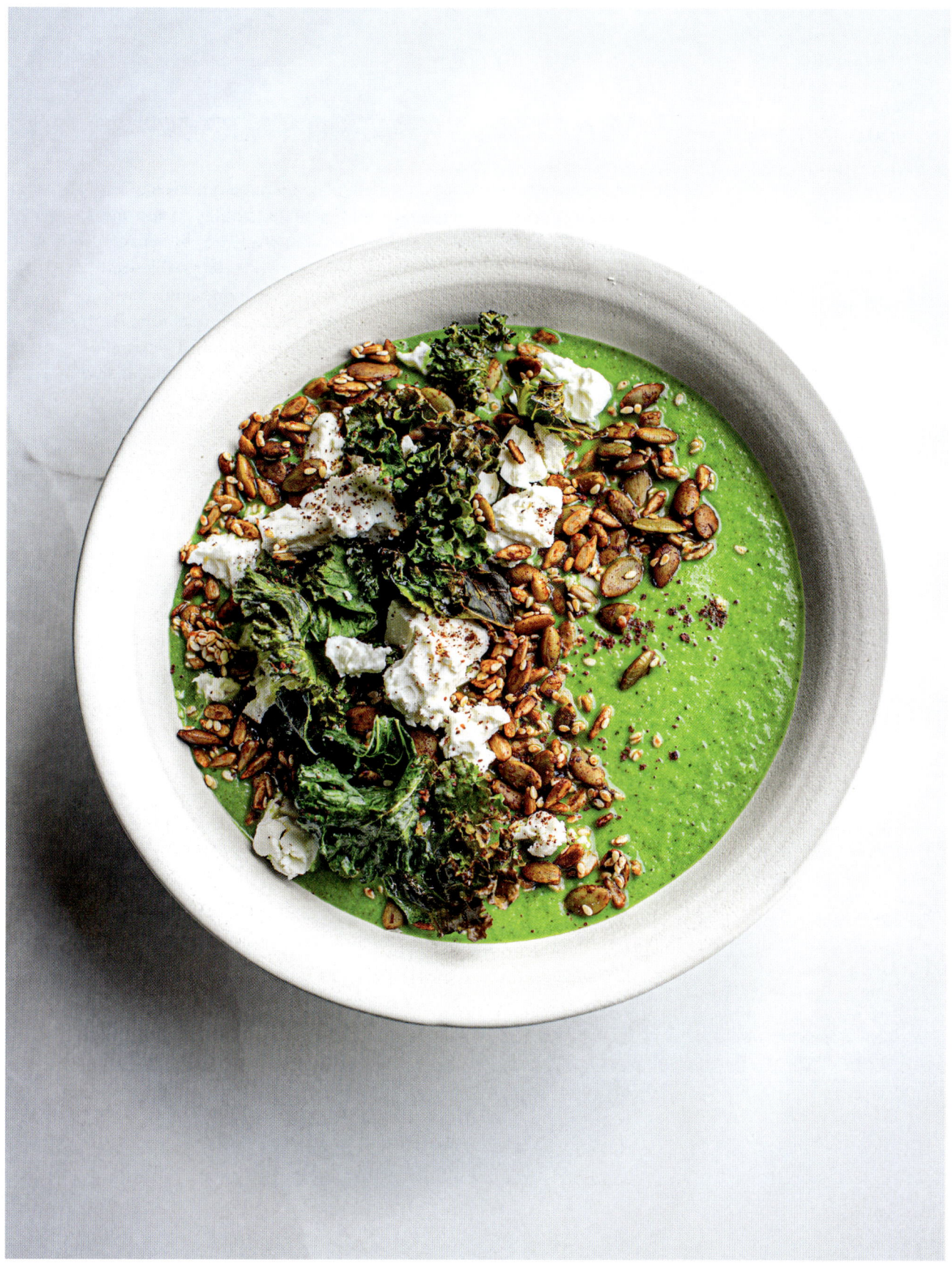

PER SERVING
PROTEIN: 40G
FIBRE: 9G
PLANT POINTS: 12.75

SERVES 4

400g chicken breasts, cut into bite-size cubes
2 tablespoons plain yoghurt
1 teaspoon ground turmeric
1 teaspoon ground cumin
2 teaspoons freshly grated ginger
2 garlic cloves, crushed
1 dessertspoon (10ml) tamari or soy sauce (Note, soy sauce isn't gluten-free)
zest and juice of 1 lime

Satay sauce
50ml coconut milk (see Tip)
4 tablespoons (60g) peanut butter (crunchy or smooth)
1 dessertspoon (10ml) tamari or soy sauce (Note, soy sauce isn't gluten-free)
2 teaspoons honey or maple syrup
1 teaspoon sriracha or chilli sauce, to taste
juice of 1 lime

Salad
200g red cabbage, finely sliced
200g white cabbage, finely sliced
200g mixed salad leaves
200g tomatoes, chopped
150g frozen edamame beans
200g sugar snap peas

Dressing
30ml lemon juice
½ teaspoon sea salt
30ml extra virgin olive oil
½ teaspoon mustard, e.g. Dijon (check it is gluten-free)

Tip: Freeze the rest of the tinned coconut milk in ice cube trays to use in soups and curries.

CHICKEN SATAY SKEWERS

I think we all love a dipping sauce, and when I tested this recipe with a group of my friends it proved to be such a success that everyone agreed it had to go into the book. The marinated skewers are tender and flavourful on their own, but when dipped into the sauce they are next level. Served with a crisp salad and gently cooked edamame, the dish offers a delightful medley of textures and tastes. You can sub the chicken for prawns or tofu if you prefer. These skewers also work well on a barbecue, and you can easily halve or double up the recipe.

---

1. In a bowl, combine the diced chicken, yoghurt, turmeric, cumin, grated ginger, crushed garlic, tamari or soy sauce, and lime juice and zest. Mix well to coat the chicken evenly. Cover and refrigerate for at least 30 minutes (or up to 2 hours). If using wooden skewers, soak them in water now to prevent them burning during cooking.

2. While the chicken marinates, give the tin of coconut milk a good shake, then measure out 50ml. Mix all the sauce ingredients together, or use a small food processor, until well combined and smooth. It should have a good dipping consistency.

3. Put the red cabbage, white cabbage, salad leaves and tomatoes into a large bowl. Heat a small pan of water and cook the frozen edamame beans for 3–5 minutes, adding the sugar snap peas for the last 2 minutes of cooking time. Drain immediately and run under cold water to cool and stop the cooking process. Add to the salad and toss to combine.

4. Turn your grill to a medium-hot setting. Thread the chicken onto the skewers and grill for 5–6 minutes per side, until cooked through.

5. Shake all the salad dressing ingredients together in a small jar and pour over the salad. Serve alongside the chicken skewers and dipping sauce.

Storage: This is best served immediately, but can be stored in an airtight container in the fridge for up to 3 days. The sauce may become 'set' in the fridge but will return to its original consistency when it reaches room temperature again.

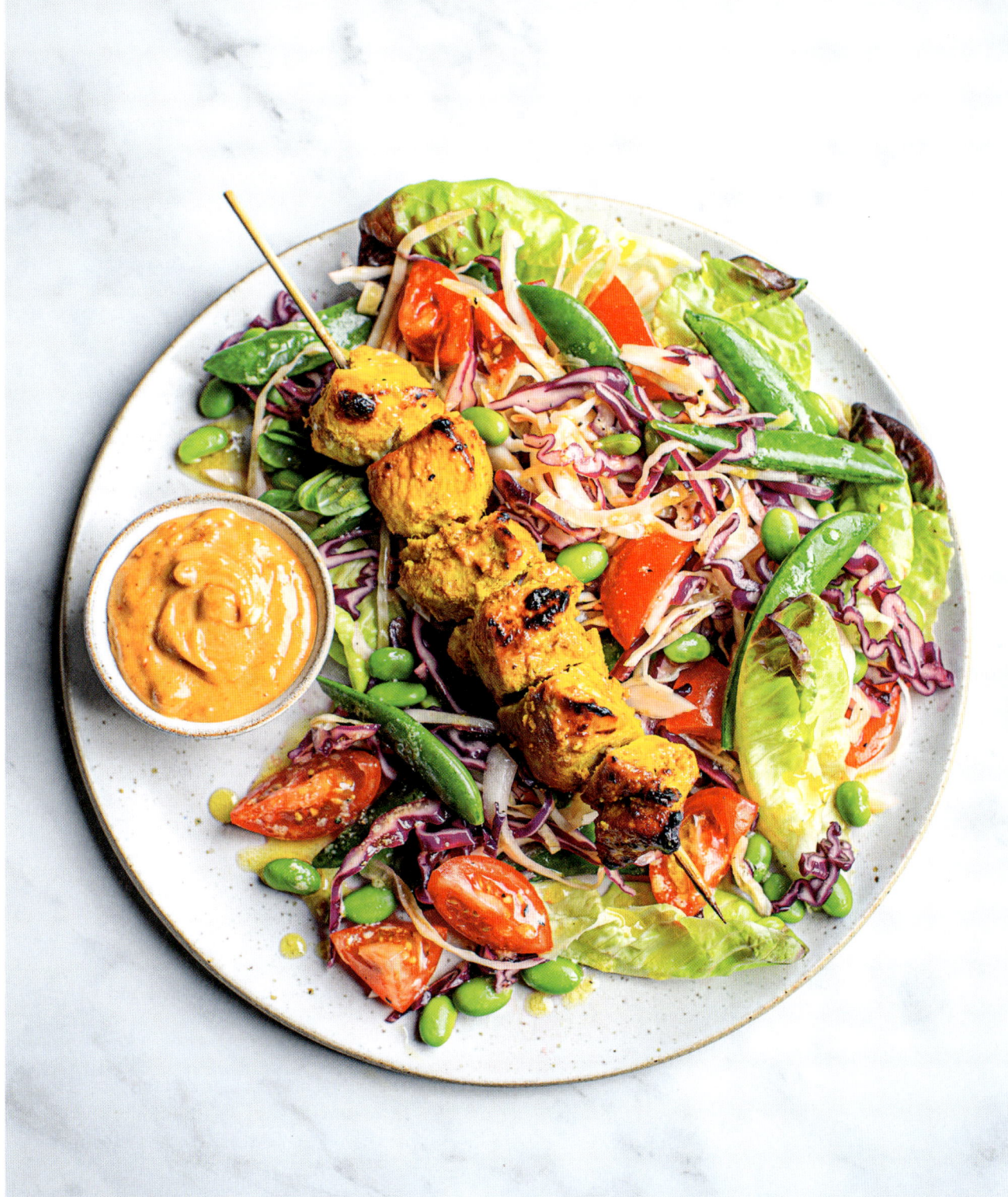

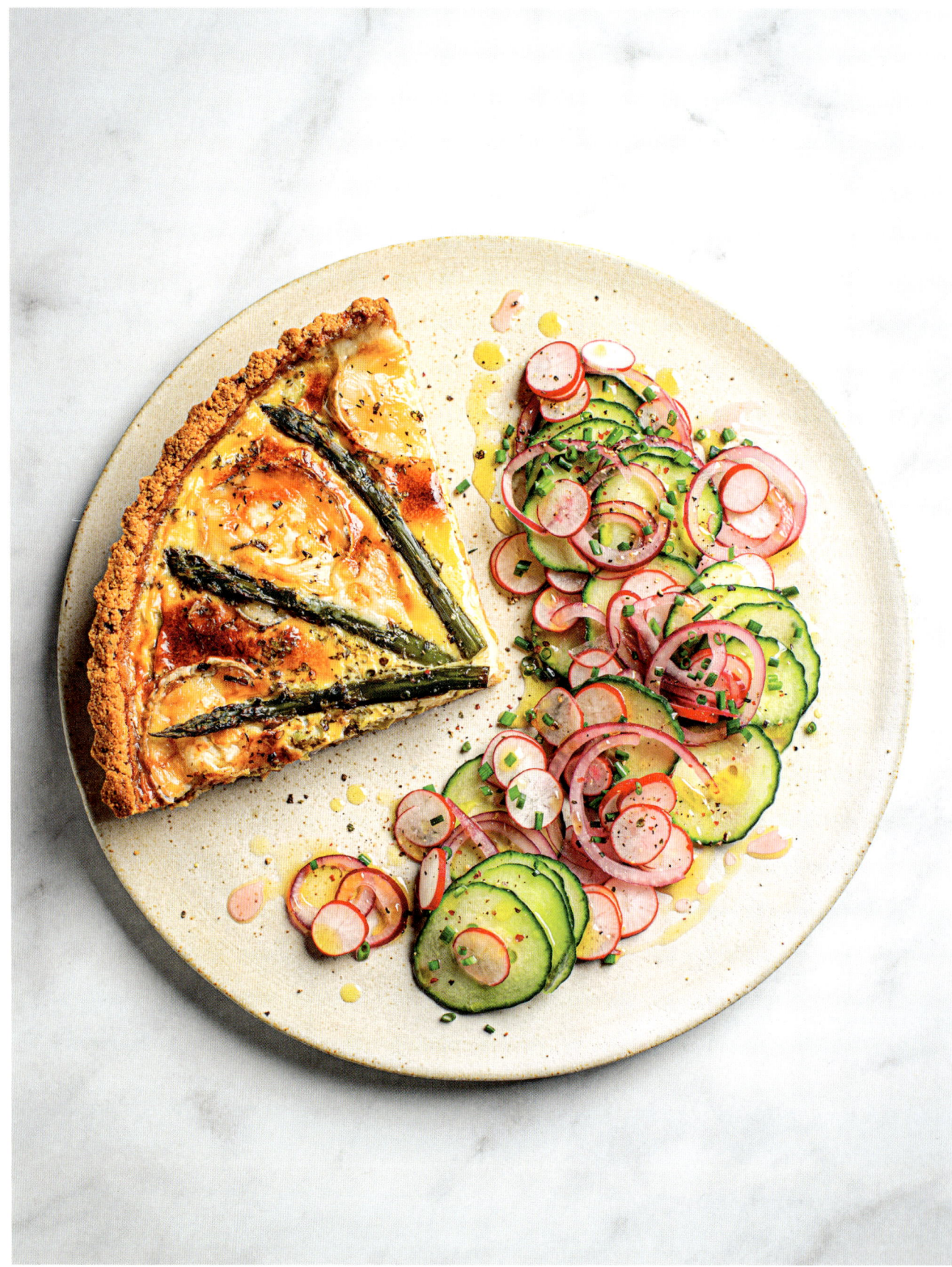

PER SERVING
PROTEIN: 35G
FIBRE: 8G
PLANT POINTS: 5.75

SERVES 4

Pastry
250g ground almonds
20g extra virgin olive oil (about 2 dessertspoons), plus extra for greasing
1 large egg
½ teaspoon baking powder
½ teaspoon sea salt
1 teaspoon dried or fresh thyme

Filling
1 red onion, finely chopped
1 tablespoon extra virgin olive oil
1 teaspoon maple syrup
150g asparagus tips
3 eggs
220g Greek yoghurt
sea salt and freshly ground black pepper
150g goat's cheese log, with rind
a small handful of chopped fresh thyme and chives

Salad
1 red onion, cut into rings
1 tablespoon apple cider vinegar
1 large cucumber, finely sliced
200g radishes, sliced
1 tablespoon extra virgin olive oil
chopped chives
sea salt and freshly ground black pepper

ASPARAGUS AND GOAT'S CHEESE ALMOND CRUST FLAN

Almond pastry might be new to you, but it is worth trying as I think it will become your new favourite 'healthy' pastry! It is just so easy to work with, is naturally gluten-free and comes with several hidden benefits. Almond pastry contains more protein and fibre, no refined carbohydrates and is more nutrient dense than regular pastry. It's also better for your blood sugars. Best of all, you do not need to roll this pastry, you can simply spread it out using the back of a spoon, making it 'fuss-free'. This flan is quite a showstopper and makes a gorgeous lunch for friends. I have a jar of dried chickpeas that I use as my baking beans and have used the same batch for a few years now. Baking beans stop the pastry from rising in the centre during cooking. Pre-cooking the pastry is a necessary step to seal it and to stop the filling from leaking through during cooking. This is a perfect Make-One-Take-One meal to enjoy the following day, too.

---

1. Start by preparing the salad. Place the red onion rings in a bowl with the apple cider vinegar and leave them to turn vibrant pink while you make the flan.

2. Preheat the oven to 180°C fan. Put all the pastry ingredients into a food processor and blend gently until the mixture comes together and holds its shape when pressed. You can also mix this by hand, but I recommend a food processor as it slightly warms and softens the pastry dough, making it easier to work with. You want the pastry to feel very malleable.

3. Grease a 22cm flan dish and line the base with a round of baking parchment. Spread the pastry evenly over the base and sides, using sweeping motions with the back of a spoon. Prick the base with a fork to allow the steam to escape while cooking. Cover the pastry with baking parchment and fill with baking beans. Bake in the oven for 10 minutes. Remove the beans and parchment, then return the flan case to the oven for another 10 minutes.

Recipe continues overleaf

ASPARAGUS AND GOAT'S CHEESE ALMOND CRUST FLAN *CONTINUED*

4. While the pastry blind bakes, sauté the chopped red onion in extra virgin olive oil and the maple syrup in a frying pan over a low heat for 10–12 minutes, until soft and caramelised.

5. Simmer the asparagus tips in a pan of salted water for about 5 minutes, until al dente, or steam if you prefer. Set aside a few spears for the top, then slice the rest and add to the onion mixture.

6. In a food processor, or by hand in a bowl, gently mix the eggs and Greek yoghurt, and season with salt and pepper. Stir in the caramelised onion and sliced asparagus. Pour the mixture into the pre-baked pastry case.

7. Cut 50g of the goat's cheese into cubes and scatter over the filling. Slice the remaining cheese into rounds and arrange with the reserved asparagus on top. Sprinkle with chopped thyme and chives.

8. Bake the flan for 35–40 minutes until golden and fully set in the centre. Allow to cool slightly before serving.

9. Once the red onions are pickled, combine them with the cucumber, radishes, extra virgin olive oil, chopped chives, and some salt and pepper. Toss the salad gently and serve alongside the warm or cooled flan.

Make-One-Take-One: Store the flan in an airtight container in the fridge for up to 2 days. Reheat individual flan portions in the oven or in an air fryer at 180°C for 7–8 minutes, or enjoy cold. The salad is best served fresh but can be stored in the fridge for up to 24 hours.

PER SERVING
PROTEIN: 32G
FIBRE: 8G
PLANT POINTS: 6.5

SERVES 4
8 eggs
200g feta, crumbled
50g baby spinach,
  roughly chopped
a pinch of nutmeg
sea salt and freshly
  ground black pepper
extra virgin olive oil,
  for greasing ramekins

Raw broccoli salad
1 large head of broccoli
  (stem included), cut into
  small bite-size pieces
2 red peppers, diced
1 large apple, skin left
  on, diced
20g dried cranberries
50g roasted hazelnuts

Dressing
2 tablespoons extra virgin
  olive oil
2 tablespoons apple
  cider vinegar
1 teaspoon Dijon mustard
  (check it is gluten-free)
sea salt and freshly ground
  black pepper

Option: For a fibre boost, serve with a portion of my Grain and Lentil Healthy Carb Mix (page 159). Note, this contains gluten.

SOUFFLÉ MADE SIMPLE, WITH BROCCOLI, HAZELNUT AND CRANBERRY SALAD

This is a recipe that I have been using for over ten years. Traditional soufflés can be finicky to make, and while my version is not made to a traditional soufflé recipe, the word 'soufflé' actually comes from the French verb 'souffler', which means to 'blow' or 'puff' – something these definitely do while they are in the oven. A bain-marie is essential and is a way of cooking soufflés more gently, the warm water allowing for a more uniform temperature and keeping the soufflés from drying out at the edges. The soufflé itself is low in fibre, so I have teamed it up with a raw broccoli salad. The broccoli marinates in the dressing, which means it will taste just as good the following day.

---

1. Preheat the oven to 180°C fan. First, make the broccoli salad. You want to make the salad first because the longer the broccoli sits in the dressing, the more it softens, which improves the taste and texture of the salad.

2. In a large bowl, mix all the dressing ingredients together. Add the broccoli, red peppers, apple, cranberries and roasted hazelnuts, reserving a few hazelnuts to sprinkle on top at the end. Toss in the dressing and leave to sit while you get on with the soufflés.

3. Crack the eggs into a small food processor. Add the crumbled feta, spinach and nutmeg, and season with salt and pepper. Process just enough to combine the ingredients, but don't over-process, as the eggs could become too 'thin' and this will affect the consistency of the final soufflés. (You can also use a stick blender for this stage.)

4. Grease 4 ramekins with a little olive oil. Divide the soufflé mixture among them and place the ramekins in a larger baking dish.

Recipe continues overleaf

SOUFFLÉ MADE SIMPLE, WITH BROCCOLI, HAZELNUT AND CRANBERRY SALAD *CONTINUED*

5. Pour hot water into the dish until it comes halfway up the sides of the ramekins, creating a bain-marie.

6. Bake for 20–25 minutes, until the soufflés are puffed up, golden on top and set in the centre. Allow to cool slightly.

7. Run a small knife around the edges and turn out onto a plate. Serve with the delicious broccoli salad.

Make-One-Take-One: Store the salad in an airtight container in the fridge for up to 3 days. The souffles will keep in an airtight container in the fridge for up to 2 days. Reheat gently in an oven at 180°C fan or in an air fryer at 180°C for 5 minutes.

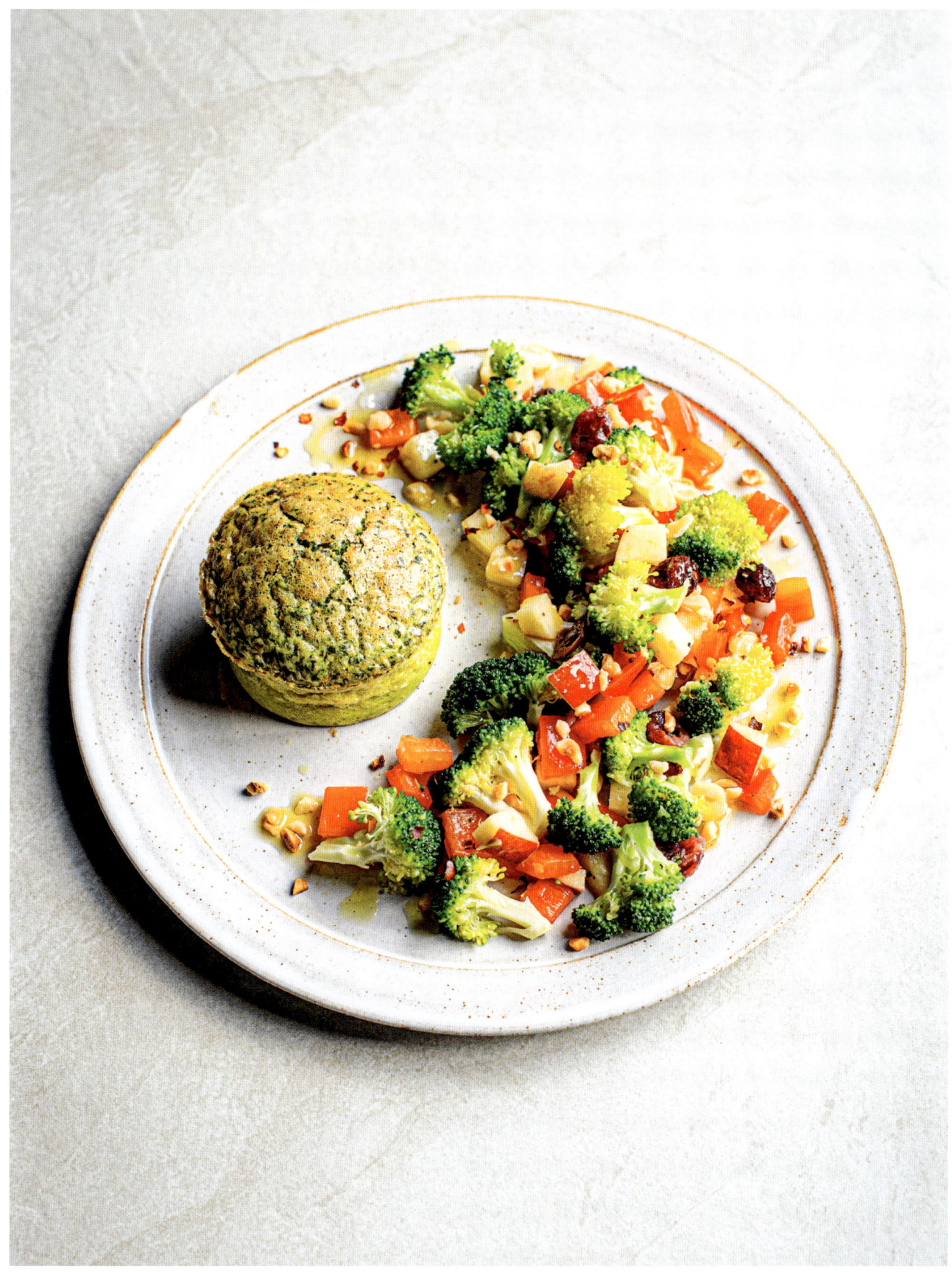

PER SERVING
PROTEIN: 25G
FIBRE: 15G
PLANT POINTS: 12.5

SERVES 4
1 medium onion, finely diced
2 garlic cloves, finely chopped
1 tablespoon extra virgin olive oil
a thumb-sized piece of fresh ginger, peeled and finely grated
1 thumb-sized piece of fresh turmeric, peeled and finely grated (or 1 level teaspoon dried turmeric)
500g carrots, scrubbed and finely diced
500g butternut squash, peeled and cubed
30g cashew nuts
zest and juice of 1 orange
600ml vegetable stock
freshly ground black pepper

To serve (per serving)
¼ quantity Whipped Feta and Bean Dip (opposite) and 30g Rosemary and Sea Salt Seeded Crackers (page 261)

Tip: Add a few chilli flakes if you want to add some heat.

SUNSHINE SOUP

Naturally rich in beta-carotene, this soup has a dazzling orange colour which contributes to its nutritional value. It is a fantastic autumnal recipe when pumpkins and squashes are in season and is a real bowl of sunshine on a cold day. When choosing a butternut squash, look for one with a longer stem and a smaller bulb. This means it is easier to chop and prepare, as you get more flesh and fewer seeds. For a balanced meal, I have paired the soup with my Whipped Feta and Bean Dip (opposite) and Rosemary and Sea Salt Seeded Crackers (page 261), to boost both fibre and protein. This can become a high-fibre lunch, so if you want to lower the fibre or are building up slowly to more fibre, feel free to swap the crackers for my quick flatbreads (page 262) or swap the dip for hummus (page 269). Also see page 157 for more on how I make my soups balanced, and my favourite soup toppings.

---

1. In a deep saucepan, gently sauté the onion and garlic in the extra virgin olive oil over a medium heat for 3–4 minutes, until soft and fragrant.

2. Add the ginger, turmeric, carrots, butternut squash, cashew nuts and orange zest, and stir for 1–2 minutes.

3. Pour in the vegetable stock, season with black pepper, and cover. Simmer for 20–25 minutes, until the vegetables are soft.

4. Once cooked, allow the soup to cool slightly. Blend until smooth, using a stick blender or food processor. Stir in the orange juice and adjust the consistency with a splash of water or stock if needed.

5. Taste and adjust the seasoning before serving. Serve with my Whipped Feta and Bean Dip (opposite) and 30g of Rosemary and Sea Salt Seeded Crackers per serving (page 261).

Storage: This soup will keep for up to 3 days in an airtight container in the fridge and can be frozen for up to a month.

PER SERVING
PROTEIN: 26G
FIBRE: 12G
PLANT POINTS: 5.5

SERVES 4
1 x 400g tin or jar of cannellini beans, rinsed and drained (240g drained weight)
200g feta
30g Parmesan (or vegetarian hard cheese), finely grated
1 garlic clove, crushed
1 tablespoon lemon juice
a small handful of fresh coriander
sea salt and freshly ground black pepper

To serve (per serving)
a thick slice of toasted sourdough bread (around 100g)
around 250g of vegetable crudités (e.g. carrot, celery, cucumber and red pepper)

WHIPPED FETA AND BEAN DIP

This quick and easy dip comes together in minutes using a food processor, making it perfect for busy days or last-minute entertaining. Packed with protein and fibre, it's a smart addition to meals and snacks, helping keep you feeling fuller for longer while supporting your nutritional goals. Enjoy it with the Sunshine Soup (opposite) and Rosemary and Sea Salt Seeded Crackers (page 261), or spread it thickly on toasted sourdough and serve with crudités for a quick lunch. Serve with gluten-free bread to make this completely gluten-free.

1. Put the beans, feta, Parmesan, garlic, lemon juice, coriander, and some salt and pepper into a food processor. Blend on a medium speed until well combined but still retaining a slightly chunky texture. If the mixture is too thick, add a little water, 1 tablespoon at a time, blending between each addition, until you reach the desired consistency.

2. Spread on toasted sourdough with the vegetables on the side.

Storage: Store in an airtight container in the fridge for up to 3 days.

LUNCH 175

PER SERVING
PROTEIN: 28G
FIBRE: 14G
PLANT POINTS: 12.5

SERVES 4 (MAKES 12 BALLS)
220g dried red lentils
500ml cold filtered water
2 tablespoons extra virgin olive oil
1 medium red onion, finely diced
2 garlic cloves, crushed
1 teaspoon sweet paprika
½ teaspoon hot chilli powder
1 large handful of spinach
2 tablespoons tomato purée
60g ground red lentils (see Tip), 60g gluten-free (or regular) rolled oats, 60g chickpea flour, or regular flour (Note, this won't be gluten-free)
sea salt and freshly ground black pepper

Lemon tahini dressing
30g tahini
2 tablespoons tamari
2 tablespoons apple cider vinegar
juice of 1 lemon (or 50ml Sicilian lemon juice)
1 garlic clove
10g fresh ginger
1 tablespoon toasted sesame oil

To serve
4 Chickpea Pancake Wraps (page 265)
crunchy, chopped salad (e.g. endive, celery, tomatoes, radish or red cabbage)
sauerkraut or kimchi

Tip: To make red lentil flour, grind raw red lentils for around 30 seconds in a powerful blender or coffee grinder.

RED LENTIL POLPETTE WITH CHICKPEA WRAPS

Polpette are Italian-style meatballs, but these ones are plant-based so you can also think of them a little like lentil falafels. They are very versatile – try them in a chickpea wrap with crunchy salad, as part of a larger salad (aim for around 200–250g vegetables per serving) or as a protein top-up in soup (page 157). They're baked, not fried, giving you time to prep your sides while they cook.

---

1. First, make the batter for the wraps (page 265). While the batter is resting, start on the polpette.

2. Put the red lentils into a pan with the water. Bring to the boil, then reduce the heat and simmer for 10 minutes until almost cooked but still holding their shape. Drain well and let cool slightly.

3. Meanwhile, preheat the oven to 210°C fan. Grease a baking sheet, or line it with baking parchment.

4. Heat the oil in a frying pan and sauté the onion and garlic over a medium-high heat until soft. Stir in the paprika and chilli powder, cook for 1 minute, then add the spinach and let it wilt slightly for 1 minute. Remove from the heat and stir in the tomato purée, ground lentils (or alternative), and season with salt and pepper. Mix well and allow to cool slightly.

5. Roll the mixture into 12 balls (or 16 if you like them a little smaller). Bake them on the prepared baking sheet for 20–25 minutes until golden and crispy on the outside.

6. While the polpette are cooking, finish making the wraps.

7. Blend the dressing ingredients in a small blender (or use a stick blender), until smooth and creamy. Add a little water if required.

8. Top each pancake with a spoonful of dressing, 3 warm polpette and salad. Drizzle over the rest of the dressing. Add some sauerkraut or kimchi for extra plant points and gut-friendly benefits.

Storage: Store the cooked polpette in an airtight container in the fridge for up to 3 days or freeze for up to 3 months. Reheat in the oven at 180°C fan for 10 minutes, until piping hot throughout.

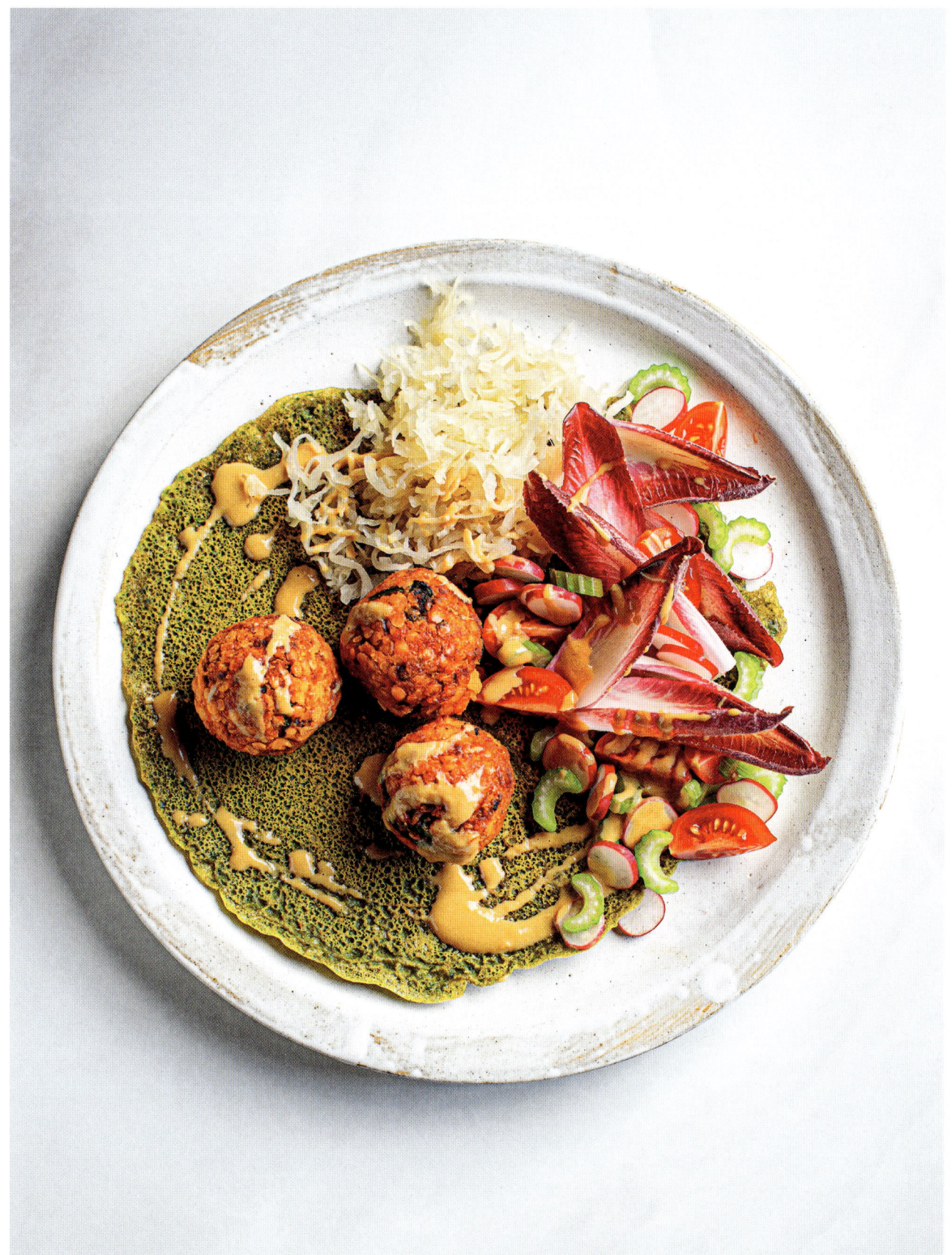

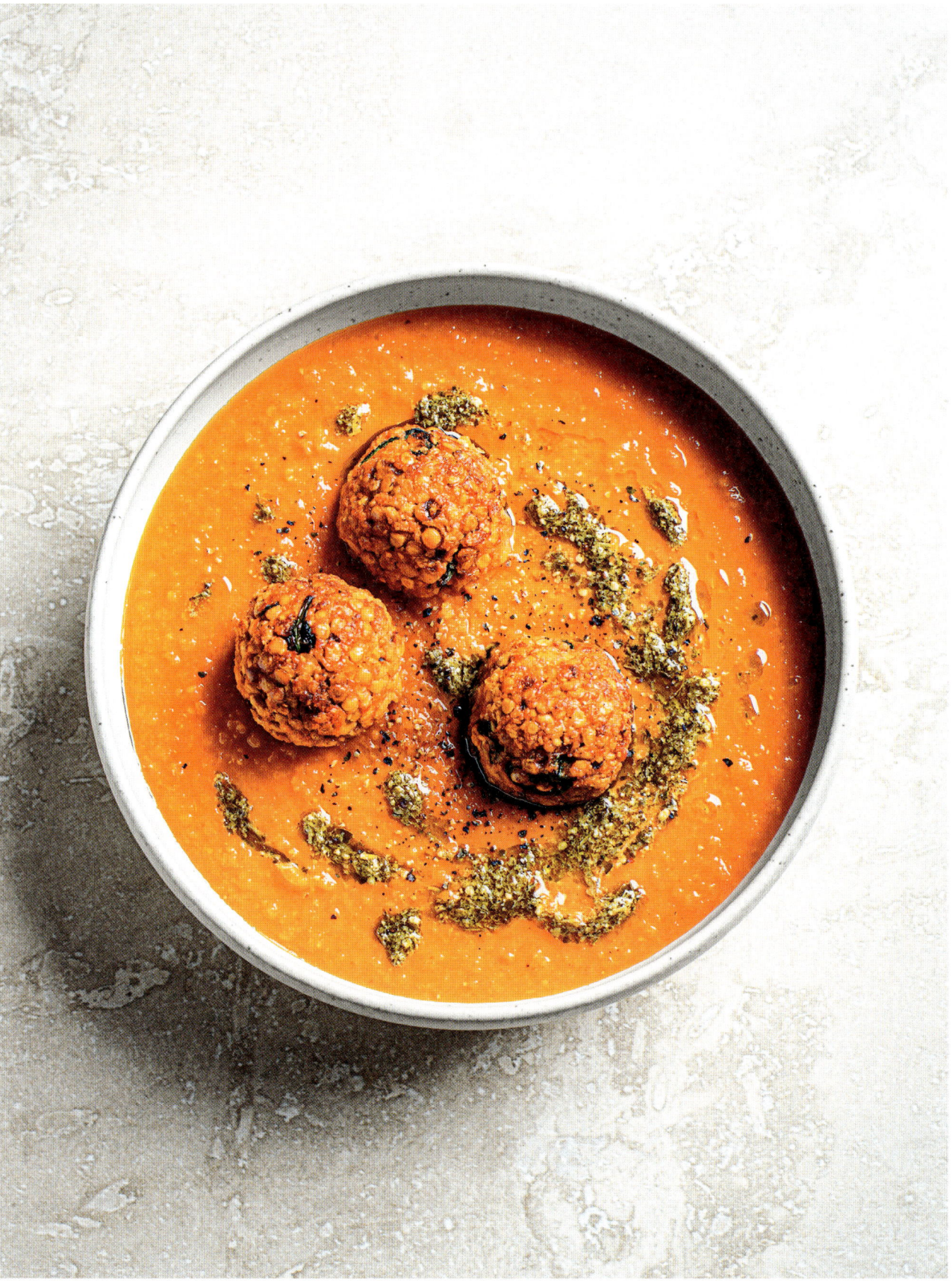

PER SERVING
PROTEIN: 25G
FIBRE: 15G
PLANT POINTS: 7.25

SERVES 4
1 tablespoon extra virgin olive oil
1 onion, finely diced
2 garlic cloves, crushed
4 large carrots, finely diced
400g fresh vine tomatoes, roughly chopped, or 1 x 400g tin of chopped tomatoes
50g dried red lentils
1 tablespoon tomato purée
400ml vegetable stock
¼ teaspoon cayenne pepper
sea salt and freshly ground black pepper

To serve
warm Red Lentil Polpette (page 176), 3 per bowl
a swirl of Green Pesto (page 205) (or vegetarian pesto)

Tip: Top up the protein further with a sprinkling of feta.

TOMATO AND CARROT SOUP WITH RED LENTIL POLPETTE

This is one of the most popular soup recipes that I share in clinic. It's often the first recipe people choose when they join my programmes, and it's one I personally make on repeat. It's simple, comforting and easy to adapt. Here, I've paired it with the Red Lentil Polpette on page 176 to top up the protein and turn it into a more filling meal, but you can add any protein you choose to this soup. I also love it with pan-fried halloumi cubes, or simply finished with crumbled feta for a quick and nourishing lunch. See page 157 for more topping ideas. You can easily make this dish dairy-free and vegan, by using a vegan pesto.

---

1. Heat the extra virgin olive oil in a large saucepan over a medium heat. Add the onion and sauté for around 5 minutes, until starting to soften. Add the garlic and cook for another 2 minutes.

2. Stir in the carrots and tomatoes and sauté for a further 2 minutes. Add the red lentils, tomato purée, stock, cayenne pepper and some salt and pepper. Simmer gently for 20 minutes, until the lentils and vegetables are tender.

3. Remove from the heat and allow to cool a little, then blend until smooth using a stick blender or food processor. Adjust the seasoning if needed, and warm through again before serving.

4. For piping-hot polpette, reheat them in the oven at 180°C fan for 10 minutes or in an air fryer at 180°C for 5–6 minutes.

5. Serve the soup, topped with warm polpette and a swirl of pesto.

Storage: Store the soup and polpette separately in airtight containers in the fridge for up to 3 days. The soup is suitable for freezing for up to 3 months; defrost and reheat until piping hot.

PER SERVING
PROTEIN: 30G
FIBRE: 14G
PLANT POINTS: 15.5

STICKY PEANUT TOFU POKE BOWL

I don't think any cookbook is complete without a poke bowl! What I love about poke bowls is that there are no set rules. The word 'poke' is derived from a Hawaiian word meaning to slice or cut, so while a traditional poke bowl might contain raw fish and rice, as long as there is plenty of chopping involved, I think anything goes! This recipe uses all plant proteins, to show it is possible to reach 30g of protein using plant-based ingredients alone. The two most important elements in a poke bowl, for me, are colour and flavour. You can freestyle with the vegetables, or use what you already have in the fridge. Aim for around 200–250g of vegetables per person. The tofu can be swapped for halloumi if preferred.

SERVES 4

Tofu
280g firm, plain tofu
1 tablespoon chickpea (gram) flour or cornflour
1 tablespoon tamari or soy sauce (Note, soy sauce isn't gluten-free)
1 teaspoon honey (or maple syrup)
1 tablespoon toasted sesame oil
a pinch of chilli flakes

Salad
100g quinoa (dry weight), or 250g cooked quinoa
100g frozen edamame beans
120g red or white cabbage, or a mix, finely sliced
1 red pepper, diced
1 yellow pepper, diced
200g tomatoes, chopped
2 carrots, grated or julienned
12 radishes, sliced
100g cucumber, diced
½ avocado, diced

Dressing
100g peanut butter
2 tablespoons tamari or soy sauce (Note, soy sauce isn't gluten-free)
2 tablespoons apple cider vinegar
juice of 1 lime
2 garlic cloves, crushed
20g fresh ginger, peeled and finely grated
1 tablespoon toasted sesame oil
2 tablespoons sriracha sauce

To serve
1 teaspoon sesame seeds
chopped coriander

1. You can cook the tofu in the oven or in an air fryer. If using the oven, preheat to 180°C fan. Line a baking sheet with baking parchment.

2. Cut the tofu into bite-size squares and press them gently with a clean tea towel to remove the excess water. In a bowl, toss the tofu with the chickpea flour or cornflour, then add the tamari, honey, sesame oil and chilli flakes. Spread on the lined baking sheet and bake for 20–25 minutes, until golden and crisp outside and soft inside. Alternatively, cook in an air fryer at 180°C for 15 minutes.

3. Meanwhile, cook the quinoa in a pan of simmering water for 15 minutes. Add the frozen edamame for the last 4 minutes. Drain and rinse under cold water.

4. To make the dressing, combine all the ingredients in a food processor or use a stick blender. Add around 75ml of water and blend until smooth.

5. Serve the vegetables, quinoa and edamame with the tofu, coriander and a sprinkle of sesame seeds. Drizzle generously with the peanut dressing.

Make-One-Take-One: Store the salad ingredients in an airtight container in the fridge for up to 3 days. Keep the dressing in a separate jar. Assemble just before serving.

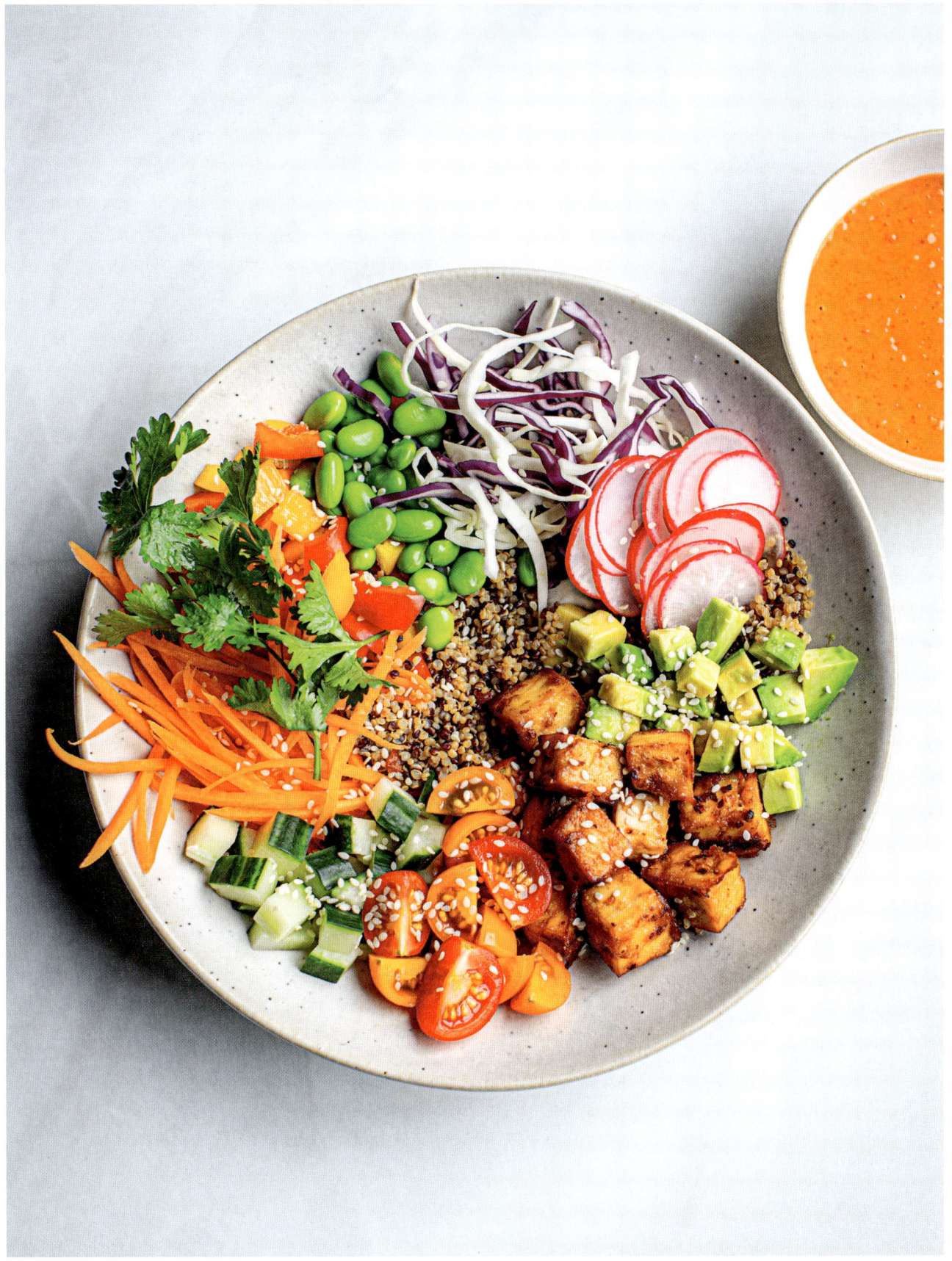

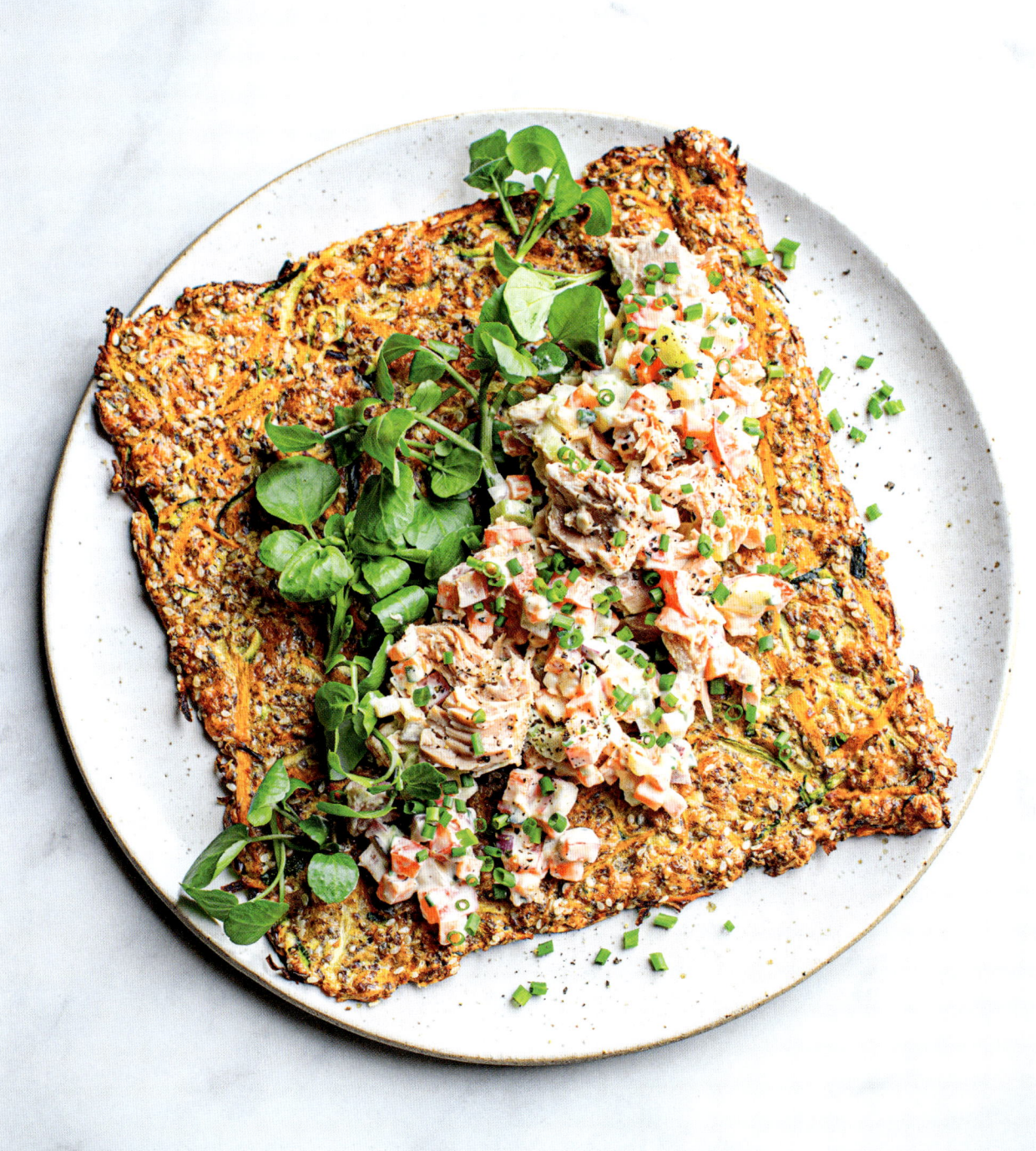

PER SERVING
PROTEIN: 33G
FIBRE: 8G
PLANT POINTS: 9.75

SERVES 4

Wrap
1 large carrot, grated (about 100g)
1 courgette, grated (about 150g)
200g hard mozzarella or Cheddar, grated
50g milled flaxseeds
10g chia seeds
30g sesame seeds
2 eggs
1 teaspoon dried oregano, or other herbs of your choice
sea salt and freshly ground black pepper

Filling
1 tin of tuna in water or oil, drained (around 160g)
1 stick of celery, finely chopped
1 large red pepper, finely diced
1 medium carrot, finely diced
½ red onion, finely diced
1 tablespoon Dijon mustard (check it is gluten-free)
75g Greek yoghurt
1 tablespoon chopped fresh chives
sea salt and freshly ground black pepper

To serve
a handful of watercress (per serving)

MOZZARELLA AND VEGETABLE SEEDED WRAPS WITH TUNA SALAD

This is a recipe where the wrap is not just a convenient carrier for the filling, it quickly becomes an important part of the meal, contributing protein, fibre and plant points. The wraps can be made in advance and used for packed lunches, or for a quick meal when time is short. You can use any filling you like, but my tuna and vegetable mix works so well with the melted cheese in the wrap. Including extra vegetables in both the wrap and the filling helps to increase the fibre content. If you prefer, you can substitute the Greek yoghurt with mayonnaise. For a change you can swap out the tuna for cooked chicken.

1. Preheat the oven to 180°C fan and line a large baking tray, or two smaller trays, with baking parchment.

2. Squeeze out the excess water from the carrot and courgette using kitchen paper.

3. Mix all the wrap ingredients in a large bowl and season well with salt and pepper. Divide the mixture into 4 equal portions and spoon them onto the lined baking tray(s). Flatten each portion with wet hands or use the back of a spoon to form rectangles approximately 20cm x 15cm. Alternatively, roll the mixture between two sheets of baking parchment and transfer to the baking tray(s).

4. Bake in the oven for 20–25 minutes, or until golden brown and crisp. Allow to cool completely.

5. While the wraps are cooking, prepare the filling. Mix the drained tuna with the vegetables, mustard, Greek yoghurt and chives, and season with salt and pepper.

6. To assemble, place a layer of watercress on each wrap, add the tuna mixture and roll up carefully.

Storage: Store the wraps in an airtight container in the fridge for up to 2 days. If not eating immediately, reheat in an air-fryer at 160°C for 3–4 minutes or warm through in a dry frying pan.

PER SERVING
PROTEIN: 29G
FIBRE: 14G
PLANT POINTS: 10.5

SERVES 4

1 onion, finely chopped
1 tablespoon extra virgin olive oil
2 garlic cloves, crushed
4 carrots, diced (around 400g)
2 red peppers, diced
1 small sweet potato (around 200g), peeled and diced
1 apple, peeled, cored and diced
1 teaspoon ground turmeric
2 teaspoons curry powder
1 teaspoon ground cumin
1 teaspoon sweet paprika
½ teaspoon ground cinnamon
100g dried red lentils
600–700ml hot, good-quality vegetable stock
1 tablespoon tomato purée
sea salt and freshly ground black pepper

Protein-rich topping

200g halloumi, cubed (or firm tofu, if preferred)
1 x 400g tin or jar of chickpeas, rinsed and drained (240g drained weight)
75g sunflower seeds
1 tablespoon extra virgin olive oil
1–2 tablespoons fajita spice mix (see below)
fresh coriander leaves, chopped

**Fajita spice mix (or use a ready-made mix)
makes 1 small jar**

½ tablespoon hot chilli powder
2 tablespoons sweet paprika
1 tablespoon ground cumin
1 tablespoon garlic powder (optional)
½ tablespoon ground coriander
1 tablespoon dried oregano

SPICY LENTIL SOUP WITH HALLOUMI AND CHICKPEAS

Soups are a great way of getting more vegetables into our diet; however, soup with bread can often leave us feeling unsatisfied, as we miss out on the extra protein. Spiced halloumi, chickpeas and seeds are a fun way to add a protein-rich topping to your soup, guaranteed to leave you feeling fuller for longer. It gives texture and flavour and turns a simple soup into a complete meal. If you prefer, you can use tofu instead of halloumi. I love packing this soup into a food flask (add the topping with the soup or keep it separate) for a balanced lunch on the go. See page 157 for more on how to make soups more balanced, and my favourite soup topper ideas.

---

1. In a heavy-based saucepan, gently sauté the onion in the extra virgin olive oil for 5 minutes, until softened. Add the garlic and cook for a further 2 minutes. Add the carrots, red peppers, sweet potato and apple. Stir-fry for 2 minutes, then add the turmeric, curry powder, cumin, paprika and cinnamon. Cook for 2 minutes to allow the flavours to develop.

2. Add the lentils, 600ml of the hot stock, the tomato purée, and season with salt and pepper. Simmer gently for 20 minutes, or until the vegetables and lentils are soft, stirring occasionally. Adjust the consistency, if necessary, by adding more of the stock. Leave the soup 'chunky', or you can part-blend with a stick blender for a smoother consistency.

3. To prepare the topping, fry the halloumi cubes, chickpeas and sunflower seeds in a heavy-based frying pan with 1 tablespoon of extra virgin olive oil and 1–2 tablespoons of the fajita spice mix over a medium heat for 6–8 minutes, until crispy and golden.

4. Ladle the soup into bowls, top with the crispy protein mix and sprinkle with fresh coriander to serve.

Make-One-Take-One: Store the soup and toppings separately in airtight containers in the fridge for up to 3 days. Freeze for up to 3 months. Defrost before reheating in a pan until piping hot. Add the protein-rich topping to the soup while reheating, or warm it separately in an air fryer at 160°C for 5 minutes, or in a frying pan without extra oil.

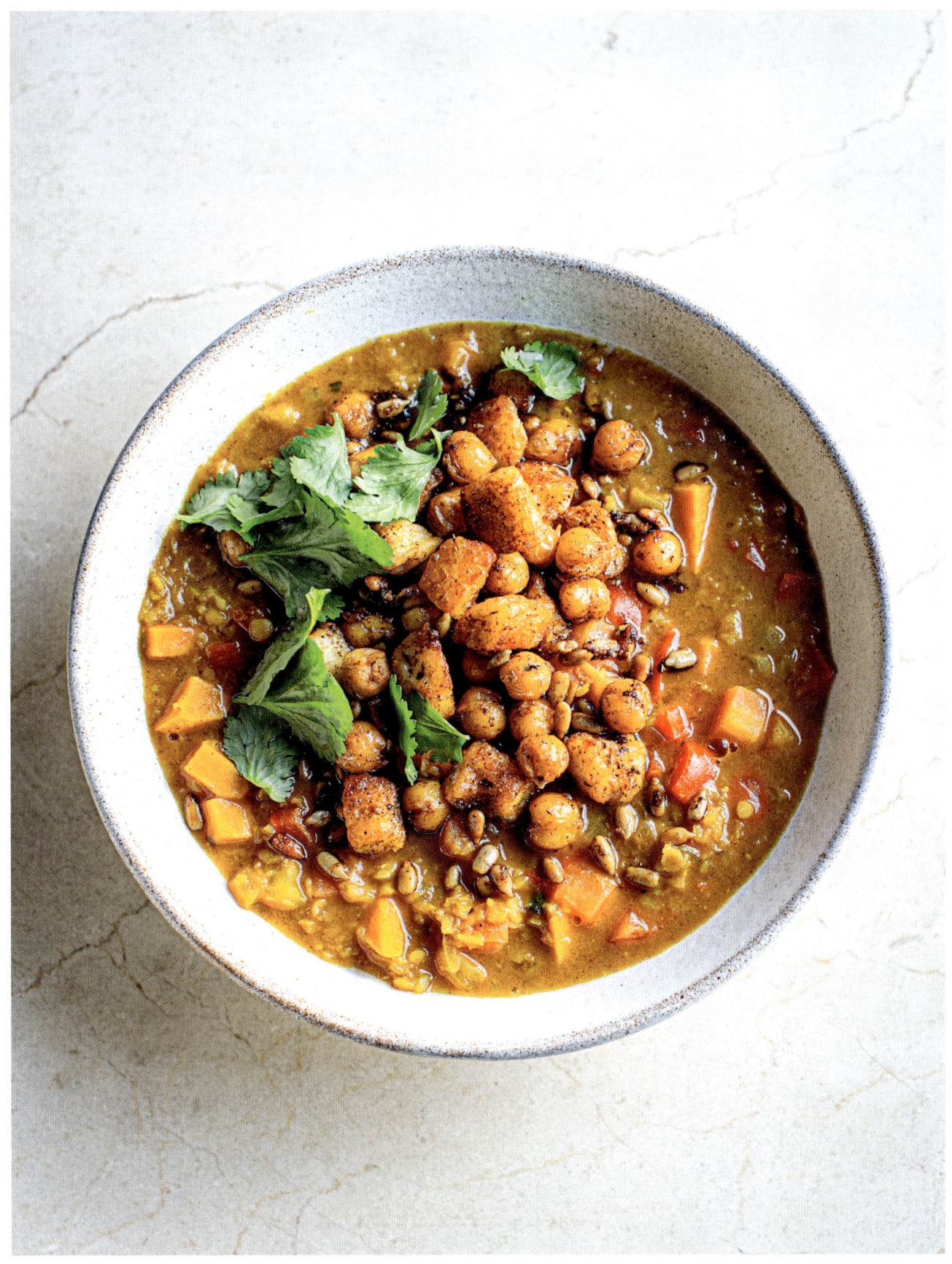

PER SERVING (TRADITIONAL)
PROTEIN: 33G
FIBRE: 7G
PLANT POINTS: 5.25

SERVES 4

Main salad
2 skinless chicken breasts (around 300g)
1 tablespoon extra virgin olive oil
2 medium romaine lettuces, chopped
250g cherry tomatoes, quartered
½ cucumber, thinly sliced

'Croutons'
1 x 400g tin or jar of chickpeas, rinsed and drained (240g drained weight)
1 tablespoon extra virgin olive oil
50g Parmesan, grated
1 teaspoon garlic powder
a pinch of sea salt

To serve
chopped chives
a few shards of Parmesan
Traditional Caesar Dressing or Lighter Caesar Dressing (page 188)

For a protein top-up: add 1 boiled egg per serving, which will add 6g protein.

For extra fibre and healthy fats: add some sliced avocado.

CHICKEN CAESAR SALAD WITH PARMESAN CHICKPEA CROUTONS

Classic Caesar salad is delicious, but can often be a high-calorie option, so I have given the traditional Caesar salad an upgrade! In this version, the fibre content has been increased by swapping croutons for cheesy chickpeas, which make the salad more balanced and nutritious. Chickpeas are rich in fibre, magnesium and folate, and they also release their energy slowly between meals. There are two dressing options on page 188: the traditional version, which is still a much healthier option compared to shop-bought, and an even lighter alternative (made with yoghurt) for those aiming to reduce their energy intake. Swap the anchovies for 1 tablespoon of capers in the dressing if you prefer.

---

1. To make the 'croutons', preheat the oven to 220°C fan. Thoroughly dry the chickpeas, using kitchen paper. Spread on a baking tray, drizzle with the extra virgin olive oil, and sprinkle with the Parmesan, garlic powder and salt. Roast for 25 minutes, or until golden and crisp.

2. Meanwhile, make your dressing of choice (see overleaf).

3. Cut the chicken into bite-size pieces. Heat the extra virgin olive oil in a heavy-based frying pan and sauté the chicken over a medium heat for 5–6 minutes, or until fully cooked and lightly browned.

4. Assemble the salad by combining the chopped romaine, cherry tomatoes, cucumber, chicken and chickpea 'croutons'. Garnish with chopped chives and Parmesan shards and drizzle with your choice of Caesar dressing.

Make-One-Take-One: Store the salad ingredients in an airtight container in the fridge for up to 3 days. Keep the dressing in a separate jar. Assemble just before serving.

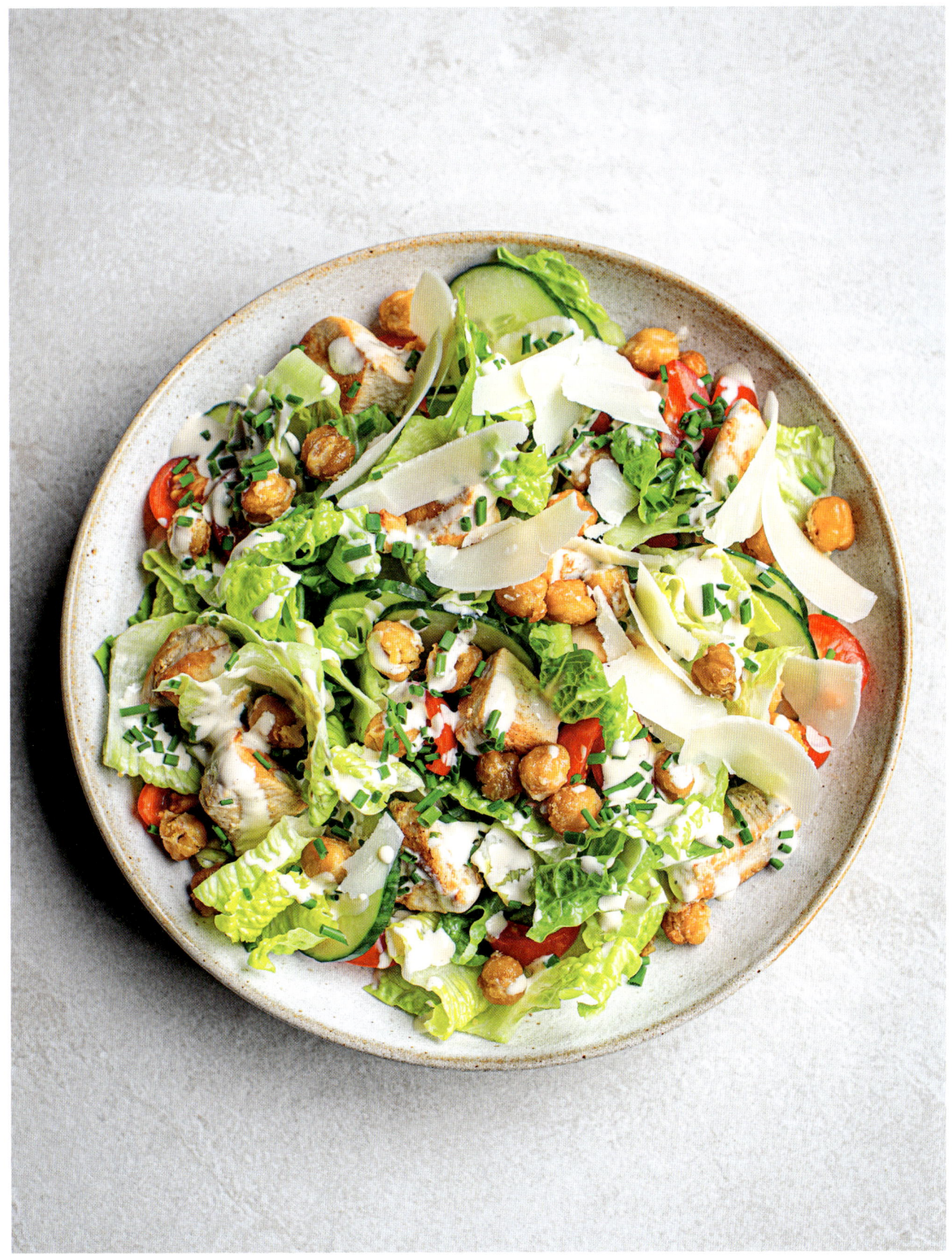

PER 40G SERVING
PROTEIN: 3G
FIBRE: 0G
PLANT POINTS: 0.75

MAKES 10 SERVINGS (40G PER SERVING)

2 eggs
juice of 1 lemon
2 garlic cloves
1 teaspoon Worcestershire sauce (gluten-free version)
4 anchovy fillets (tinned or from a jar)
150ml neutral oil, e.g. cold-pressed rapeseed oil or avocado oil (or a 50:50 blend with extra virgin olive oil)
sea salt and freshly ground black pepper, to taste
50g Parmesan, grated

TRADITIONAL CAESAR DRESSING

A neutral oil such as cold-pressed rapeseed oil or avocado oil works best, as extra virgin olive oil can impart a strong flavour due to its high polyphenol content. However, I like to use a 50:50 blend of extra virgin olive oil with cold-pressed rapeseed oil or avocado oil. You will have more dressing than you need, so store the extra in the fridge in an airtight container for up to 3 days.

---

1. Put all the ingredients except the Parmesan into a small blender or a tall jar suitable for a stick blender. Blend until the mixture thickens and emulsifies. Add the Parmesan and blend again until smooth.

PER 50G SERVING
PROTEIN: 7G
FIBRE: 0G
PLANT POINTS: 0.5

MAKES 6 SERVINGS (50G PER SERVING)

200g Greek yoghurt
juice of 1 lemon
4 anchovy fillets (tinned or from a jar)
2 garlic cloves, crushed
1 teaspoon mustard (e.g. Dijon) (check it is gluten-free)
1 teaspoon Worcestershire sauce (gluten-free version)
50g Parmesan, grated
sea salt and freshly ground black pepper, to taste

LIGHTER CAESAR DRESSING

This is a lighter alternative dressing that works really well with the Caesar salad. You will have a some left over, which you can store in the fridge in an airtight container; use within a couple of days as a ranch-style dressing.

---

1. Blend all the ingredients together in a food processor or mix by hand (finely chop the anchovies first, if you are mixing by hand).

PER SERVING
PROTEIN: 30G
FIBRE: 12G
PLANT POINTS: 12.5

SERVES 6

500g aubergine, washed and sliced into 1–1.5cm-thick discs
2 medium onions, finely diced
3 garlic cloves
2 tablespoons extra virgin olive oil, plus extra for greasing
350g dried red lentils, or a mix of red and Puy
2 yellow peppers, finely diced
1 large carrot, grated
1 courgette, sliced into 1cm-thick discs
1 tablespoon ground ginger
¼ teaspoon ground cinnamon
1 tablespoon dried oregano
1 x 400g tin of chopped tomatoes
1 tablespoon tomato purée
sea salt and freshly ground black pepper
600–700ml vegetable stock

Cheese sauce
500–550ml milk (I used semi-skimmed cow's milk)
40g gluten-free or regular flour
a pinch each of sea salt and freshly ground black pepper
a pinch of nutmeg
120g Parmesan (or vegetarian hard cheese), grated

Dairy-free cheese sauce
500ml plant-based milk
50g gluten-free or regular flour
50g tahini
2 teaspoons vegetable stock powder or bouillon
1 tablespoon nutritional yeast
a pinch each of sea salt and freshly ground black pepper
30g sunflower seeds

To serve
mixed salad using 4 different vegetables (e.g. pepper, tomato, rocket, avocado)

VEGETABLE MOUSSAKA

This dish includes proteins from the red lentils and also the cheese sauce. I have given an option to make it dairy-free though, if you choose. If you do this, add 30g sunflower seeds to the topping to make it even more nutrient dense.

---

1. Place the aubergine slices in a steamer over a pan of boiling water for 10–15 minutes, until tender.

2. While the aubergine is steaming, sauté the onions and garlic in the extra virgin olive oil in a deep-sided frying pan over a medium heat for 4–5 minutes. Add the lentils, finely diced peppers, grated carrot and sliced courgette, and cook for a further 3–4 minutes.

3. Stir through the ginger, cinnamon and oregano. Add the tinned tomatoes and tomato purée, and season with salt and pepper. Add 600ml of the vegetable stock and simmer for around 30 minutes with a lid on, adding more stock if needed.

4. Preheat the oven to 180°C fan.

5. When the lentil mix is cooked, arrange some of the aubergine slices in the base of a greased ceramic oven dish, 25cm x 30cm. Cover with the lentil mixture, then top with more aubergine slices.

6. In a pan over a medium heat, using the all-in-one method, whisk together all the cheese sauce ingredients, except for the Parmesan, whisking all the time, until it becomes thick and creamy. Take off the heat and stir through 80g of the Parmesan, reserving the rest for the topping. For the dairy-free sauce, mix all the ingredients (apart from the sunflower seeds) in a pan and stir or whisk over a medium heat until thickened.

7. Pour the sauce over the final layer of aubergines and top with the remaining Parmesan cheese (or sunflower seeds). Bake in the oven for 30 minutes until bubbling and golden.

8. Serve with the mixed salad.

Make-One-Take-One: The moussaka will keep in an airtight container in the fridge for up to 3 days. Reheat in the oven at 160°C fan for 20–25 minutes, until piping hot.

PER SERVING
PROTEIN: 29G
FIBRE: 8G
PLANT POINTS: 8.5

BURRATA AND PEACH SALAD

This is the most colourful summer salad – it is a meal in itself for two, or can serve four as a starter. Burrata is a soft Italian cheese made from mozzarella and cream, which gives it a rich creamy centre. You can, of course, swap it for regular mozzarella if you prefer. This salad is an explosion of flavours and textures, with the sweet balsamic dressing, salty Parma ham, juicy peaches, bursts of pomegranate, crunchy nuts and rich extra virgin olive oil. (Shiny red pomegranate seeds add colour and sweetness, but you can leave them out if you don't have any, and it will still be delicious.) If the sun is out and you fancy some alfresco dining, this salad is the perfect choice.

**SERVES 2
(OR 4 AS A STARTER)**

2 ripe peaches, sliced
1 shallot, finely sliced
200g cherry or baby plum tomatoes, halved
80g mixed salad leaves, washed
1 bunch of basil, roughly torn
150g burrata (or mozzarella)
80g Parma ham
25g mixed pecan nuts and/or pumpkin seeds
2 tablespoons pomegranate seeds

Dressing
2 tablespoons extra virgin olive oil
2 tablespoons balsamic vinegar

To serve
a small slice of toasted seeded sourdough (about 50g per serving)

1. To make the dressing, whisk the extra virgin olive oil and balsamic vinegar together in a small bowl.

2. Arrange the peach slices, shallot, tomatoes, mixed leaves and basil on serving plates or a large platter. Cut into the burrata, revealing the creamy centre, and add to the salad along with the Parma ham.

3. Scatter over the pecan nuts and/or pumpkin seeds and the pomegranate seeds. Drizzle over the dressing just before serving. Enjoy with crispy sourdough bread.

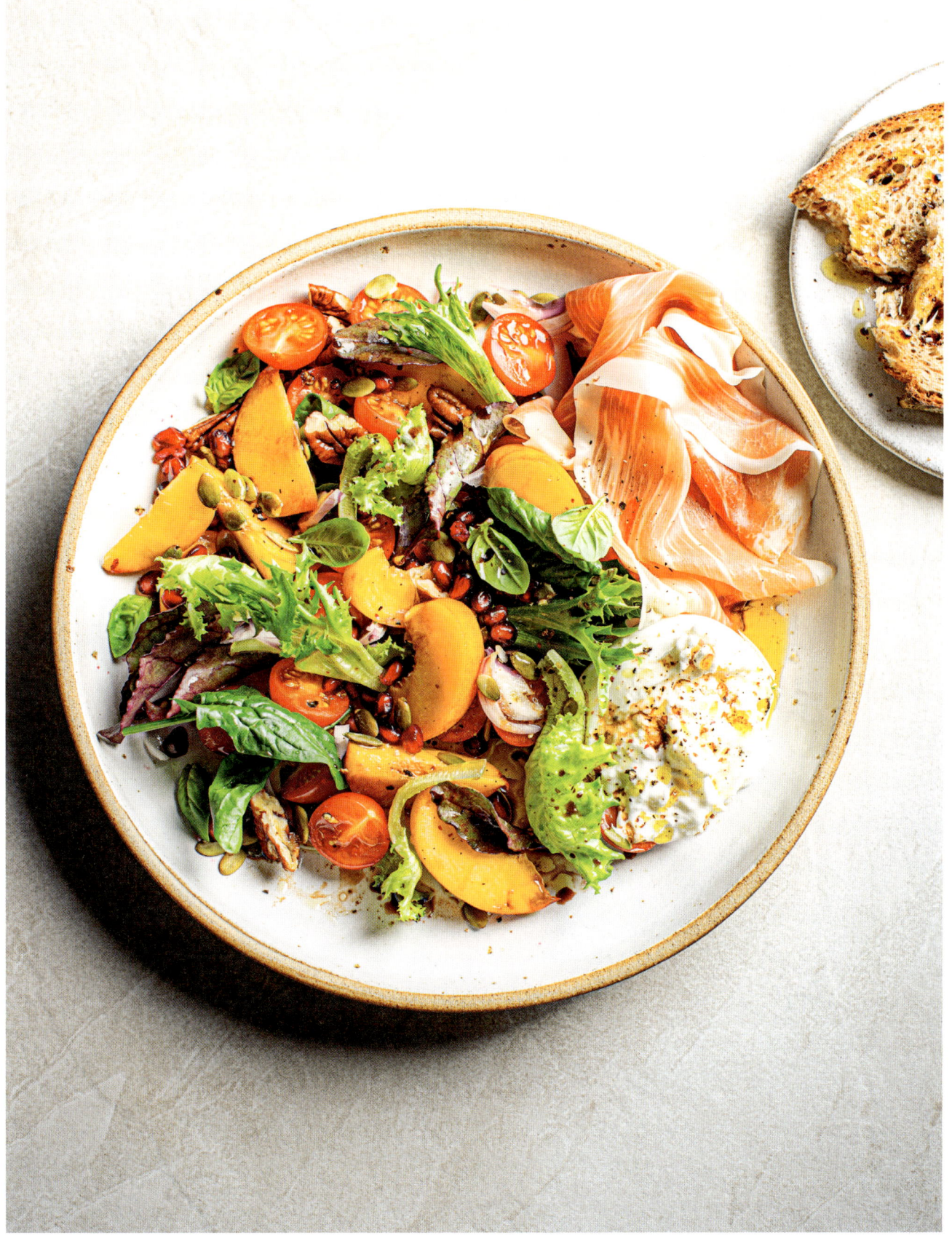

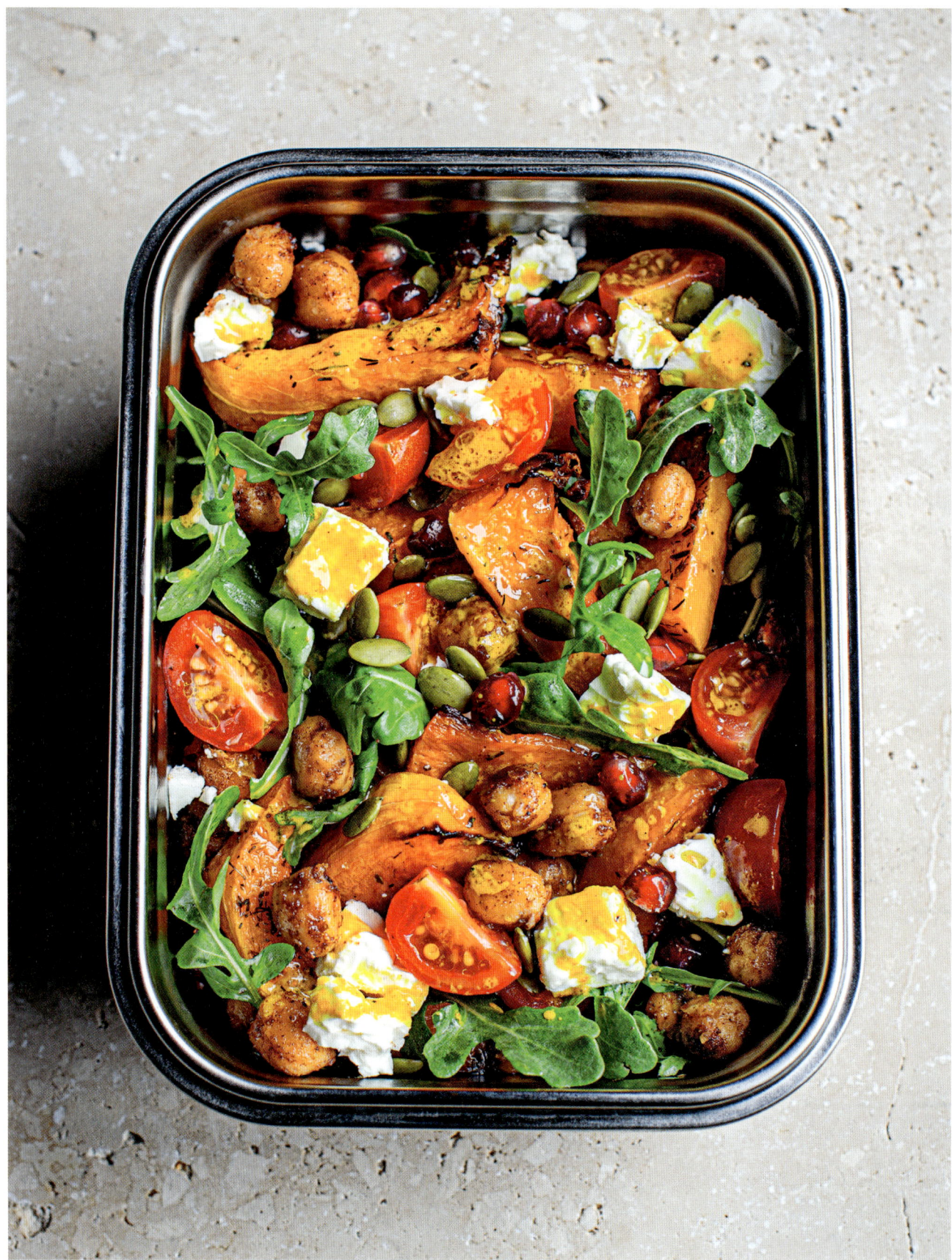

PER SERVING
PROTEIN: 23G
FIBRE: 15G
PLANT POINTS: 6.5

SERVES 4

1 butternut squash
2 tablespoons extra virgin olive oil
a few sprigs of fresh thyme or 1 teaspoon dried thyme
2 x 400g tins or jars of chickpeas, rinsed and drained (480g drained weight)
3 teaspoons harissa spice mix (ready-made or make your own, see Tip)
½ teaspoon sea salt
freshly ground black pepper, to taste
120g rocket
4 fresh tomatoes, chopped
200g feta
25g pumpkin seeds
50g fresh pomegranate seeds

Turmeric dressing

2 tablespoons extra virgin olive oil
2 tablespoons lemon juice
1 level teaspoon mustard e.g. Dijon (check it is gluten-free)
1 teaspoon ground turmeric
sea salt and freshly ground black pepper

Tips:
You can make your own harissa with 1 teaspoon of ground cumin, 1 teaspoon of paprika and 1 teaspoon of mild chilli powder.

To add another 5g protein to your plate, serve with a slice of seeded bread or sourdough.

ROASTED BUTTERNUT SALAD WITH WARM TURMERIC DRESSING

My daughter Issi has always loved this salad, so it is fitting that it finds a place in this book. We like to eat it slightly warm or at room temperature, rather than cold from the fridge. The thing I love about this salad is that it works all year round. This is down to the dressing, which is made with warming turmeric. The turmeric has the ability to lift the flavour of the butternut squash, making this salad a pleasure to eat, even on a cold day. You can chop and change the cheese you use. Issi likes hers with feta, but I also like it with Manchego or fried halloumi. Choose your favourite, but if you're in doubt, follow Issi's lead!

---

1. Preheat the oven to 200°C fan. Peel the butternut squash, remove the seeds, and slice into thick wedges. Arrange on a roasting tray, drizzle with 1 tablespoon of the extra virgin olive oil, and add the thyme. Toss to coat in the oil and herbs, then roast for 35 minutes, until tender and golden at the edges.

2. While the squash roasts, heat the remaining 1 tablespoon of extra virgin olive oil in a frying pan over a medium-high heat. Add the chickpeas and the harissa spice mix and cook gently for 5–8 minutes, until heated through and slightly crisp at the edges. Season with salt and pepper, then set aside.

3. Once the squash is out of the oven, let it cool for about 30 minutes.

4. Toss the roasted butternut with the chickpeas, then divide among four plates or bowls. Fold through the rocket and chopped tomatoes, then crumble over the feta, and scatter over the pumpkin seeds and pomegranate seeds.

5. Combine the dressing ingredients in a jar and shake vigorously. Drizzle over the salad just before serving.

Storage: Store the salad and dressing separately in airtight containers in the fridge for up to 2 days. The salad can be served chilled or at room temperature. The dressing may thicken, so allow to reach room temperature before serving.

PER SERVING
PROTEIN: 30G
FIBRE: 11G
PLANT POINTS: 14

SERVES 2

175g smoked mackerel fillets
50g cream cheese
¼ red onion, finely diced
1 tablespoon horseradish cream
a pinch of chilli flakes
1 tablespoon chopped fresh coriander, dill or parsley
zest of 1 orange
1 tablespoon freshly squeezed orange juice

To serve

500g fresh salad vegetables (e.g. red pepper, red cabbage, rocket, tomato or cucumber)
2 thin slices of Seed and Nut Loaf (page 253)
a drizzle of extra virgin olive oil
lemon wedges

MACKEREL PÂTÉ

This creamy, protein-rich pâté works brilliantly for lunch, but I will often have it for breakfast too! Smoked mackerel is quite rich, so balancing it out with the cream cheese softens the flavour, and the orange adds a little sweetness. You can make the texture as smooth or as chunky as you like. Feel free to use tinned mackerel instead of smoked, which would make this a great store-cupboard recipe. You can prepare the pâté in advance and store it in the fridge in an airtight container.

---

1. Remove the skin and any bones from the mackerel fillets. Flake the mackerel into a bowl, then add the cream cheese, diced red onion, horseradish, chilli flakes, herbs and the orange zest and juice. Mix until combined, retaining some of the texture.

2. Slice the salad vegetables and arrange them on the side of the plate. Serve the pâté with Seed and Nut Loaf slices, and drizzle with extra virgin olive oil. Squeeze over a little lemon juice, if desired.

Storage: Store in an airtight container in the fridge for up to 2 days.

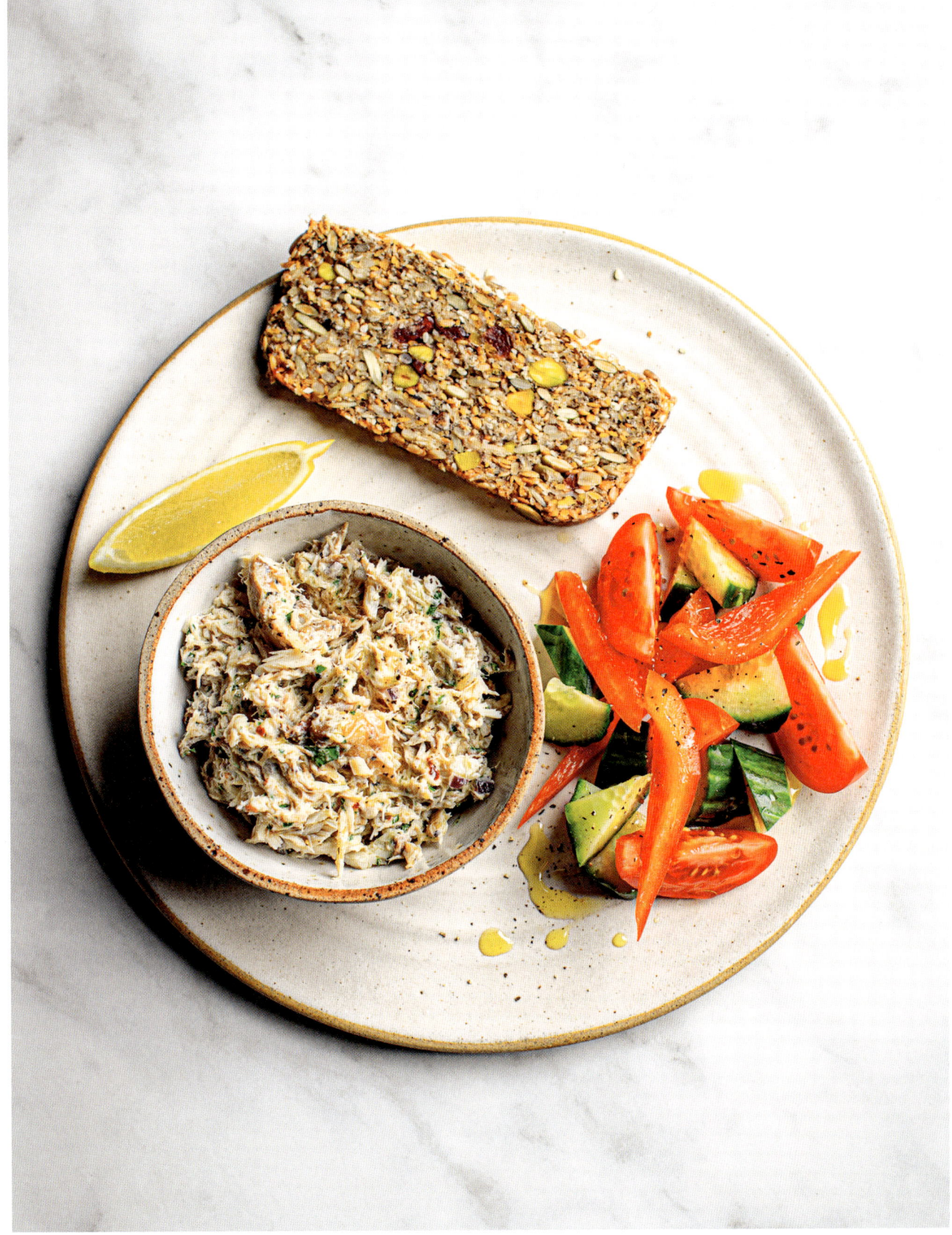

PER SERVING
PROTEIN: 29G
FIBRE: 12G
PLANT POINTS: 7.5

SERVES 2

75g dried Puy lentils (or 150g cooked)
4 purple or white spring onions, sliced
50g baby spinach
150g cooked beetroot, sliced
100g salad leaves
150g goat's cheese log
1 large pear, cored and sliced
30g raw or lightly toasted walnuts
microgreens, to garnish (optional)

Dressing
1 tablespoon extra virgin olive oil
1 tablespoon apple cider vinegar
½ teaspoon mustard (I used Dijon) (check your mustard is gluten-free)

PEAR AND GOAT'S CHEESE SALAD WITH TOASTED WALNUTS

I always enjoy pairing goat's cheese with fruit and nuts. I love the tangy, salty cheese together with the natural sweetness of the fruit and the crunch of nuts; for me it is a winning combination. This salad is simple to prepare and makes a perfect light lunch. It is also very transportable, for lunch on the go. The lentils top up the fibre and the protein, making the dish more satisfying, but you can swap them out for another grain or some seeded bread if you prefer. Beetroot gets its colour from the high concentration of plant pigments called anthocyanins, which act as antioxidants in the body. Beetroot is also a rich source of folate (vitamin B9), which is essential for healthy red blood cell formation.

1. Cook the lentils in a pan of simmering salted water for around 20–25 minutes with the lid on, until just al dente. Drain in a sieve and rinse under cold water.

2. Mix the dressing ingredients together in a small bowl or shake in a jar until emulsified.

3. Wash and prepare the vegetables and salad leaves. Put them into a large bowl or divide between two plates. Add the cooled lentils and toss gently to combine.

4. Slice the goat's cheese into bite-size pieces and arrange over the salad with the sliced pear and walnuts.

5. Drizzle over the dressing. Add microgreens on top for a splash of colour, if using.

Storage: Best assembled just before eating. Store the components separately in airtight containers in the fridge for up to 2 days.

PER SERVING
PROTEIN: 29G
FIBRE: 14G
PLANT POINTS: 10.25

SERVES 4

2 tablespoons extra virgin olive oil
1 large onion, finely sliced
3 garlic cloves, crushed
1 carrot, diced
1 stick of celery, chopped
800g fresh ripe tomatoes, or 2 x 400g tins of chopped tomatoes
200g dried red lentils
500–800ml vegetable stock (see Note, below)
2 bay leaves
4 tablespoons tomato purée
sea salt and freshly ground black pepper
1 x 400g tin or jar of butter beans, rinsed and drained (240g drained weight)

Topping
2 tablespoons Green Pesto (page 205) (or vegetarian pesto)
75g hard cheese, such as Cheddar or Parmesan (or vegetarian hard cheese)

Dairy-free option:
swap out the cheese for 25g of my Savoury Seed Mix (page 136) per serving

To serve
4 thin slices (50g each) of dark sourdough or gluten-free bread, toasted

Note: The amount of stock you need depends on if you use fresh or tinned tomatoes. Start with less and add more as needed.

TOMATO AND BUTTER BEAN SOUP

This soup is a complete meal that is satisfying and filling – and perfect for batch cooking. Increasing the amount of beans in our diet is so good for our gut health. The skins of the beans contain insoluble fibre that helps to absorb water and keep our gut moving, and the middle of the bean contains gel-like soluble fibre, which slows down digestion (keeping you feeling fuller for longer) while doubling as a fuel source to power up your gut microbes. I have topped up the plant protein with grated melted cheese so that you won't have to think about food all afternoon. If you'd prefer a dairy-free option, swap the cheese for my Savoury Seed Mix (page 136), using around 25g per portion, and use a vegan pesto.

1. Heat the extra virgin olive oil in a large saucepan over a medium heat. Gently sauté the onion for about 5 minutes, until softened. Add the garlic and cook for another 2 minutes. Stir in the carrot and celery and cook for 4–5 minutes, until beginning to soften.

2. Add the tomatoes and cook for around 5 minutes, stirring occasionally, until they start to break down.

3. Next, add the lentils, 500ml of the stock, the bay leaves and tomato purée, and season with salt and pepper. Simmer with the lid on for 20–25 minutes, until the soup is thick and the lentils are fully cooked. Add more stock to reach your favourite consistency.

4. Allow to cool slightly, then remove the bay leaves and blend until smooth using a stick blender or food processor. Add the drained butter beans, stir through and heat until piping hot. Divide among bowls and drizzle with the pesto.

5. Grate the cheese over the top just before serving (or, to make it plant-based, use 25g of savoury seed mix per portion instead of the cheese). Serve with toasted bread.

Make-One-Take-One: Store in an airtight container in the fridge for up to 3 days. Freeze for up to 3 months. Defrost and reheat thoroughly.

PER SERVING
PROTEIN: 30G
FIBRE: 8G
PLANT POINTS: 9

SERVES 4

100g dried freekeh (or 200g cooked)
a little sea salt or vegetable stock powder or bouillon
a drizzle of extra virgin olive oil (optional)
400g halloumi, drained and cut into 1cm-thick slices

Salsa
150g pomegranate seeds
¼ red onion, finely diced
100g cucumber, finely diced
¼ red chilli, deseeded and finely diced
zest and juice of 1 lime
1 rounded tablespoon chopped fresh herbs, e.g. mint and coriander
sea salt and freshly ground black pepper

Salad
1 orange
120g rocket leaves
200g cooked baby beetroot, quartered
½ red onion, finely sliced

Dressing
2 tablespoons extra virgin olive oil
2 tablespoons apple cider vinegar or lemon juice

To serve
a few drops of pomegranate molasses or balsamic vinegar

HALLOUMI SALAD WITH POMEGRANATE SALSA

Freekeh traditionally comes from the Middle East and is harvested from young green durum wheat. It uses ancient processing methods, involving roasting the wheat and rubbing it to remove the 'chaff' or dry outer layer. It can have a distinct smoky flavour if it is roasted over an open flame, but mostly now has a milder taste. Freekeh needs to be brought more into the spotlight, as it contains slightly more fibre and protein than other similar grains. This is the perfect healthy carb to add to this salad, and it works well with the salty cheese and sweet pomegranate. You can swap freekeh for bulgur wheat or quinoa if you prefer. The pomegranate salsa is a generous side dish that really complements the salty halloumi.

1. Put the freekeh into a pan of simmering water seasoned with a little sea salt or vegetable stock powder or bouillon. Cover and cook over a medium heat for 15–20 minutes, until tender. Drain and leave to cool.

2. Heat a non-stick or heavy-based frying pan over a medium heat. You can add a drizzle of extra virgin olive oil if you like, though halloumi usually cooks well in a dry pan. Lay the halloumi slices in a single layer in the pan and fry for 2–3 minutes on each side, until golden brown and crisp. Remove from the heat.

3. Whisk together the extra virgin olive oil and apple cider vinegar (or lemon juice) to make the dressing.

4. Combine all the salsa ingredients and season with salt and pepper to taste.

5. For tender orange pieces, peel the orange using a paring knife, and remove the skin surrounding the orange segments. Arrange the rocket, orange segments, beetroot, red onion and cooked freekeh on plates or a large platter. Drizzle over the dressing. Top with grilled halloumi, spoon over the pomegranate salsa and finish with a few drops of pomegranate molasses or balsamic vinegar.

Storage: The salsa can be stored in an airtight container in the fridge for up to 2 days. The freekeh can be cooked in advance and stored in an airtight container in the fridge for up to 3 days.

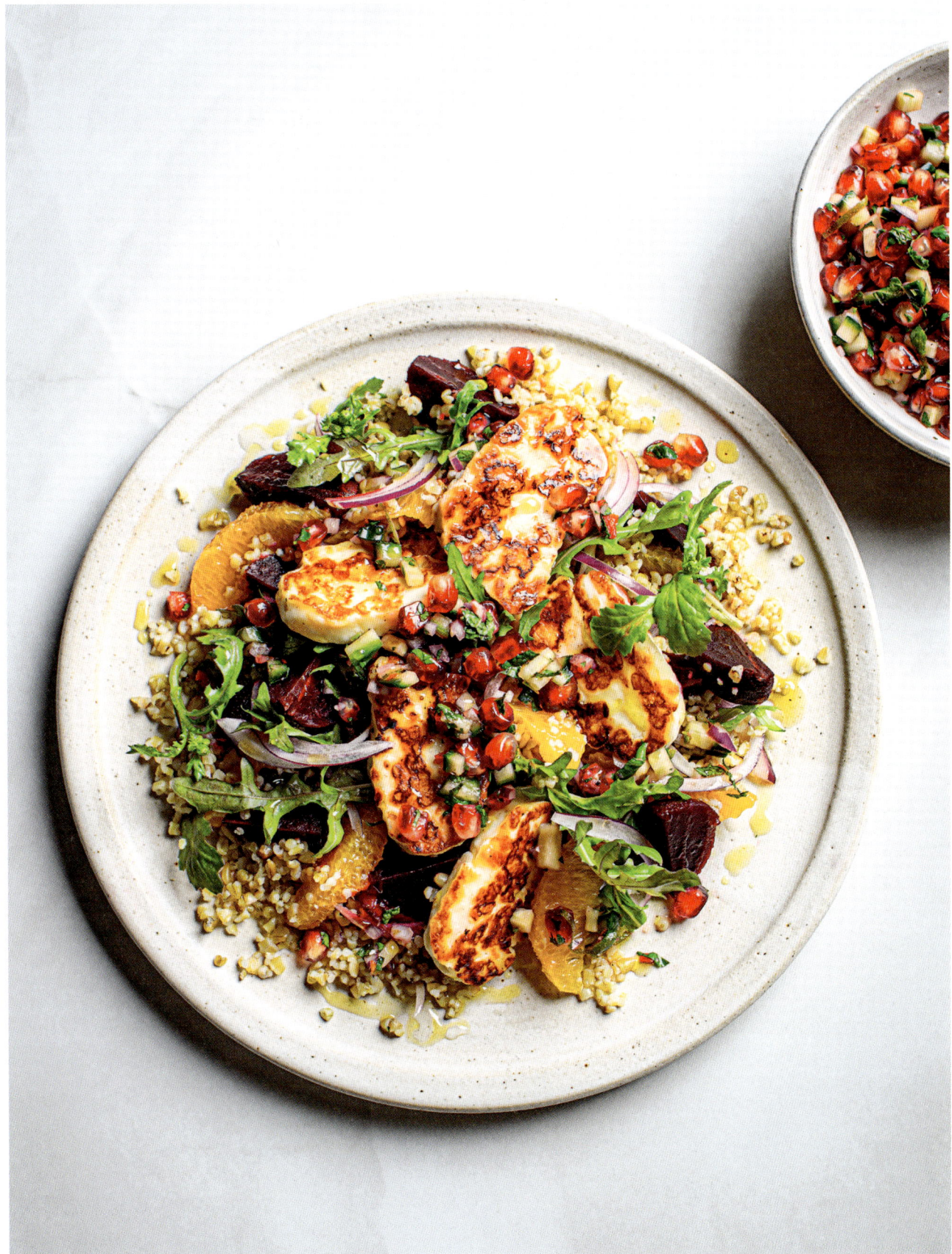

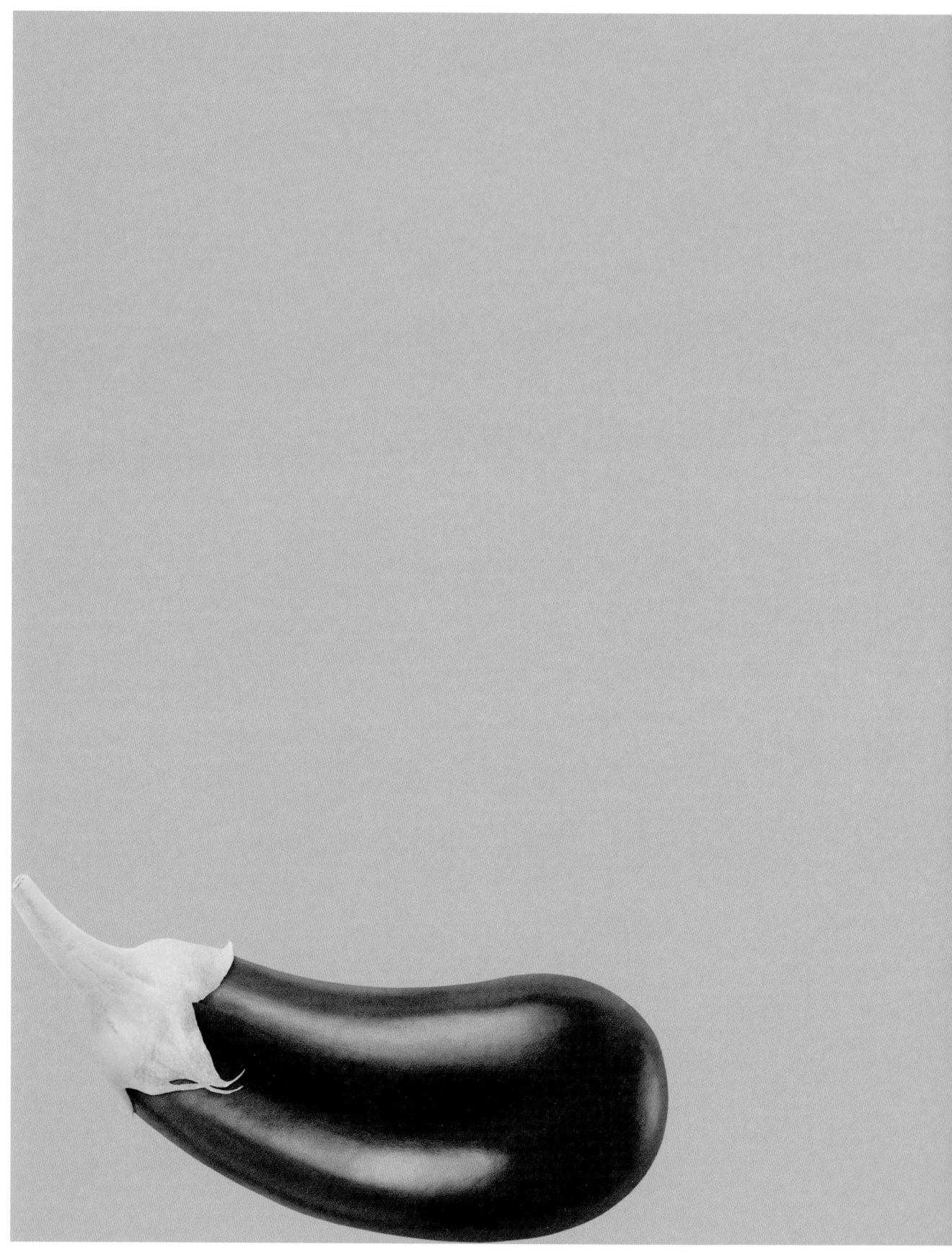

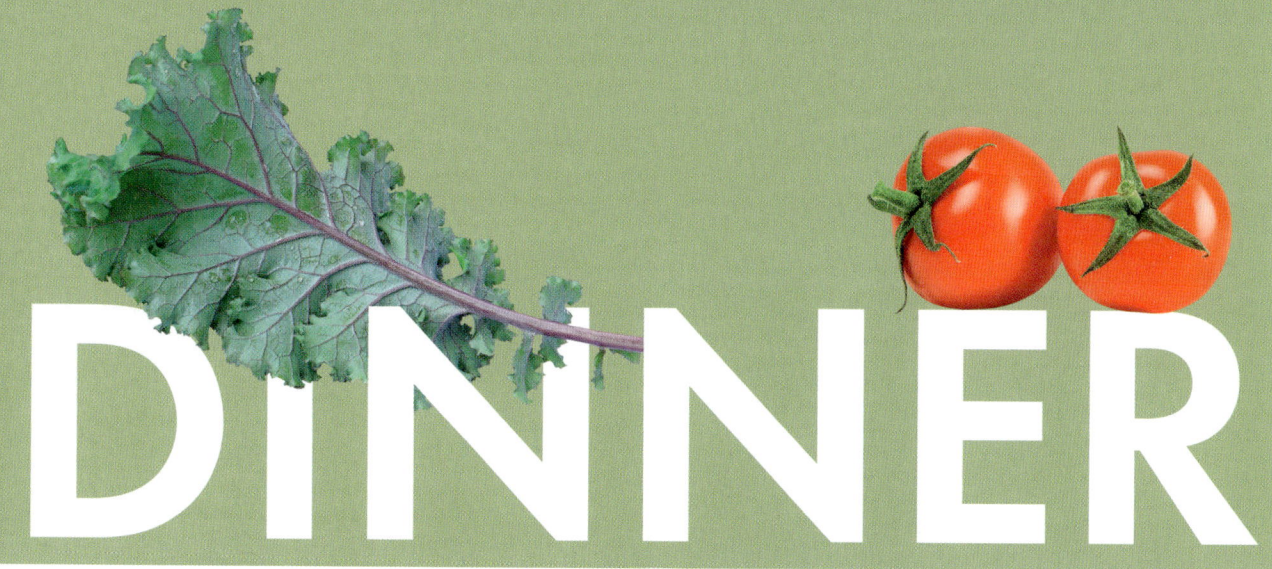

Getting your evening meal right is key. It needs to provide sufficient nutrition to keep you full and satisfied and to keep your blood sugar levels stable overnight. We're looking to leave a 12 to 14-hour gap before we eat breakfast (see page 72), so we need to be eating the right foods in the correct proportion – and we don't want to spend ages in the kitchen ending up eating too late.

All my recipes have been developed with simplicity in mind. I want you to feel like you can just throw some healthy ingredients together to create a delicious meal, and I want you to enjoy a variety of flavours and ingredients throughout the week, so you can begin to really start to enjoy your mealtimes. To achieve this, I've used lots of herbs and spices in my recipes, as well as punchy dressings, marinades and sauces to maximise taste without adding to the cooking time. Try the Prawn Fishcakes with Soba Noodle Salad and Wasabi Dipping Sauce (page 206), Pork Loin with Smoky Beans (page 240), Firecracker Chicken (page 208) or Sticky Trout with Salad (page 231), which are full of flavour and may become your new favourite recipes!

When it comes to creating balance, tucking into a double beef patty with cheese in a lettuce leaf wrap might give you up to 60g of protein, but it will be missing fibre and will not offer much of a buffet for the trillions of guests living in your gut. It's also a large portion of animal protein lacking the valuable benefits of plant proteins. Conversely, a vegetable curry with rice – but without any beans, tofu or lentils – might seem like a healthy, large plate of food, but although it will help you meet your fibre targets, it is likely to also short-change your body of the protein that helps to slow down your digestion and keep you energised.

We need both the fibre and the protein together and that's what my recipes provide, packing around one third (10g) of our daily fibre needs into each meal and one third of our protein (30g) – sometimes more! And because we are getting plenty of our fibre and protein from legumes, wholegrains, vegetables, seeds and nuts, we are also getting the right amount of healthy carbohydrates and fats simultaneously.

I'm always looking for ways to increase the plant protein and fibre in my recipes with healthy swaps and alternatives, such as in the Rustic Butter Bean 'Gnocchi' (page 224), which uses butter beans instead of potato and flour gnocchi, the Shepherdess Pie, made with lentils, with a cheesy bean and parsnip mash (page 221) and the Beef Chilli with Lentils and Chocolate (page 219). You really won't notice the swap!

You may notice that there are a few recipes in this chapter that don't include a healthy carbohydrate. Although I don't agree with going low-carb because we can often miss out on the fibre that comes with the carbohydrates (see pages 37–38), I didn't want to add an extra carb just for the sake of it. The odd meal that is lower in carbohydrates is certainly not going to do us any harm, especially when I have perfectly balanced the fibre for you.

Halve the recipes if you need to, batch-cook or jump in feet first with the Make-One-Take-One concept, marked at the top of the recipes, such as in the Chicken and Yellow Pea Curry with Cauliflower 'Pilau' Rice (page 215) or the Cauliflower and Broccoli Cheese (page 227). I encourage you to plan and prep ahead so you can enjoy knowing there is always something healthy in the fridge or freezer for those days when you are short of time.

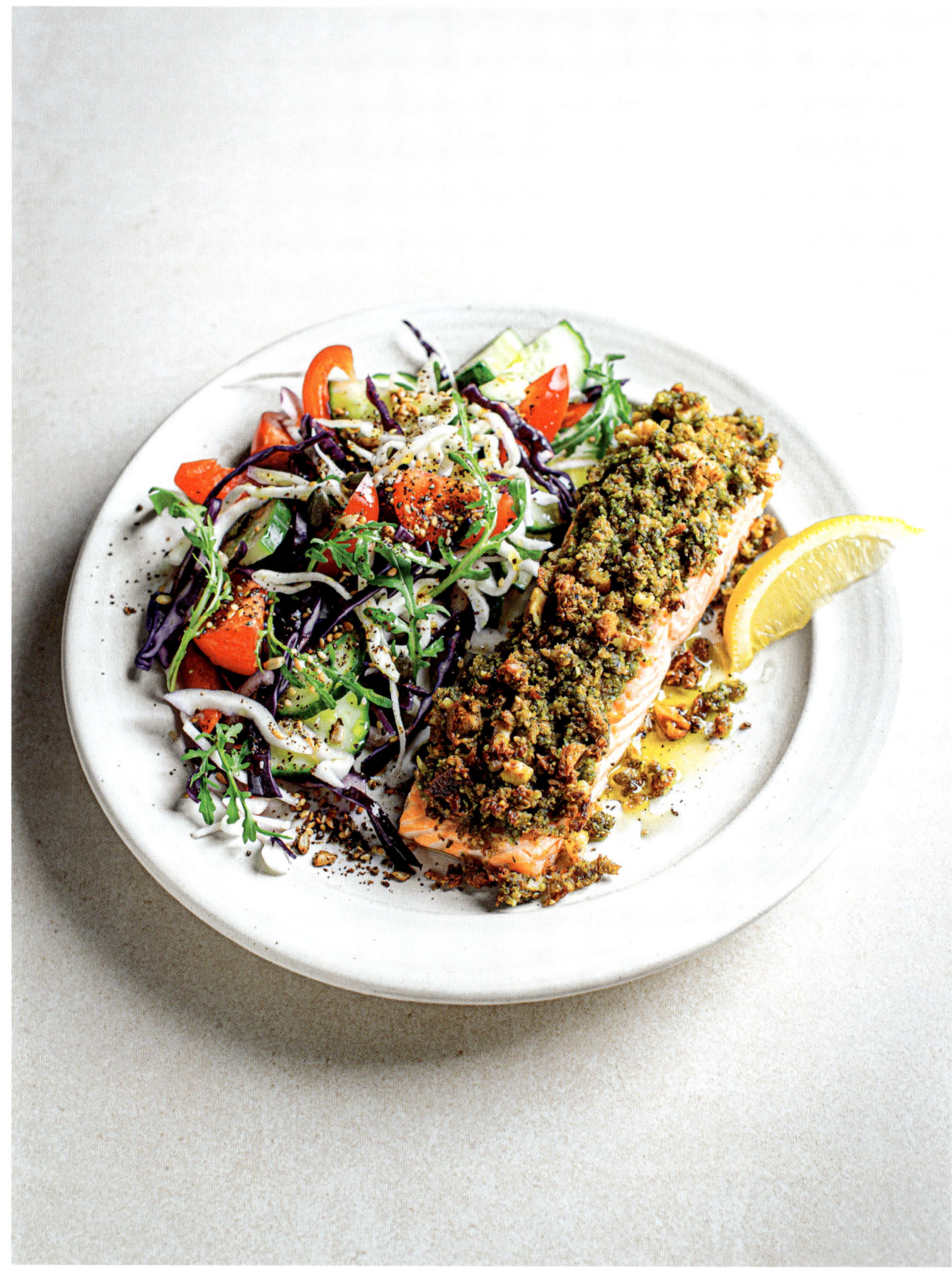

PER SERVING
PROTEIN: 37G
FIBRE: 10G
PLANT POINTS: 15

SERVES 4

160g wholegrain sourdough or rye bread
50g walnut halves, crushed
100g walnut and basil pesto (see below)
2 tablespoons lemon juice
4 x 100g salmon fillets, preferably wild

Green walnut and basil pesto (makes 1 large jar)
80g Parmesan, grated (see Tip)
80g basil leaves
50g walnut halves
2 garlic cloves, peeled
150ml extra virgin olive oil
½ teaspoon sea salt

For garnish
10g mixed Savoury Seed Mix per serving (see page 136) or mixed seeds

To serve
a large mixed salad (200–250g per serving) to create half a plate of vegetables: for example, red and white cabbage, rocket, tomatoes, yellow pepper, cucumber, red onion, with a simple oil and vinegar dressing and sprinkle of the Savoury Seed Mix (page 136) for extra crunch and fibre
lemon wedges

Tip: To make the pesto suitable for vegetarians, use a vegetarian hard cheese instead of Parmesan.

PESTO AND WALNUT CRUST SALMON

This can be a speedy mid-week meal or makes an impressive showstopper for entertaining, simply by doubling up the crust ingredients and swapping the salmon fillets for half a side of salmon (increase the cooking time to 25–35 minutes, depending on the thickness). It tastes delicious cold as a Make-One-Take-One idea. It can also be cooked in an air fryer. I think of my air fryer as a mini convection oven for times when I don't want to heat the whole oven for smaller amounts of food. I use a silicone liner, to protect the food and also to keep the inside of my air fryer in pristine condition. I always like to have a jar of my green pesto in an airtight container in the fridge, as it is just so versatile, but you can use ready-made pesto if you are short on time. To keep your pesto vibrant green, add a layer of olive oil on top before storing.

1. If you are cooking your salmon in the oven, preheat the oven to 180°C fan. Line a baking tray or dish with baking parchment.

2. To make the pesto, put the grated Parmesan into a food processor with the basil, walnuts, garlic, extra virgin olive oil and sea salt. Blend until smooth and creamy. Transfer to a clean, dry glass jar.

3. Put the bread into the food processor and pulse until it forms fine breadcrumbs. Stir in the crushed walnuts, pesto and lemon juice.

4. Place the salmon fillets, skin side down, on the lined baking tray or ceramic dish. Divide the breadcrumb mixture between the fillets and press it down to form a thick crust.

5. Bake in the oven for 18–20 minutes, until the crust is golden and the salmon is just pale pink and cooked through in the centre – or cook for around 10–12 minutes in an air fryer at 175°C.

6. Serve with a large mixed salad on the side and a lemon wedge to squeeze over the top.

Make-One-Take-One: Store the salmon in an airtight container in the fridge for up to 2 days. The pesto will keep, covered in a layer of oil, in an airtight container in the fridge, for up to 2 weeks.

PER SERVING
PROTEIN: 36G
FIBRE: 8G
PLANT POINTS: 9.25

PRAWN FISHCAKES WITH SOBA NOODLE SALAD AND WASABI DIPPING SAUCE

I am a huge fan of fishcakes, but I don't like them to be weighed down with too much potato. This version, inspired by traditional Thai fishcakes, is potato-free and is made from a mix of white fish and prawns. They are delicious on their own but my wasabi dipping sauce adds a cool flavour to cut through the chilli. You can adapt this recipe to use any fish you like. It also works well with a mix of salmon and white fish. Adjust amount of fresh chilli to your taste.

SERVES 4

Prawn fishcakes
2 garlic cloves, crushed
3cm piece of fresh ginger, grated
300g white fish (e.g. cod or hake)
150g frozen raw tiger prawns, defrosted
2 tablespoons tamari or soy sauce (Note, soy sauce isn't gluten-free)
2 teaspoons fish sauce
a handful of fresh coriander, finely chopped
1 red chilli, finely chopped (or ¼ teaspoon chilli flakes)
4 spring onions, chopped
30g sesame seeds
2 tablespoons toasted sesame oil
lime wedges, to serve

Soba noodle salad
120g (100% buckwheat) soba noodles
4 carrots, julienned or grated
½ red cabbage, finely sliced
4 spring onions, chopped
200g mixed salad leaves
1 fresh red chilli, finely chopped

Dressing
juice of 1 lime
1 tablespoon tamari or soy sauce (Note, soy sauce isn't gluten-free)
2 tablespoons toasted sesame oil
1 teaspoon maple syrup (optional)

Wasabi dipping sauce
150g Greek yoghurt
1 garlic clove, crushed
1 teaspoon wasabi paste
1 tablespoon lime or lemon juice

1. Put the garlic and ginger into a food processor along with the remaining fishcake ingredients (apart from the sesame seeds and sesame oil) and pulse a few times until well combined but still slightly chunky. Roll the mixture into 8 balls and flatten each one slightly. Coat both sides with the sesame seeds.

2. Heat the sesame oil in a frying pan over a medium heat and fry the fishcakes for 2–3 minutes on each side, until golden and cooked through. Keep warm while you make the salad.

3. Cook the soba noodles according to the packet instructions, then drain and rinse under cold water to stop them sticking as they cool.

4. In a small bowl, whisk together the lime juice, tamari or soy sauce, sesame oil and maple syrup, if using, to make the dressing.

5. In a large bowl, combine the noodles, carrots, red cabbage, spring onions, mixed leaves and chopped chilli. Mix through the dressing and gently combine until well coated.

6. Mix the ingredients for the wasabi dipping sauce in a small bowl.

7. Serve the fishcakes with the noodles, the wasabi dipping sauce on the side, and a squeeze of lime.

Storage: Store the cooked fishcakes and wasabi yoghurt dip in separate airtight containers in the fridge for up to 2 days. Reheat the fishcakes gently in a frying pan or in an air fryer for 3–4 minutes at 160°C. Not suitable for freezing.

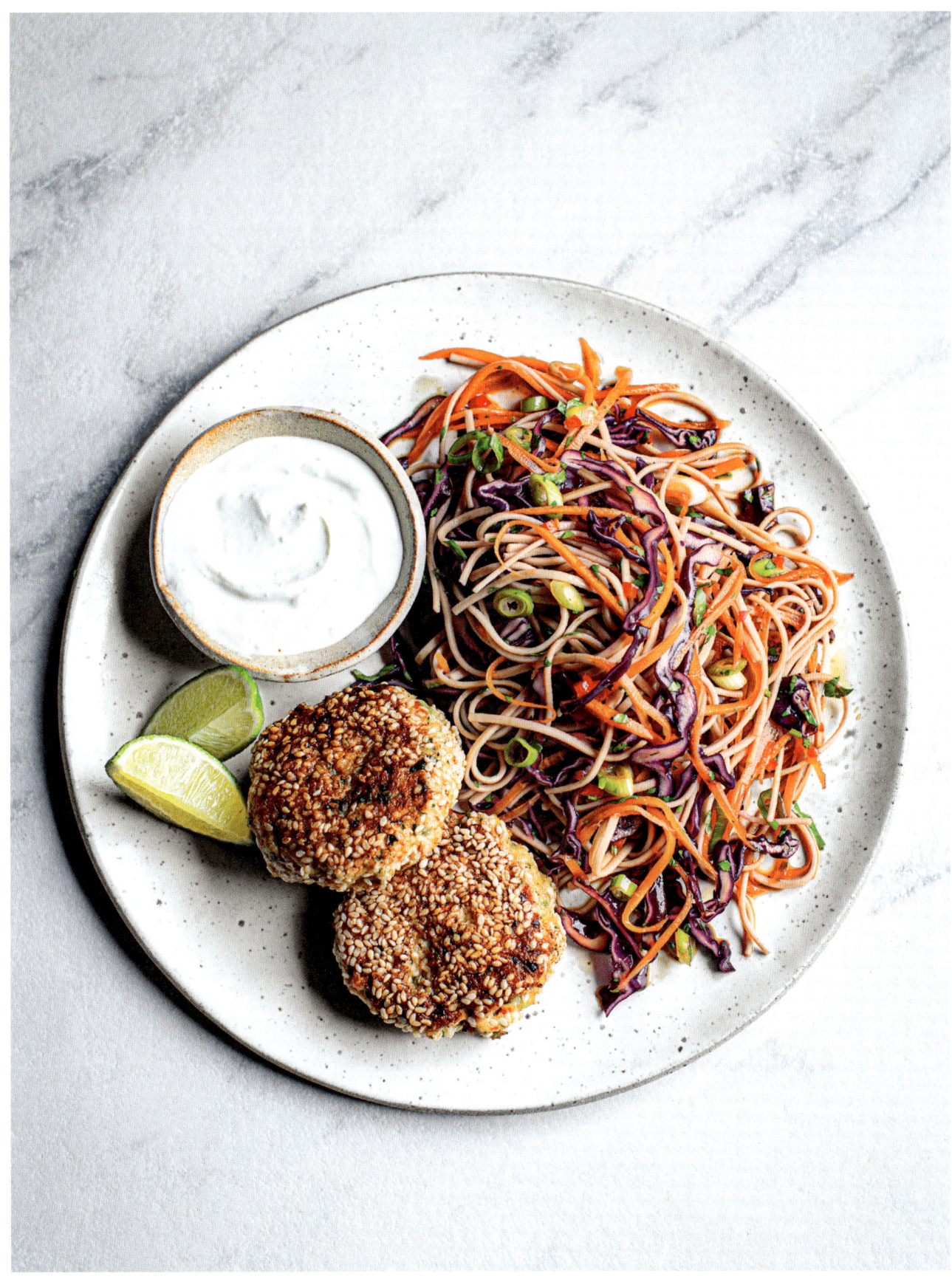

PER SERVING
PROTEIN: 39G
FIBRE: 9G
PLANT POINTS: 7.75

SERVES 4

200g red or black rice
3 chicken breasts (around 400g)
25g cornflour
1 tablespoon toasted sesame oil

Firecracker sauce
juice of 2 oranges
2 tablespoons sriracha sauce
a thumb-sized piece of fresh ginger, peeled and finely grated
4 garlic cloves, crushed
1 tablespoon tomato purée
1 tablespoon toasted sesame oil
2 teaspoons tamarind paste
1 tablespoon tamari or soy sauce (Note, soy sauce isn't gluten-free)
1 teaspoon lemon juice

Vegetables
3 red peppers, finely sliced
500g broccoli spears, roughly chopped
1 tablespoon toasted sesame oil
a dash of vegetable stock (or water)

To serve
20g mixed white and black sesame seeds
2 chopped spring onions

FIRECRACKER CHICKEN

I love firecracker chicken, but in restaurants this dish can be high in sugar and is often unbalanced, with too much rice and not enough protein, vegetables and fibre. So, in my true no-nonsense style, I have decided to give this recipe a healthy Triple 30 makeover by going back to basics. Rather than use sugar, I have used oranges to add a touch of sweetness. I have also reduced the rice serving to the perfect portion size and chosen red or black rice, which have a nutty texture, are slower acting on blood sugars, and contain extra plant pigments called anthocyanins. Feel free to use any rice you like though. I want to give you new ideas and options to jazz up your everyday cooking, but having adaptations can help the recipes fit into your everyday life too! The vegetable side dish is necessary to keep your fibre up, so make sure to include it.

---

1. Rinse the rice and place it in a saucepan with double the volume of water and a pinch of sea salt. Bring to the boil, then reduce to a simmer and cook gently according to the packet instructions, usually around 25–35 minutes, until tender.

2. While the rice cooks, cut the chicken into bite-size cubes and coat with the cornflour. In a small bowl, mix together all the sauce ingredients and set aside.

3. Heat 1 tablespoon of toasted sesame oil in a heavy-based frying pan over a medium heat. Add the chicken and cook for 3–4 minutes, until just golden. Pour over the sauce and cook for 6–7 minutes, stirring regularly, until the sauce thickens and the chicken is fully cooked through.

4. Meanwhile, in a wok or frying pan, stir-fry the red peppers and broccoli in 1 tablespoon of toasted sesame oil with a dash of vegetable stock (or water) over a medium heat for 4–5 minutes, until just tender, but still vibrant.

5. Serve the chicken with the rice and vegetables. Sprinkle over the sesame seeds and chopped spring onions to finish.

Storage: Leftover chicken can be stored in an airtight container in the fridge for up to 2 days. Reheat until piping hot.

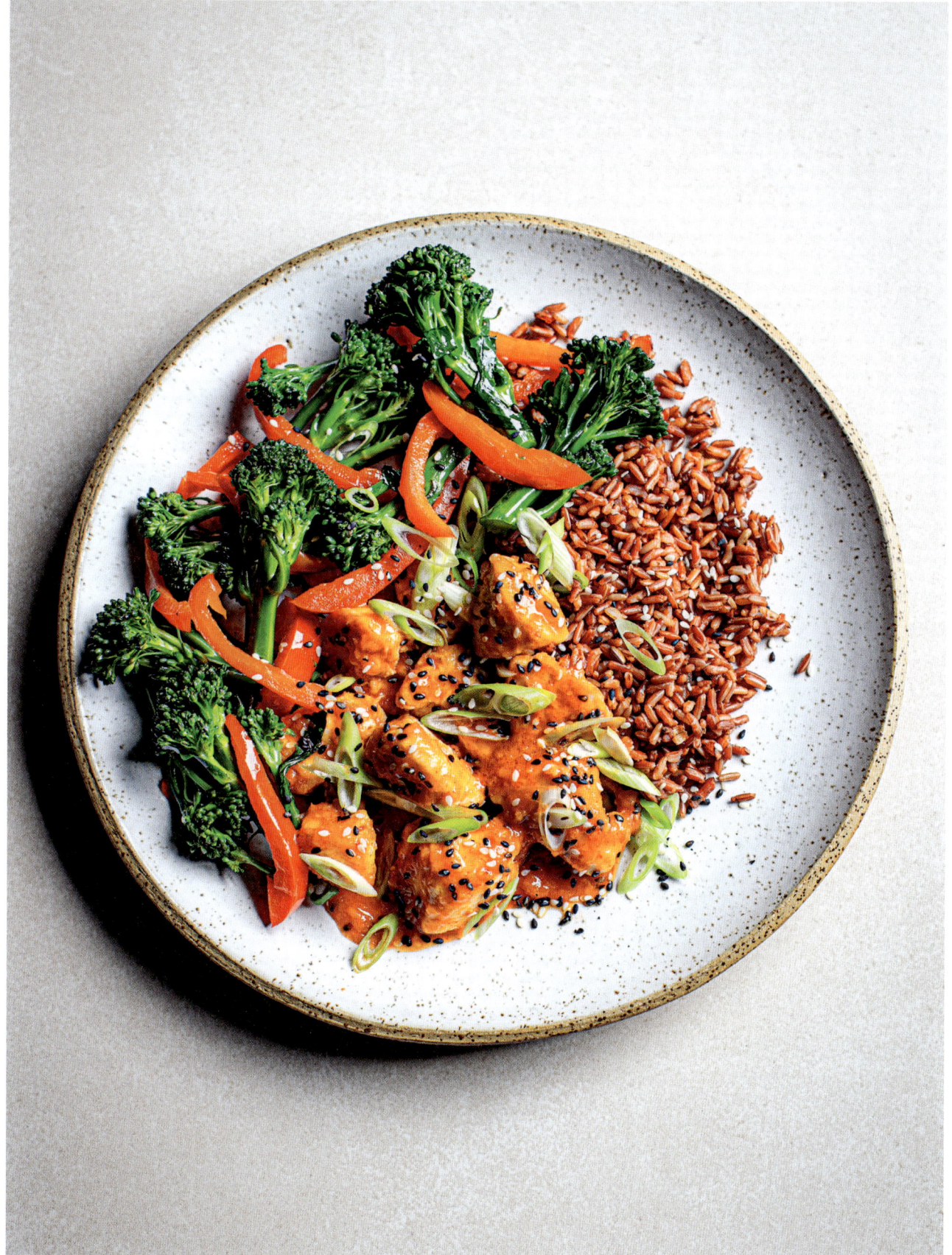

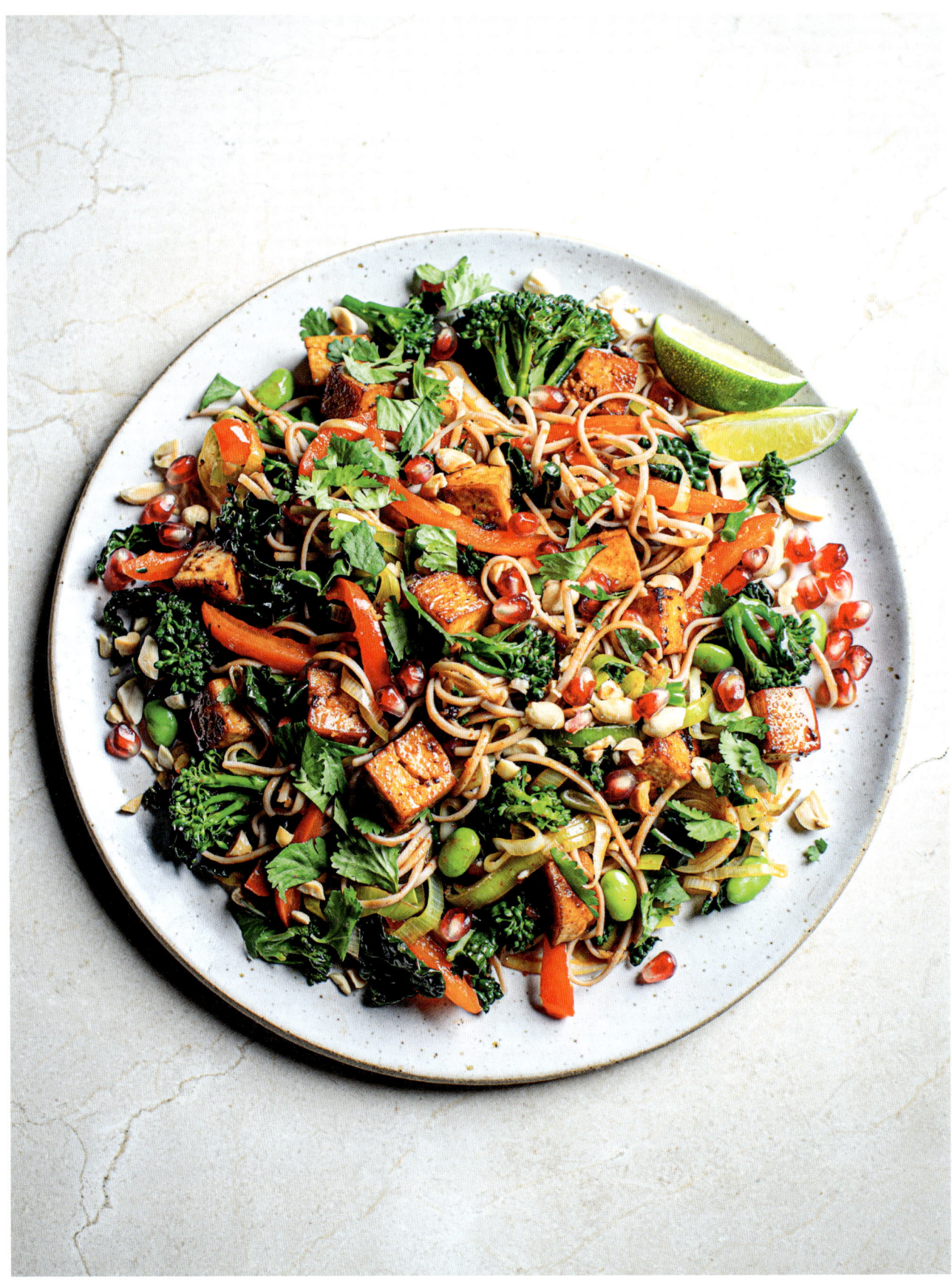

PER SERVING
PROTEIN: 31G
FIBRE: 13G
PLANT POINTS: 12

SERVES 4

280g firm, plain tofu
180g (100% buckwheat) soba noodles
100g frozen edamame beans, defrosted

Marinade
50ml tamari or soy sauce (Note, soy sauce isn't gluten-free)
5cm piece of fresh ginger, peeled and finely grated
2 teaspoons sriracha sauce
3 garlic cloves, crushed
1 tablespoon toasted sesame oil

Vegetables
1 tablespoon toasted sesame oil
2 small leeks, finely sliced
150g cavolo nero, de-stalked and chopped
200g Tenderstem broccoli, roughly chopped
2 red peppers, sliced

To serve
50g peanuts, crushed
1 large bunch of coriander, leaves chopped
50g pomegranate seeds
1 lime, cut into wedges

STICKY TOFU NOODLES

Tofu is the perfect food for taking on flavours, especially those used in Asian cooking, transforming it into the star of the show and a delicious mid-week meal. I like my tofu to be crispy around the edges and soft inside. As a bonus, tofu is rich in plant polyphenols called phytoestrogens, which can have a mild balancing effect on our own natural hormone rhythm. Soba noodles are naturally gluten-free and are made from buckwheat, which is closely related to the rhubarb plant, rather than being a true grain.

1. You can cook the tofu in the oven or in an air fryer, or you can pan-fry it in a little extra sesame oil. If you are using your oven, preheat it to 180°C fan; or heat your air fryer to 180°C. If you are cooking in the oven, line a baking sheet with baking parchment.

2. Mix the marinade ingredients together in a small bowl.

3. Drain the tofu and pat dry with kitchen paper. Chop into bite-size cubes and put in a shallow bowl or dish. Pour over half of the marinade and mix thoroughly.

4. Spread on the lined baking sheet and bake for 20–25 minutes, until golden and crisp outside and soft inside. Alternatively, cook in an air fryer at 180°C for 15 minutes. Or gently fry on the hob in extra sesame oil for 8 minutes until crispy on all sides, turning frequently. Keep warm while you finish cooking the rest of the dish.

5. Heat a large pan of water and when it comes to a simmer, add the noodles. Cook according to the packet instructions, adding the edamame beans to the water for the last 3 minutes of cooking. Drain the noodles and edamame in a sieve and run under cold water to prevent the noodles from sticking and to prevent overcooking.

6. Gently sauté the vegetables in the remaining sesame oil in a large frying pan or a wok over a medium heat until softened. Stir through the remaining marinade, the noodles and edamame beans.

7. To serve, top the dish with the crispy tofu, crushed peanuts, coriander, pomegranate seeds and lime wedges to squeeze over.

Storage: Store leftovers in an airtight container in the fridge for up to 2 days. Not suitable for freezing.

PER SERVING
PROTEIN: 27G
FIBRE: 12G
PLANT POINTS: 7.25

SERVES 6

2 large aubergines, diced (around 750g)
4 tablespoons extra virgin olive oil
a pinch of sea salt

Dhal

1 tablespoon extra virgin olive oil
1 large onion, finely chopped
4 garlic cloves, crushed
a thumb-sized piece of fresh ginger, peeled and finely grated
1 teaspoon mustard seeds
1 teaspoon ground turmeric
2 teaspoons garam masala
1 teaspoon ground cumin
½ teaspoon hot chilli powder
250g dried red lentils
1 x 400g tin of chopped tomatoes
2 tablespoons tomato purée
400–500ml vegetable stock
sea salt and freshly ground pepper
500g frozen peas

To serve

chopped fresh coriander
a pinch of chilli flakes
1 large spoonful of Greek yoghurt per serving
my Gluten-free Flatbreads or Simple Flatbreads (page 264 or 262)

LENTIL, PEA AND CRISPY AUBERGINE DHAL

Aubergine is such a delicious vegetable if cooked well, but many people avoid it because they worry about its texture. This recipe changes everything! Cooking it at a higher heat in the oven allows the aubergine to caramelise, creating golden, crispy cubes with a creamy centre. Serve the dhal with wholegrain, black or red rice, or my Simple Flatbreads (page 262) to mop up the sauce. This also works beautifully as a summer salad, paired with barbecued meats and served at room temperature.

1. Preheat the oven to 220°C fan and line a baking tray with baking parchment. Spread the diced aubergine on the lined baking tray and drizzle with the extra virgin olive oil. Sprinkle with salt and mix well. Roast for 25–30 minutes, until the skins are golden and crispy and the flesh is soft and creamy when gently pressed with a fork.

2. Meanwhile, heat 1 tablespoon of extra virgin olive oil in a large, heavy-based saucepan over a medium heat. Gently sauté the chopped onion for about 5 minutes, until translucent. Add the garlic, ginger and spices and cook 2 minutes. Stir in the red lentils, tinned tomatoes, tomato purée and 400ml of the vegetable stock. Season with salt and pepper. Cover and simmer for 20 minutes, or until the lentils are soft but still holding their shape. Add more stock if needed.

3. Add the frozen peas and simmer for 5 minutes, until the peas are bright green. (If preparing ahead, add the peas and remove the pan from the heat, then reheat gently when ready to serve.)

4. Spoon the dhal into bowls and pile the crispy aubergine on top. Garnish with plenty of chopped coriander, chilli flakes and a spoonful of Greek yoghurt. Serve with warm flatbreads, if you like.

Storage: Store the dhal and cooked aubergine in separate airtight containers in the fridge for up to 3 days. Reheat until piping hot. You can crisp up the aubergine again quickly in a dry frying pan, or for 3 minutes in an air fryer at 180°C. Suitable for freezing for up to 1 month, though the aubergine will melt into the curry.

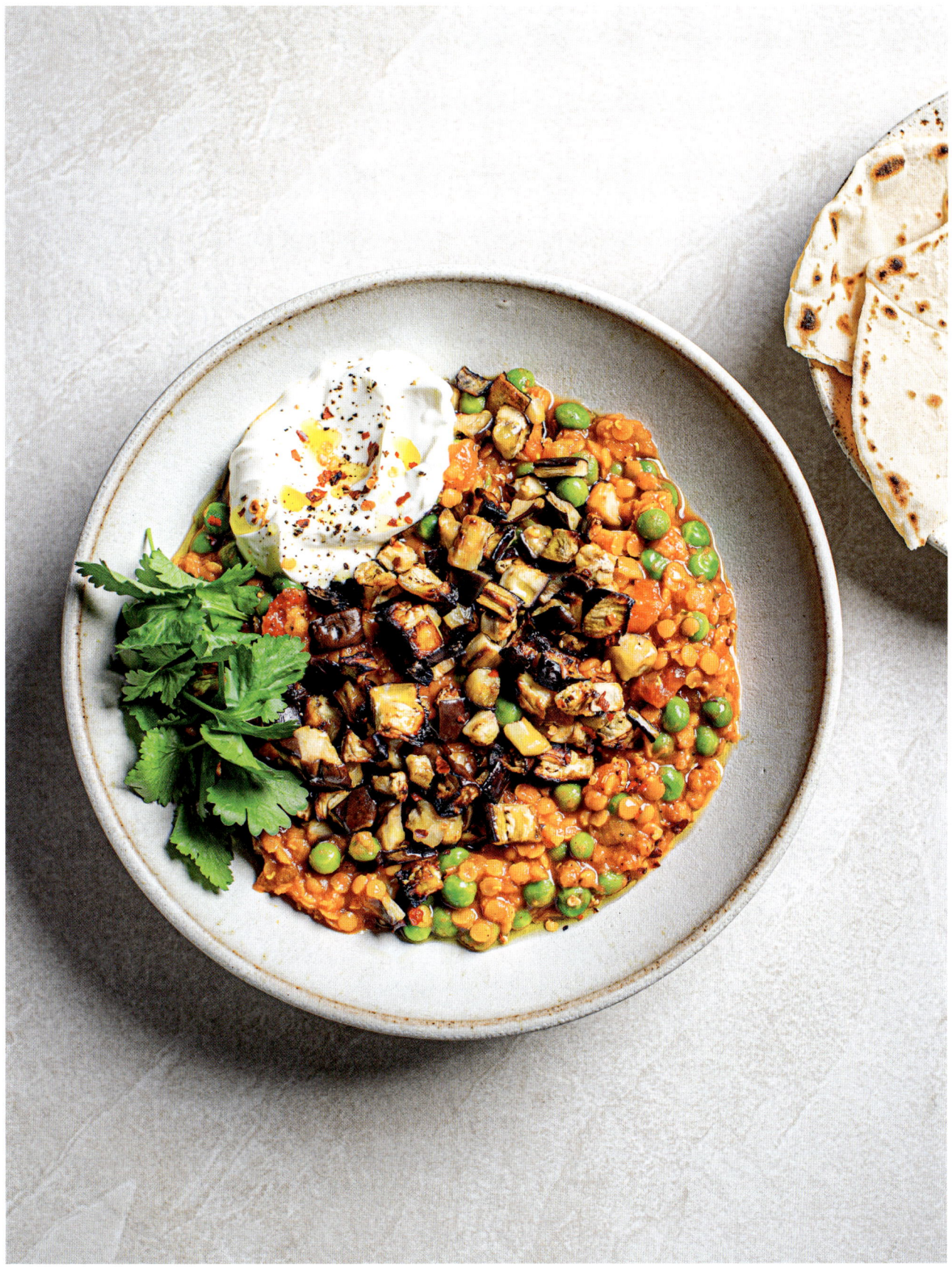

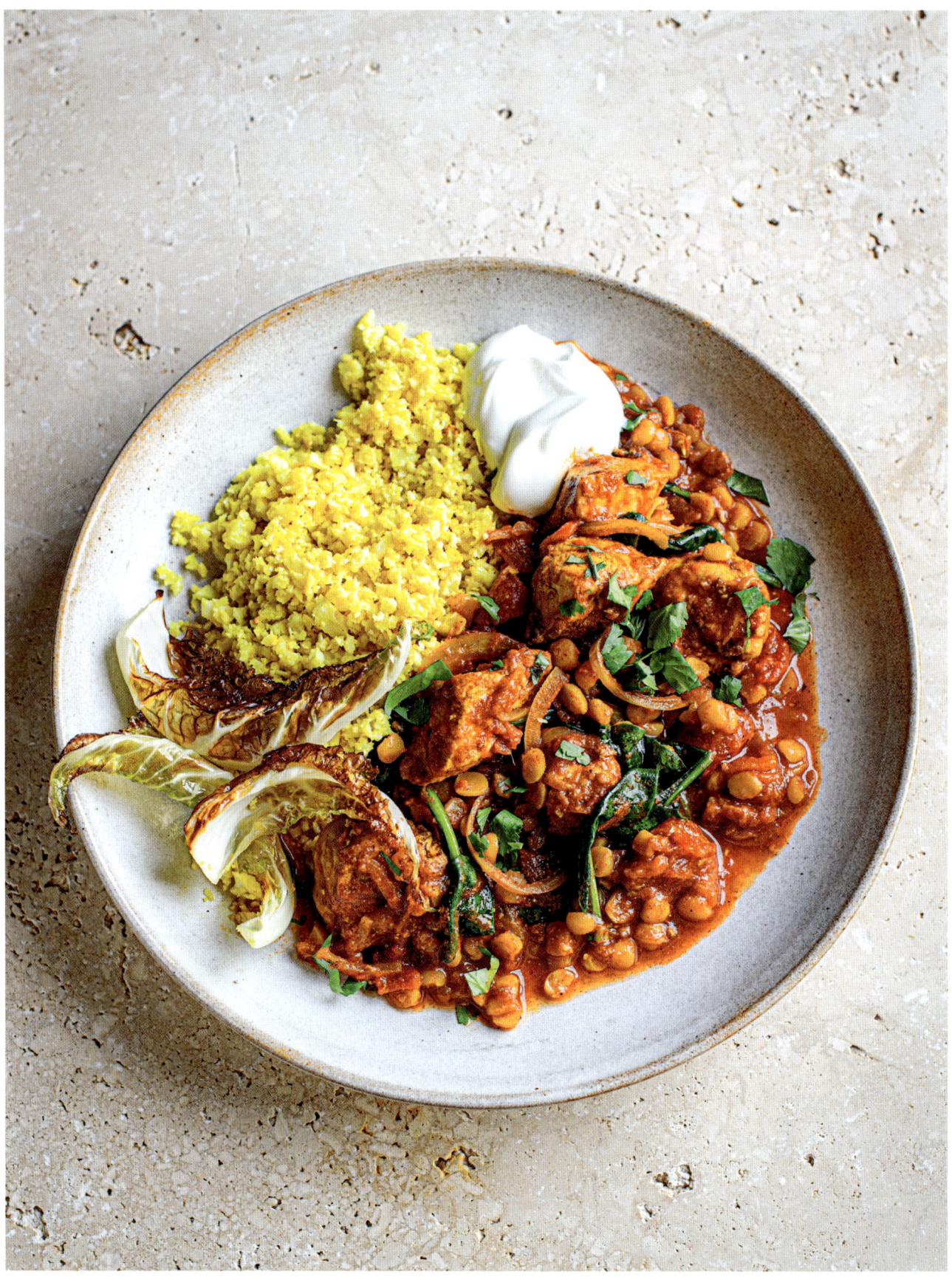

PER SERVING
PROTEIN: 31 G
FIBRE: 11 G
PLANT POINTS: 7.75

SERVES 6

Curry
3 chicken breasts (around 400g in total)
1 tablespoon extra virgin olive oil
1 red onion, thinly sliced
2 garlic cloves, crushed
2.5cm piece of fresh ginger, peeled and finely grated, or 1 teaspoon dried ginger
1 teaspoon ground turmeric
2 teaspoons ground cumin
1 teaspoon ground coriander
1 teaspoon hot chilli powder (adjust to taste)
2 teaspoons garam masala
1 tablespoon tomato purée
1 x 400g tin of chopped tomatoes
150g dried yellow split peas, rinsed
400–500ml chicken stock
120g baby spinach
sea salt and freshly ground black pepper, to taste
1 tablespoon lemon juice
100g Greek yoghurt
a handful of fresh coriander leaves, chopped

Cauliflower 'pilau' rice
1 head of cauliflower, cut into florets
½ teaspoon ground turmeric
1 tablespoon extra virgin olive oil
½ teaspoon sea salt
freshly ground black pepper

To serve
my Gluten-free Flatbreads or Simple Flatbreads (page 264 or 262) (optional)

CHICKEN AND YELLOW PEA CURRY WITH CAULIFLOWER 'PILAU' RICE

This recipe came about when I had lots of leftover chicken, which I wanted to turn into a curry. It's a great example of how adding legumes can dramatically increase the fibre content of a dish. It is filling, meets my Triple 30 principles, but is also quite low in calories (which we don't talk about much in this book!). I use fresh chicken here, but you can also use leftover cooked chicken or turkey (see Tip). Yellow split peas keep their shape while cooking, giving the curry a chunkier texture, and by adding legumes to your meals you can often cut back on the amount of meat you are using, as the ingredients go further. I have served this with cauliflower 'pilau' rice to keep the dish light, but it also works well with regular rice or my Simple Flatbreads (page 262). As this recipe serves 6, there should be some leftovers for a quick lunch the next day.

---

1. Cut the chicken into bite-size pieces. Heat the extra virgin olive oil in a large saucepan over a medium heat. Add the red onion and cook for around 5 minutes, until soft and golden. Stir in the garlic and ginger and cook for another 1–2 minutes.

2. Add the ginger, turmeric, cumin, coriander, chilli powder and garam masala. Stir and cook for 1–2 minutes to release the flavours. Add the chicken and mix well to coat in the spicy onion mixture. Cook for 5–6 minutes, until lightly browned.

3. Add the tomato purée to the pan and stir to combine. Pour in the tinned tomatoes and add the yellow split peas. Add 400ml of the chicken stock, reserving the rest to adjust the consistency later. Bring the mixture to a simmer, then cook gently with a lid on for 35–45 minutes, or until the chicken is fully cooked, the split peas are tender, and the curry has thickened to your desired consistency. Stir occasionally and add more stock if required.

4. Take the curry off the heat, then stir in the baby spinach and allow it to wilt. Season with salt and pepper.

Recipe continues overleaf

CHICKEN AND YELLOW PEA CURRY WITH CAULIFLOWER 'PILAU' RICE CONTINUED

Tip: If using leftover chicken or turkey, add the leftover meat after 20 minutes' cooking to allow time for it to absorb the sauce and the curry flavours.

5. While the curry simmers, prepare the cauliflower rice. Preheat the oven to 180°C fan and grease a large baking tray with oil. Put the cauliflower florets, turmeric, extra virgin olive oil, salt and pepper into a food processor and pulse a few times until it starts to resemble rice in texture. Alternatively, grate the cauliflower by hand.

6. Spread evenly over the oiled tray (along with some of the cauliflower leaves if you have them) and bake for 10–15 minutes, stirring once, until the cauliflower is just tender. Oven-baking the cauliflower helps prevent it from becoming soggy and produces individual grains that more closely resemble the texture of traditional rice. The turmeric gives it a lovely golden colour and a 'pilau' feel.

7. Finish the curry with lemon juice and serve with the warm cauliflower 'pilau' rice, Greek yoghurt and chopped fresh coriander. For a more substantial option, also pair with homemade flatbreads (page 262).

Make-One-Take-One: Leftover curry can be stored in an airtight container in the fridge for up to 3 days – but only if you have used fresh chicken; leftover chicken should only be reheated once. Reheat gently in a pan until piping hot. Cauliflower rice is best eaten fresh, but can be stored in the fridge for up to 2 days and reheated in a pan.

PER SERVING
PROTEIN: 40G
FIBRE: 10G
PLANT POINTS: 10

SERVES 4

2 medium leeks, finely chopped
400g closed-cup mushrooms, sliced
2 tablespoons extra virgin olive oil
4 chicken breasts (around 400g in total)
25g gluten-free (or regular) plain flour
2–3 tablespoons Dijon mustard (see Tip)
1–2 tablespoons English mustard (see Tip)
1 bunch of fresh tarragon, finely chopped
500ml hot chicken stock
sea salt and freshly ground black pepper
150ml crème fraîche

To serve
150g Grain and Lentil Healthy Carb Mix (page 159) (dry weight) (or 150g quinoa, dry weight)
300g extra vegetables (I like to use a mix of carrots and green beans)
a little extra chopped tarragon

Tip: Most English mustards contain gluten, but some brands are gluten-free, so check the ingredients if you are sensitive to gluten or wheat. Dijon mustards are mostly gluten-free, but check the label.

DIJON CHICKEN WITH TARRAGON

This dish is a firm family favourite. It's great for doubling up portions for batch cooking or for entertaining. It also makes great leftovers to take to work in a food flask. I like to pack in plenty of mushrooms and leeks, which makes the chicken go further and tops up our plant points at the same time. Be bold with the mustard, as it is the making of this dish – adjust the amounts to suit your taste.

---

1. Preheat the oven to 180°C fan. Sauté the leeks and mushrooms in 1 tablespoon of the extra virgin olive oil in a heavy-based frying pan over a medium heat for around 5 minutes, until softened. Transfer to a casserole dish.

2. Coat the chicken breasts in the flour, then add to the same heavy-based frying pan with the remaining tablespoon of extra virgin olive oil. Cook for 2–3 minutes on each side, until lightly coloured. Transfer to the casserole dish with the leeks and mushrooms.

3. Add the Dijon mustard, English mustard, chopped tarragon, hot stock, and a pinch each of salt and pepper. Put a lid on the casserole dish, or cover tightly with foil, and cook in the oven for 30–40 minutes. Keep checking the chicken to see if it is cooked, as chicken breasts can dry out quickly. Remove from the oven and let the casserole rest with the lid on for at least 15 minutes.

4. Meanwhile, cook the Grain and Lentil Mix (or quinoa) in a saucepan with plenty of salted water for around 20–25 minutes.

5. In a separate pan, cook the vegetables in a little salted water for 5 minutes, until al dente. I use as little water as possible and put a lid so the vegetables above the water lightly steam-cook.

6. Shred the chicken using two forks, then stir through the crème fraîche. Serve with the grains or quinoa and the vegetables, and garnish with a little extra tarragon.

Make-One-Take-One: Store the cooled casserole in an airtight container in the fridge for up to 2 days. Reheat gently on the hob until piping hot. Freeze before adding the crème fraîche for up to 2 months; defrost fully before reheating until piping hot.

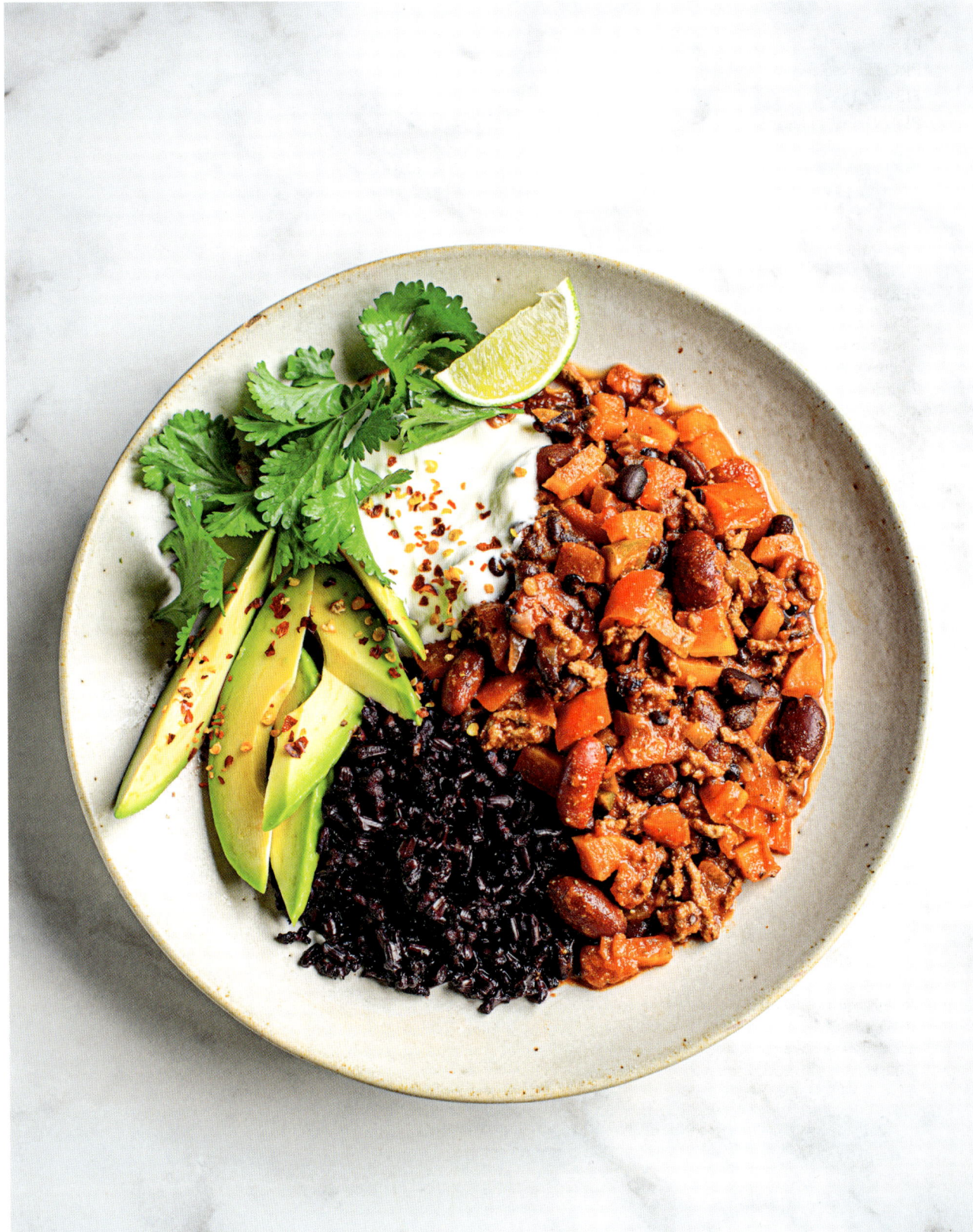

PER SERVING
PROTEIN: 25G
FIBRE: 15G
PLANT POINTS: 11.75

SERVES 10
500g beef mince
2 tablespoons extra virgin olive oil
2 large onions, chopped
4 garlic cloves, crushed
4 carrots, scrubbed and diced
4 green and red peppers, diced
2 teaspoons ground cumin
2 teaspoons ground coriander
1 teaspoon hot chilli powder (adjust to taste)
2 x 400g tins of chopped tomatoes
3 tablespoons tomato purée
250g Puy or black beluga lentils (or a mix) (dry weight)
1 x 400g tin or jar of kidney beans, rinsed and drained (240g drained weight)
1 x 400g tin or jar of black beans, rinsed and drained (240g drained weight)
500ml beef stock
40g dark chocolate (85%) or unsweetened cacao
sea salt and freshly ground black pepper

To serve (per serving)
choose your favourite sides:
30g black rice (dry weight)
cauliflower rice (page 215–216)
100g peas
a few slices of avocado
1 tablespoon soured cream
a few chilli flakes, to serve

BEEF CHILLI WITH LENTILS AND CHOCOLATE

This is no ordinary chilli. It's a flavour-packed twist on the classic that is more nourishing and more sustainable. I recommend using higher-welfare beef and combining it with extra plant proteins in the form of beans and lentils, which makes it go further. Because black and Puy lentils hold their shape well when cooked, they blend seamlessly into the meat, being virtually undetectable (so much so that my husband didn't notice them at all the first time I made this). They add extra fibre and plant diversity without compromising the texture or flavour. You'll also get more portions from the same amount of meat, which means you can keep some back for leftovers and/or freeze a few portions too. I like to use both black beans and kidney beans as well as black and Puy lentils, to boost plant points.

The last twist is the addition of dark chocolate or cacao to the chilli. This combination has deep historical roots dating back long before chilli con carne became a staple in modern kitchens. Just a small amount of cacao brings a sense of balance and complexity, against the acidity of the tomatoes and the spices. To make this recipe completely vegan, leave out the meat and use an extra 100g of lentils, replacing the beef stock with vegetable stock, and adding a little extra stock.

---

1. Heat a large heavy-based frying pan over a medium heat. Dry-fry the beef mince for 4–5 minutes, until browned and the fat begins to render, breaking up the mince with a wooden spoon. If using lean mince, add a little oil to prevent sticking. Once browned, transfer to a plate and set aside.

2. In the same pan, heat the extra virgin olive oil. Sauté the onions for about 5 minutes until softened. Add the garlic, carrots and peppers, and cook for 2 minutes. Stir in the cumin, coriander and chilli powder and cook for another minute to release the flavours.

3. Return the beef to the pan along with the tinned tomatoes, tomato purée, lentils, kidney beans, black beans and beef stock. Stir well and bring to a gentle simmer.

Recipe continues overleaf

BEEF CHILLI WITH LENTILS AND CHOCOLATE CONTINUED

4. Cover and cook over a low heat for 45 minutes to 1 hour, stirring occasionally to prevent it sticking to the pan. You may need to add a little more stock or hot water during the cooking time, depending on how much water the lentils are absorbing and how much steam has been lost from the pan. I like to keep the lid ON for the first 25 minutes to allow the ingredients to retain the heat, but you may like to have the lid on tilt for the second half of cooking to allow some of the steam to escape and to ensure the chilli has a richer, thicker consistency.

5. When cooked through, add the dark chocolate and mix through until melted. Season with salt and pepper, to taste.

6. While the chilli is cooking, get your sides ready. If serving with rice, cook your desired quantity in a pan of simmering salted water. Black rice takes around 35–40 minutes, with the lid on, until tender. Otherwise prepare your cauliflower 'pilau' rice (page 215). Serve with your choice of sides, and a few extra chilli flakes over the top, if you like it hot. The nutritional information shows the chilli with black rice, avocado and soured cream.

Make-One-Take-One: Cool the chilli and store in an airtight container in the fridge for lunch or dinner the next day. Freeze leftovers in individual portions for easy, nourishing meals when time is tight. Defrost fully before reheating until piping hot.

PER SERVING
PROTEIN: 26G
FIBRE: 20G
PLANT POINTS: 17.75

SERVES 6
1 tablespoon extra virgin olive oil
2 red onions, finely chopped
2 garlic cloves, crushed
3 medium carrots, diced
2 sticks of celery, diced
250g dried lentils (black, green, or a mix of both)
1 bay leaf
4 sprigs of fresh thyme
1 x 400g tin of chopped tomatoes
2 tablespoons tomato purée
2 tablespoons balsamic vinegar (see Tip)
400–500ml vegetable stock
sea salt and freshly ground black pepper

Cheesy parsnip mash
250g sweet potatoes, peeled and diced
250g parsnips, peeled and diced
1 x 400g tin or jar of white beans (e.g. cannellini or butter beans), rinsed and drained (240g drained weight)
150g mature Cheddar, grated
a splash of milk, if needed, to loosen

To serve
sautéed spring greens, Savoy cabbage, green beans or broccoli
1 tablespoon Savoury Seed Mix (page 136)

Tip: Instead of balsamic vinegar, you can use Worcestershire sauce for extra flavour, although it will no longer be vegetarian. If you are gluten-free choose a gluten-free version.

SHEPHERDESS PIE WITH CHEESY BEAN AND PARSNIP MASH

Shepherd's pie is the ultimate comfort food, but I wanted to make a vegetarian version that doesn't compromise on the flavour. I have packed in plenty of vegetables, but to ensure the dish still delivers on protein – which can be trickier when cooking with beans or lentils – I created a deliciously cheesy mash with white beans in place of potato, and sprinkled my Savoury Seed Mix (page 136) over the top for extra crunch. While lentils contain plenty of fibre, they are not particularly high in protein and generally need propping up with another protein-rich food at the same meal. Adding foods into a recipe can help even out the proportions of nutrients and make your meal perfectly balanced. This is now a high-fibre meal due to all the beans and lentils, so if you are still getting used to more fibre in your diet, replace the beans in the mash with 500g cooked potatoes, or just enjoy a smaller portion.

---

1. Heat the extra virgin olive oil in a large heavy-based frying pan or hob-proof casserole dish over a medium heat. Sauté the onions for around 5 minutes until soft and translucent, then add the garlic and cook for a further 2 minutes.

2. Add the diced carrots and celery and continue cooking for another 3–4 minutes, stirring regularly. Stir in the lentils, bay leaf, thyme, chopped tomatoes, tomato purée and balsamic vinegar.

3. Add the stock and season with salt and pepper, then stir to combine. Bring to a gentle boil, cover and simmer for 20 minutes, stirring occasionally. The lentils should still be al dente, as they will finish cooking in the oven. The mixture should be thick and stiff to prevent the filling from bubbling up through the mash during baking. If it is looking too dry, adjust the consistency with more water.

Recipe continues overleaf

SHEPHERDESS PIE WITH CHEESY BEAN AND PARSNIP MASH *CONTINUED*

4. Meanwhile, preheat the oven to 180°C fan and bring a large pan of salted water to the boil. Add the sweet potatoes and parsnips and cook for about 10 minutes, until just tender. Drain well and allow the steam to evaporate. Mash together with the white beans and 100g of the Cheddar to create a smooth, creamy mash. A food processor can be used for a finer texture. Add a splash of milk, if needed to loosen the mixture.

5. Either leave the filling in the casserole dish or transfer it to an ovenproof baking dish. Spread the mash evenly over the top and sprinkle with the remaining 50g of grated cheese.

6. Bake in the oven for 25–30 minutes, until the top is golden and crisp. Serve with sautéed Savoy cabbage, green beans or broccoli. Sprinkle with the seed mix just before serving, for added crunch.

Storage: Portion leftovers into airtight containers and store in the fridge for up to 2 days. Reheat in the oven for 20–25 minutes at 180°C fan until piping hot again. Freeze for up to 1 month; defrost fully before reheating.

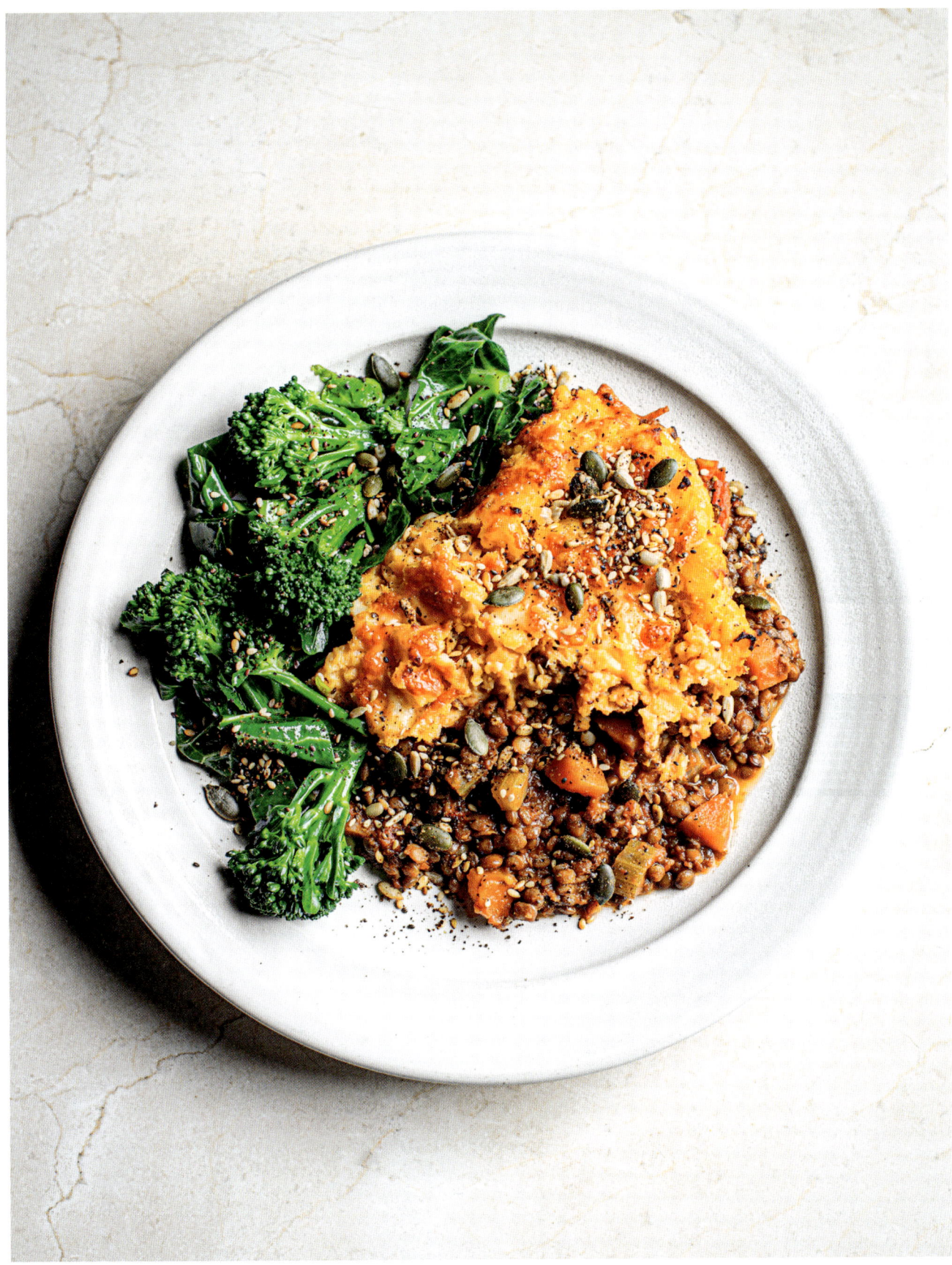

PER SERVING
PROTEIN: 29G
FIBRE: 17G
PLANT POINTS: 7

SERVES 2

1 tablespoon extra virgin olive oil
1 red onion, finely diced
2 garlic cloves, crushed
1 carrot, finely diced
1 courgette, finely diced
1 x 400g tin or jar of butter beans, with their water
1 x 400g tin of chopped or cherry tomatoes
1 tablespoon tomato purée
120g baby spinach
a handful of fresh parsley, chopped
juice of ½ lemon
sea salt and freshly ground black pepper

To serve
50g Parmesan (or vegetarian hard cheese), finely grated
100g Greek yoghurt

RUSTIC BUTTER BEAN 'GNOCCHI'

Swapping out traditional potato gnocchi for butter beans results in a meal that is equally comforting but with added nutritional benefits. Butter beans are a fantastic alternative to gnocchi and bring a wealth of health to your plate. Not only are they naturally gluten- and wheat-free, making them ideal for those with dietary restrictions, but they're also excellent for balancing blood sugar levels. Packed with soluble fibre and protein, butter beans contain more fibre than most other beans, to help keep you feeling full for longer, while promoting better digestion. This butter bean swap is one that you can use in your everyday cooking to replace not only gnocchi, but also sometimes pasta. Bolognese, for example, works perfectly with butter beans instead of spaghetti and is a quick and easy win.

1. Heat the extra virgin olive oil in a cast-iron cooking pot, deep-sided frying pan or heavy-based saucepan over a medium heat. Add the red onion and sauté for about 5 minutes, until soft. Stir in the garlic and carrot and cook for 2–3 minutes. Add the courgette and continue cooking for another 4–5 minutes, until all the vegetables are tender. (Add the courgette slightly later if you prefer it firmer.)

2. Tip in the butter beans with their water, followed by the tinned tomatoes and tomato purée. Stir to combine, then cover and simmer gently for 5–6 minutes over a low heat.

3. Stir in the spinach and allow it to wilt. Add the parsley and lemon juice and season with salt and pepper to taste.

4. Divide between serving bowls. Top with the Parmesan and swirl over the Greek yoghurt before serving.

Storage: Best eaten fresh but leftovers can be stored in an airtight container in the fridge for up to 2 days. Reheat in a pan on the hob until piping hot. Suitable for freezing without yoghurt or cheese.

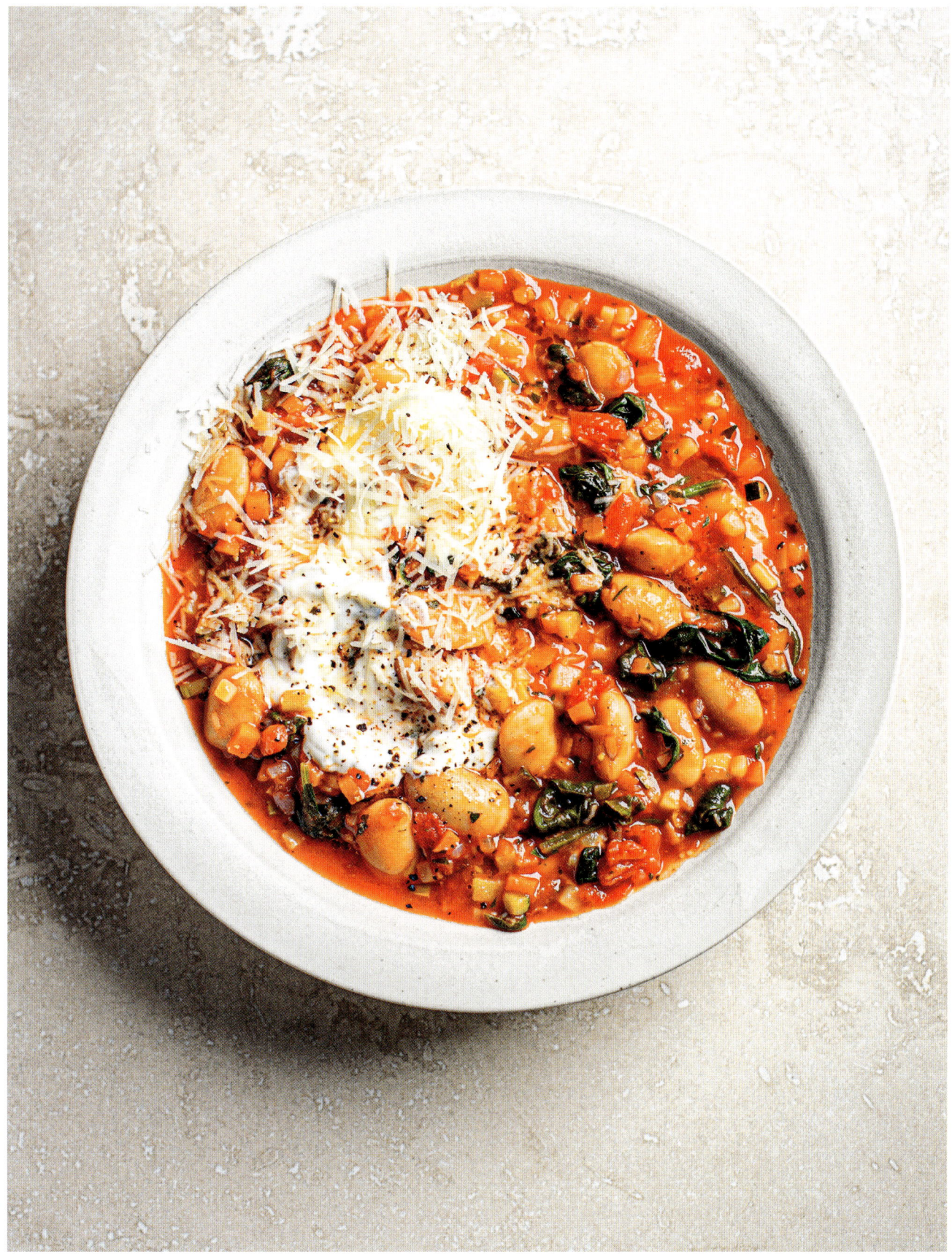

PER SERVING
PROTEIN: 37G
FIBRE: 8G
PLANT POINTS: 5

PRAWN AND TOMATO PASTA

You won't find a much easier or more delicious mid-week prawn pasta dish than this! Packed with protein from the prawns and fibre from the carrots and broccoli, it offers a balanced meal that's satisfying, but straightforward to prepare. Julienned, spiralised or thickly grated carrot also reduces the need for extra pasta, and, as a bonus, squeezes in another plant point.

SERVES 2

1 tablespoon extra virgin olive oil
½ red onion, finely chopped
3 garlic cloves, crushed
1 x 400g tin of cherry tomatoes, or 400g cherry tomatoes, roughly chopped
1 tablespoon tomato purée
1 teaspoon sweet paprika
a pinch of chilli flakes
100g broccoli, cut into small bite-size pieces
100g dried pasta (e.g. spaghetti), or red lentil pasta
150g carrots, julienned, spiralised or coarsely grated
200g frozen large raw prawns, defrosted
sea salt and freshly ground black pepper

To serve
40g Parmesan, finely grated
a handful of rocket

1. Heat the extra virgin olive oil in a heavy-based frying pan over a medium heat and sauté the onion gently for around 5 minutes. Add the crushed garlic and cook for 2 minutes. Stir through the cherry tomatoes, tomato purée, paprika and chilli flakes. Add the broccoli and simmer over a low-medium heat for around 10 minutes, until the vegetables are tender and the sauce has thickened.

2. Meanwhile, cook the pasta in boiling salted water according to the packet instructions (usually 8–10 minutes). Drain when al dente, reserving a little pasta water, just in case you need it at the end to loosen the sauce.

3. Add the carrots and prawns to the pasta sauce and cook for 3–4 minutes, until the carrots are just tender and the prawns are cooked through.

4. Stir the drained pasta through the sauce and combine well, loosening the sauce with a little of the reserved pasta water if needed. Season with salt and pepper, to taste. Sprinkle with Parmesan and rocket to serve.

Storage: Best served fresh. Leftovers can be stored in an airtight container in the fridge for up to 2 days. Reheat gently in a pan with a splash of water until piping hot. Not suitable for freezing.

PER SERVING
PROTEIN: 39G
FIBRE: 11G
PLANT POINTS: 6.25

SERVES 4
200g dried red lentil or green pea pasta
1 large head of cauliflower (around 500g), cut into small bite-size pieces (including the stalks)
1 large head of broccoli (around 500g), cut into small bite-size pieces (including the stalks)

Cheese sauce
1 tablespoon extra virgin olive oil or butter
40g gluten-free (or regular) flour
550ml milk of choice (I used semi-skimmed cow's milk)
1 heaped teaspoon mustard (English, Dijon or both!) (see Tip)
1 tablespoon Worcestershire sauce (use a gluten-free version if you are gluten-free) (or balsamic vinegar if vegetarian)
150g mature Cheddar, grated
50g Parmesan (or vegetarian hard cheese), grated
sea salt and freshly ground black pepper

Topping
20g pumpkin seeds
20g sunflower seeds
10g white or black sesame seeds
chilli flakes, to taste (optional)

Tip: Most English mustards contain gluten, but some brands are gluten-free, so check the ingredients if you are sensitive to gluten or wheat. Dijon mustards are mostly gluten-free, but check the label.

CAULIFLOWER AND BROCCOLI CHEESE

Macaroni cheese was my absolute favourite after-school supper. My mum always made it with a crunchy breadcrumb and cheese topping, and it always arrived in a blue and white patterned Pyrex dish! So, forty years on, this is my twist on the classic macaroni cheese to give you a lighter, more balanced version that boosts the fibre and adds some extra plant diversity to your plate.

If you want to make it dairy-free, swap the cheese for nutritional yeast (to taste) and a tablespoon of tahini (for an earthy flavour). While red lentil or green pea pasta boost fibre (about double that of white pasta) and protein, you can use any pasta you like. It's perfect on its own, but a crisp green salad is always a welcome extra.

---

1. Preheat the oven to 180°C fan. Bring a large pan of salted water to the boil. Add the pasta and cook for 5–6 minutes, until just al dente. In the final 3 minutes of cooking, add the cauliflower and broccoli. The vegetables should be al dente, as they will continue to cook in the oven. Drain together in a colander and rinse briefly under cold water to stop the cooking process. Drain and leave to steam-dry.

2. To make the sauce, return the pan to the hob. Heat the extra virgin olive oil or butter over a medium heat, then stir in the flour to form a paste. Cook for 3 minutes, stirring continuously. Whisk in the milk gradually, to prevent lumps, continuing until the sauce is thick and smooth. Remove from the heat. Stir in the mustard, Worcestershire sauce (or balsamic vinegar), Cheddar and Parmesan. Season with salt and pepper. I like to keep the sauce a little thicker, as it usually becomes thinner when cooked in the oven with the vegetables.

3. Combine the pasta, vegetables and sauce in an ovenproof dish until everything is evenly coated. Sprinkle over the seeds and chilli flakes, if using. Bake for 30 minutes, until bubbling and golden.

Make-One-Take-One: Store leftovers in an airtight container in the fridge for up to 2 days. Reheat in the oven at 180°C fan until hot throughout. Not suitable for freezing.

PER SERVING
PROTEIN: 33G
FIBRE: 7G
PLANT POINTS: 5.25

CREAMY LEMON PASTA WITH SALMON BITES

I've added plenty of vegetables to this simple salmon pasta dish that is light in texture, yet still creamy and satisfying. Peas are one of my favourite ways to top up the protein and fibre. Feel free to use a bit more cream cheese if you like it extra creamy, otherwise the 60g works well as long as you are eating immediately. Cream cheese should be just one ingredient – milk – so read the packaging to check there are no unnecessary additives. You can use a garlic and herb cream cheese if you prefer. I opted for wholewheat pasta, but green pea or red lentil pasta will boost the fibre some more.

SERVES 4

350g salmon fillets, preferably wild
a handful of fresh parsley, chopped
sea salt and freshly ground black pepper
2 tablespoons extra virgin olive oil
200g good-quality wholewheat pasta
200g frozen peas
3 shallots or 1 onion, finely diced
2 garlic cloves, crushed
2 large courgettes, cut into batons
60g full-fat soft cream cheese
zest and juice of 1 lemon

To serve
watercress or rocket

1. Put the salmon, parsley and a little salt and pepper into a food processor and pulse until combined but still a little chunky. Shape the mixture into 12 bite-size patties and flatten them slightly.

2. Heat the extra virgin olive oil in a frying pan over a medium heat. Cook the salmon patties for 2–3 minutes on each side, until golden and cooked through. Remove from the pan and keep warm.

3. Meanwhile, cook the pasta in a pan of salted water according to the packet instructions. Add the frozen peas in the final 2 minutes of cooking. Drain the pasta and peas, reserving a little pasta water to loosen the sauce later, if needed.

4. In the same frying pan, gently sauté the shallots or onion over a medium heat for about 5 minutes, until softened. Add the garlic and cook for 2 minutes. Add the courgette batons and cook until just tender. Stir in the cream cheese until smooth. Add the drained pasta and peas to the pan, along with the lemon juice and zest. Stir well, adding a little of the reserved pasta water if the sauce needs loosening, or a little extra cream cheese. Season to taste.

5. Return the salmon bites to the pan and allow them to warm through. Serve with watercress or rocket.

Storage: Best served fresh. Leftovers can be stored in an airtight container in the fridge for up to 2 days. Reheat gently in a pan with a splash of water to prevent the sauce from drying out.

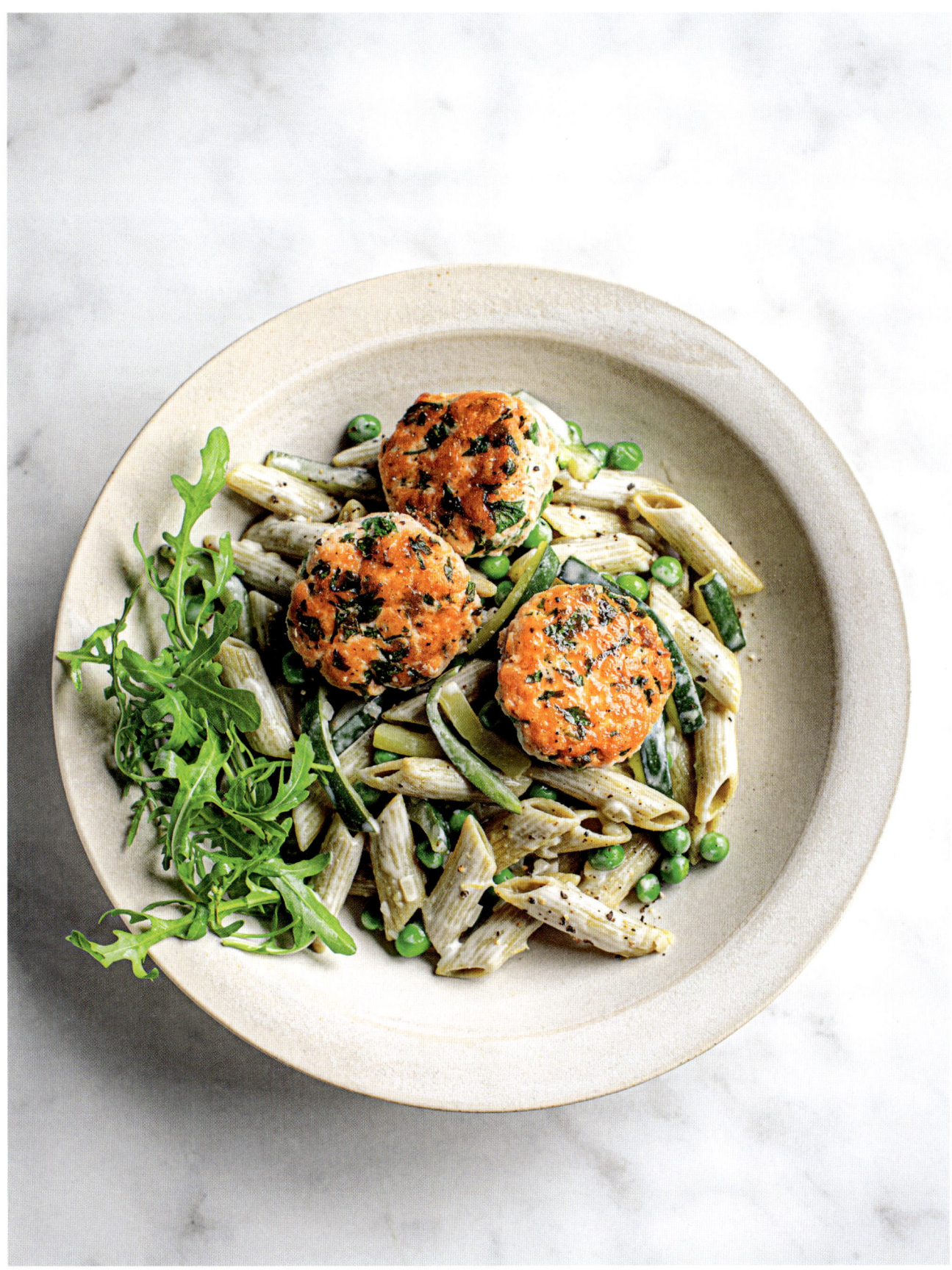

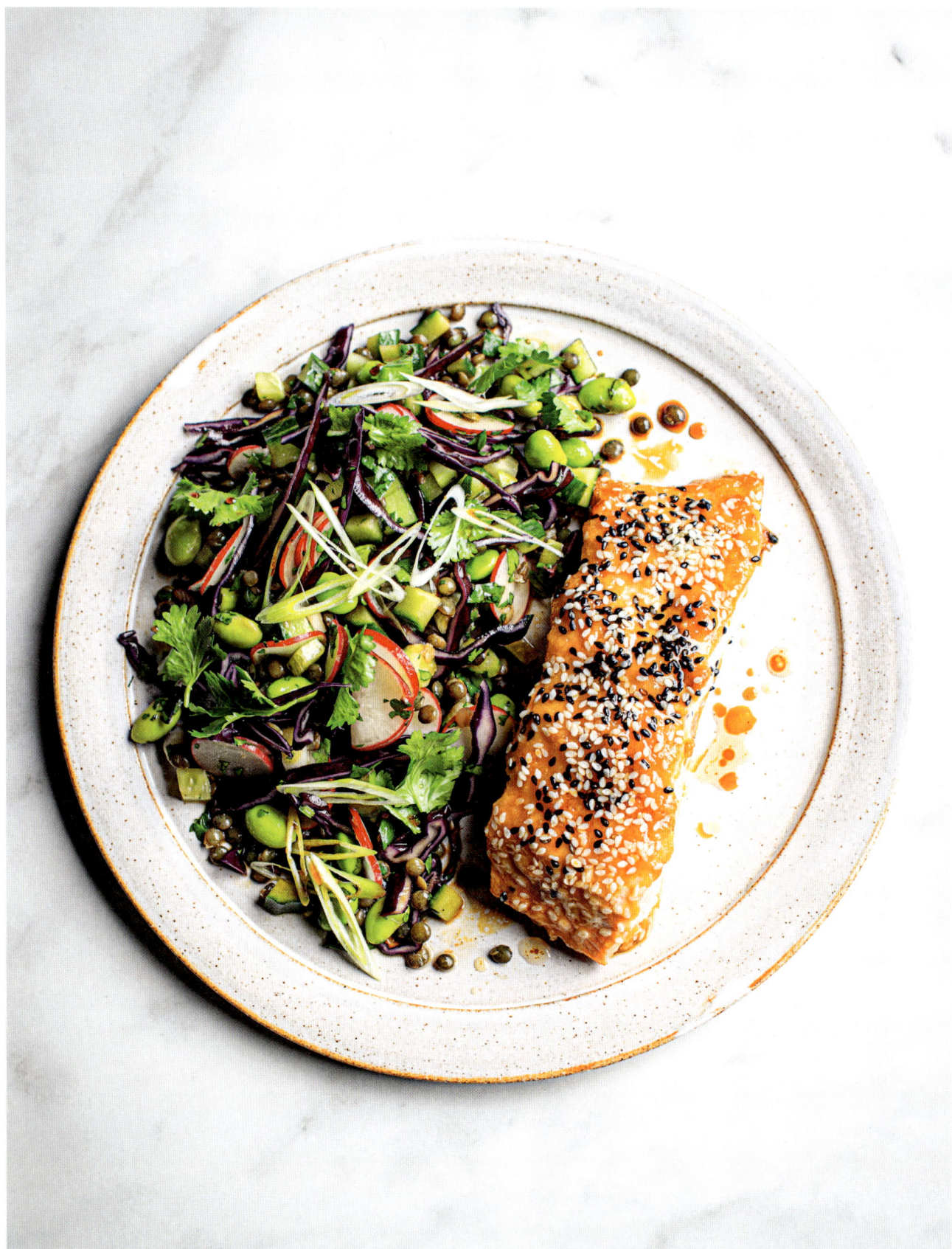

PER SERVING
PROTEIN: 38G
FIBRE: 9G
PLANT POINTS: 8.25

SERVES 4

4 trout or salmon fillets
4 teaspoons sesame seeds (white, black or a mix)

Glaze
20ml toasted sesame oil
4 garlic cloves, crushed
30g fresh ginger, peeled and finely grated
10ml lemon juice
2 teaspoons maple syrup or honey
2 teaspoons miso paste (light or dark)

Salad
150g edamame beans
100g dried black or green lentils (or 200g ready-cooked)
vegetable stock or water, for cooking the lentils
8 spring onions, finely sliced
400g cucumber, diced
150g radishes, sliced
200g red cabbage, finely shredded
a handful of fresh coriander, chopped

Salad dressing
2 tablespoons tamari or soy sauce (Note, soy sauce isn't gluten-free)
20ml toasted sesame oil
2 tablespoons filtered water

To serve (optional)
fresh coriander, chopped
spring onions, chopped

STICKY TROUT WITH SALAD

This is the perfect Make-One-Take-One meal. It's great for a simple supper and works well, chilled the next day, either packed up to take into the office or to enjoy at home as a stress-free lunch. The combination of the miso and maple syrup makes a slightly sticky glaze which works so well with the fish. It's probably my favourite trout recipe, but it works just as well with salmon. Serve it warm with vegetables or cold with this vibrant, crunchy salad. The glaze would also work with tofu if you wanted a plant-based version.

1. Preheat the oven to 180°C fan. Mix together all the glaze ingredients. Place the trout or salmon fillets, skin-side down, in a lightly greased ovenproof dish and pour over the glaze, ensuring all the fish is well coated. Keep the fillets slightly apart to allow even cooking. Sprinkle with the sesame seeds and bake for 18 minutes, until cooked through. (The fish can also be cooked in an air fryer at 180°C for 8–12 minutes.)

2. If using frozen edamame beans, boil for 3 minutes, then rinse under cold water to stop the cooking process and keep their colour.

3. If using dried lentils, simmer them in vegetable stock or water for 20–25 minutes with the lid on until tender. Drain, rinse under cold water, and allow to cool. If using ready-cooked lentils, warm them briefly in stock or water, then drain and allow to cool.

4. Mix the lentils with the edamame beans and the chopped salad vegetables. Combine the salad dressing ingredients in a small bowl, by mixing with a fork. Serve the freshly dressed salad with the warm, sticky trout. Drizzle over the dressing for eating immediately. Top with extra coriander and spring onions, if you like.

Make-One-Take-One: Leftover salad and trout can be stored in airtight containers in the fridge for up to 2 days. Keep any extra dressing in a separate pot and add just before serving.

PER SERVING
PROTEIN: 36G
FIBRE: 10G
PLANT POINTS: 13.5

TANDOORI CHICKEN SALAD WITH RAITA

Tandoori chicken is traditionally cooked in a clay tandoor oven, but while my version is cooked at a lower temperature in a regular oven it still delivers on taste. I swapped out the rice for my Grain and Lentil Healthy Carb Mix (page 159), so that once you make up a jar, you get to use it in a few of my recipes! Of course, you can swap this for wholegrain rice or my Simple Flatbreads (page 262) if you prefer, but the fibre content will be slightly lower. Fresh raita makes the perfect sauce to dip the spicy chicken into. You can make your own tandoori spice mix using the recipe below, or for ease use six teaspoons of a bought tandoori masala or tandoori spice mix.

SERVES 4
4 tablespoons plain yoghurt
1 tablespoon lemon juice
400g chicken breast fillets
1 tablespoon chopped fresh coriander

Tandoori spice mix
1 teaspoon ground cumin
1 tablespoon sweet paprika
½ teaspoon garlic powder
½ teaspoon ground ginger
1 teaspoon garam masala
½ teaspoon chilli powder
¼ teaspoon ground turmeric

Raita
200g Greek yoghurt
½ cucumber, grated
2 garlic cloves, crushed
12 fresh mint leaves
sea salt and freshly ground black pepper

Grain mix
200g Grain and Lentil Healthy Carb Mix (page 159)
1 teaspoon stock powder or bouillon or ½ teaspoon salt

Salad
150g mixed salad leaves
1 large red pepper, diced
1 yellow pepper, diced
200g cherry tomatoes, chopped
½ cucumber, diced

Simple dressing
4 tablespoons extra virgin olive oil
4 tablespoons apple cider vinegar
1 teaspoon Dijon mustard
sea salt and freshly ground black pepper

1. Preheat the oven to 180°C fan. In a bowl, mix the yoghurt, lemon juice and the tandoori spice mix (or 6 teaspoons of bought tandoori masala or tandoori spice mix). Add the chicken and coat well. Cover and leave to marinate in the fridge for up to 2 hours, to allow the chicken to take up the flavours and to tenderise the meat. If you are short of time, you can skip this stage, as it will still taste good.

2. Place the chicken in an oiled ovenproof dish. Cook in the oven for 18–20 minutes, until cooked through and the edges begin to colour and char slightly.

3. Meanwhile, mix the raita ingredients together. Season to taste.

4. Put the grain and lentil mix into a saucepan with the stock powder or salt, cover with water and bring to the boil. Simmer gently for around 25 minutes, until tender, then drain away any excess liquid.

5. Assemble the salad by tossing the mixed leaves, peppers, tomatoes and cucumber in a bowl. In a jar, combine the extra virgin olive oil, apple cider vinegar, Dijon mustard and seasoning. Shake well. Serve the grain and lentil mix with the chicken. Scatter with fresh coriander and serve with the raita alongside. Pour the dressing over the salad just before serving.

Storage: Leftover chicken, salad, dressing and raita can be stored in separate airtight containers in the fridge for up to 2 days.

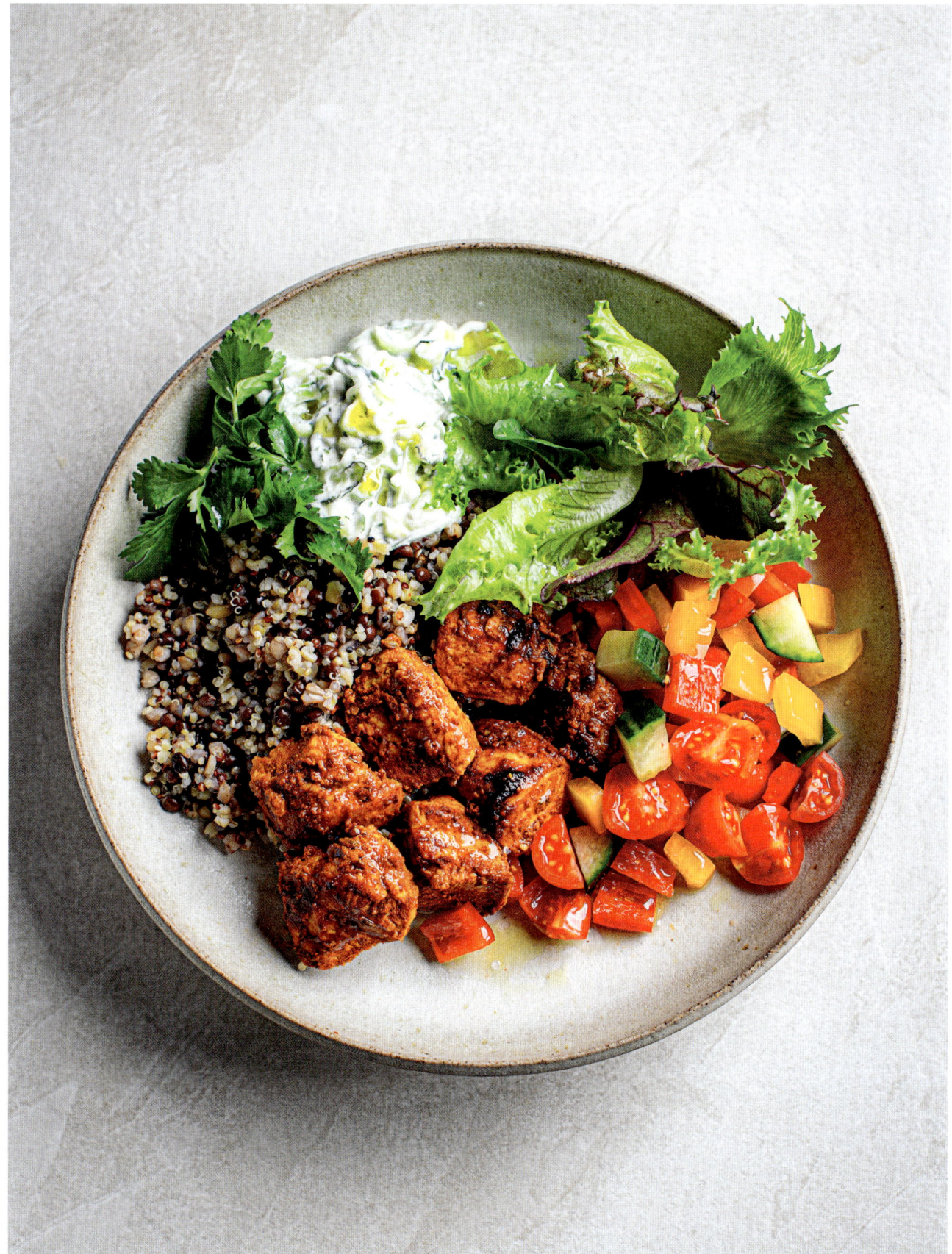

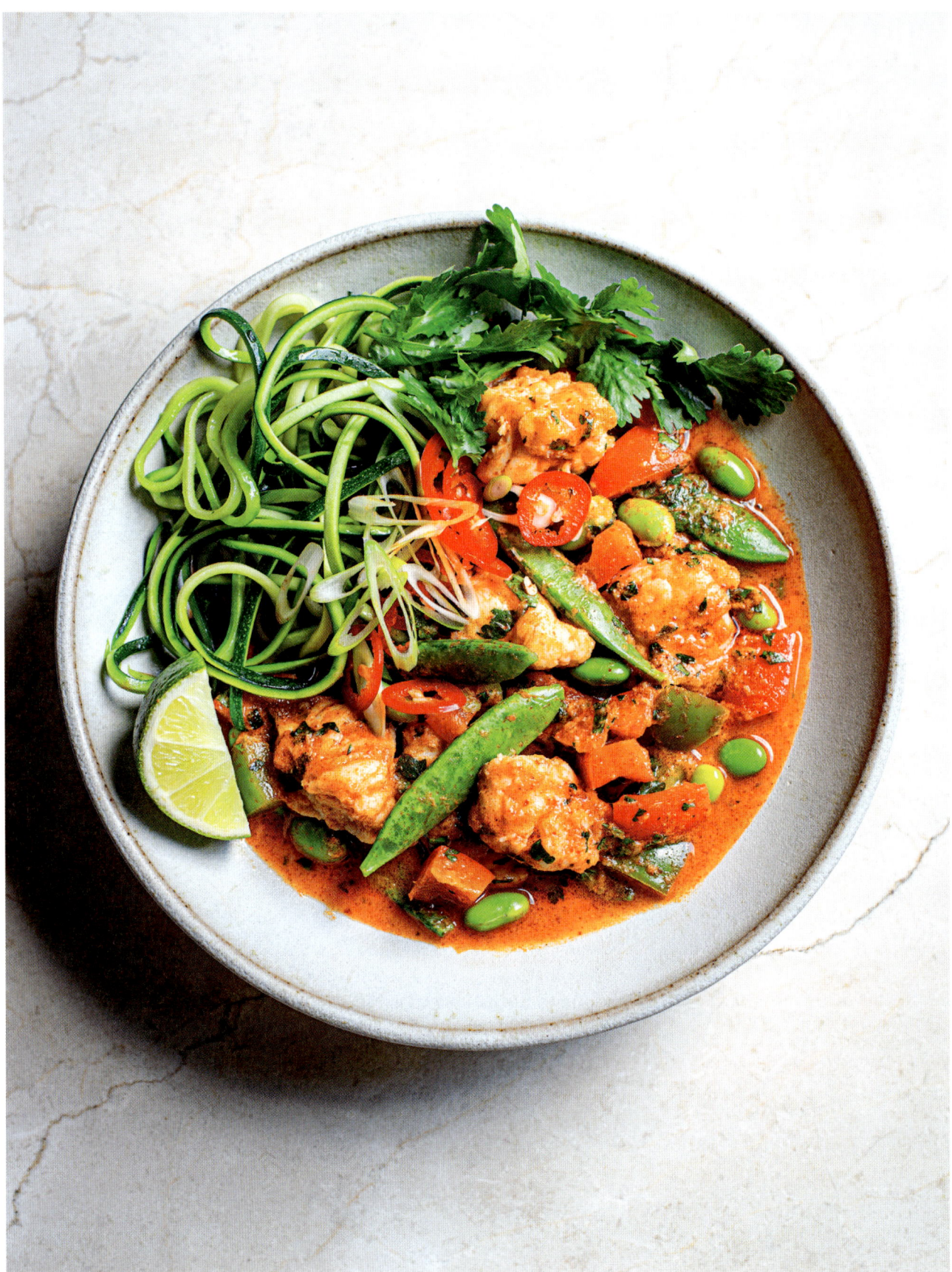

PER SERVING
PROTEIN: 27G
FIBRE: 8G
PLANT POINTS: 7.75

SERVES 4

1 tablespoon extra virgin olive oil
1 garlic clove, crushed
1 green pepper, diced
1 red pepper, diced
a thumb-sized piece of fresh ginger, peeled and finely grated
5–6 tablespoons ready-made Thai red curry paste (around 175g) (check the label, as some are more fiery than others)
1 x 400ml tin of full-fat coconut milk
2 tablespoons fish sauce (nam pla)
100g frozen edamame beans, defrosted
200g sugar snap peas
400g white fish (e.g. monkfish), cut into bite-size cubes
a handful of fresh coriander, chopped

Sesame zoodles
2 large courgettes, julienned, grated or spiralised
1 tablespoon toasted sesame oil

To serve
1 red chilli, deseeded and finely sliced
1 small bunch of spring onions, sliced
fresh coriander, chopped
1 lime, quartered

THAI FISH CURRY WITH SESAME ZOODLES

This meal is quick to prep and cook, making it the perfect mid-week dinner. I love the way rich coconut milk gently softens the chilli flavours, and I find this kind of curry lends itself well to fish. For the fish, I would recommend a thick, firm white fish such as cod, halibut or even monkfish. Monkfish can be more expensive, but holds its shape well when cooking. You can also use a mix of different fish. The vegetables add texture, fibre and sweetness to the dish. I have served my curry with zucchini noodles, but feel free to use black or red rice if you prefer. Nam pla fish sauce is made from fermented anchovies and salt, and improves the flavour, but you can easily omit it if you don't have any. You can also make this dish with prawns, chicken or tofu if you prefer, but adjust the cooking times accordingly.

---

1. Heat the extra virgin olive oil in a large saucepan over a medium-low heat. Gently sauté the garlic, peppers and ginger for 3–4 minutes, taking care not to burn them. Stir in the curry paste and cook for a further minute, then pour in the coconut milk.

2. Add the fish sauce, edamame beans and sugar snap peas. Cover and simmer over a low heat for 2 minutes, then add the fish pieces. Replace the lid and simmer very gently for about 5 minutes, or until the fish is just cooked through and the vegetables are tender. Remove from the heat and gently stir through half the coriander, being careful not to disturb the fish too much in the process.

3. Meanwhile, prepare the courgette noodles. Heat the toasted sesame oil in a heavy-based frying pan. Add the courgettes to the hot pan and flash-fry them as quickly as possible, as slower cooking can result in soggy zoodles. They should cook in less than 2 minutes.

4. Serve the curry in bowls, topped with the red chilli, spring onions, more coriander and a wedge of lime for squeezing over.

Storage: Store leftovers in an airtight container in the fridge for up to 2 days. Reheat the curry and zoodles gently until piping hot.

PER SERVING
PROTEIN: 31 G
FIBRE: 11 G
PLANT POINTS: 8.25

RED LENTIL PIZZA WITH YOGHURT AND CUCUMBER SALAD

This really is a pizza with a twist! While it's fine to enjoy a regular pizza every now and again, this gluten-free lentil-based alternative will leave you feeling energised, not sluggish, and it works very well with my cucumber salad. I usually prefer fresh mozzarella, but it can be quite moist on a pizza, so for this recipe I use grated mozzarella. Feel free to use your own favourite veggies – and don't forget to soak the lentils the night before or in the morning!

SERVES 3

Base
200g dried red lentils, soaked in water overnight, or for around 8 hours
2 tablespoons (around 15g) whole psyllium husk flakes, to bind the dough
2 tablespoons extra virgin olive oil
25ml lemon juice or apple cider vinegar
1 teaspoon baking powder
3 teaspoons dried herbs (e.g. rosemary, thyme, oregano)
1 teaspoon sea salt
freshly ground black pepper, to taste
100–150ml filtered water

Toppings
20g Green Pesto (page 205) (or vegetarian pesto)
100g finely chopped courgette
80g sliced raw asparagus, ends trimmed
80g sliced tomatoes
20g olives
150g grated mozzarella

Cucumber salad
1 large cucumber, finely sliced
30g Greek yoghurt
freshly chopped dill or chives
sea salt and freshly ground black pepper, to taste

1. Preheat the oven to 190°C fan and line a baking sheet with baking parchment.

2. Drain the soaked lentils and rinse well in a sieve. Shake off any excess water, then put them into a high-speed blender or food processor and blend until smooth.

3. Add the psyllium husk flakes, extra virgin olive oil, lemon juice or apple cider vinegar, baking powder and dried herbs, and season with salt and pepper. Blend briefly to combine, then slowly add the filtered water and process again until smooth. The mixture should resemble a thick paste. Leave to stand for 5–10 minutes to thicken.

4. Spread the lentil mixture evenly over the lined baking sheet to roughly 28cm x 20cm, using the back of a spoon.

5. Brush a thin layer of pesto over the base with a pastry brush. Arrange the courgette, asparagus, tomatoes and olives on top, leaving small gaps between the vegetables so that the base can cook through. Adding the vegetables too close together can result in a soggy base. Scatter over the grated mozzarella. Bake for 30–40 minutes, until golden and the base is fully cooked through.

6. To make the salad, mix the cucumber with the Greek yoghurt, chopped herbs, salt and pepper.

7. Serve the pizza warm, with the cucumber salad on the side.

Storage: Store leftover pizza in an airtight container in the fridge for up to 3 days. Reheat in a hot oven until piping hot. The salad is best eaten fresh, but can be stored in the fridge for up to 24 hours.

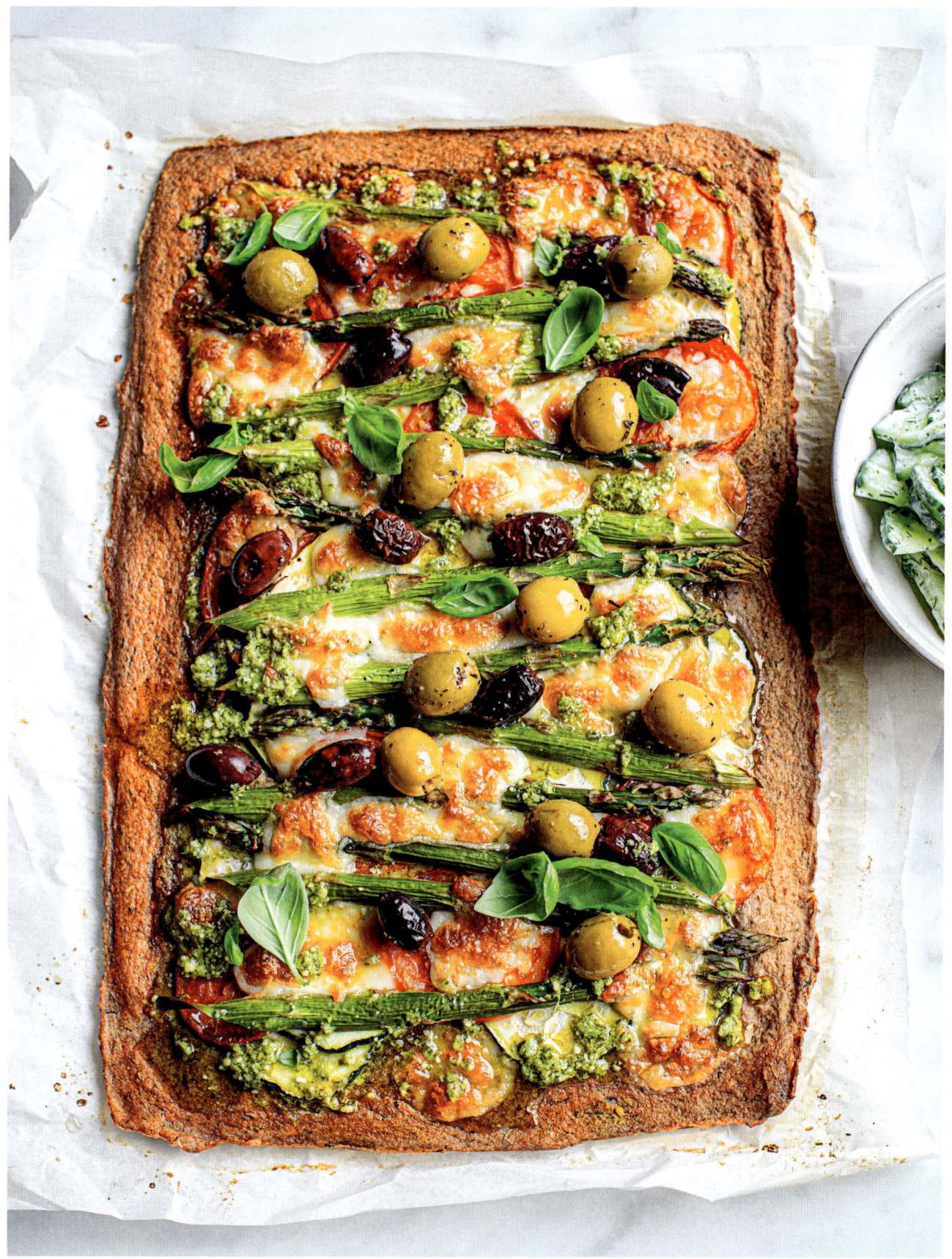

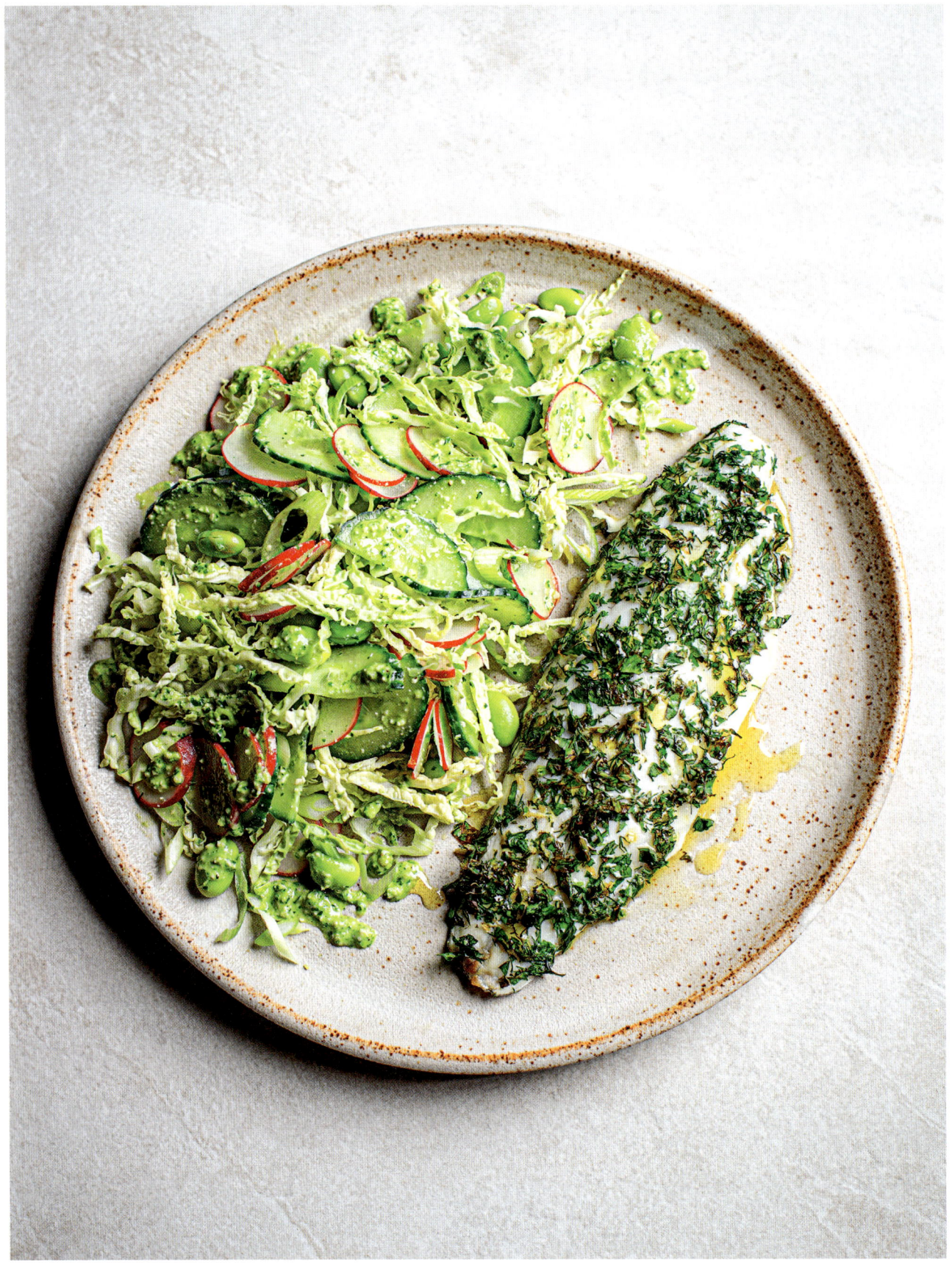

PER SERVING
PROTEIN: 32G
FIBRE: 10G
PLANT POINTS: 9.75

SERVES 4

4 sea bass or sea bream fillets (around 360g in total)
a small handful of finely chopped fresh herbs (e.g. parsley, oregano, basil, dill), or 2 teaspoons dried herbs
zest and juice of ½ unwaxed lemon
a drizzle of extra virgin olive oil

Green glow coleslaw
1 whole white cabbage, finely sliced or pulsed briefly in a food processor
150g radishes, finely sliced
1 large cucumber, finely sliced
1 small bunch of red spring onions, sliced
150g frozen edamame beans

Dressing
60g cashew nuts
2 garlic cloves, peeled
a handful of spinach or rocket
a handful of 2 or 3 different types of fresh herbs (e.g. basil, coriander, chives, parsley)
3 tablespoons nutritional yeast (around 20g), or 30g grated Parmesan (Note, if you use Parmesan, the dish won't be dairy-free)
zest and juice of 2 unwaxed lemons
50ml extra virgin olive oil
1 tablespoon apple cider vinegar
70–100ml filtered water

SEA BREAM WITH GREEN GLOW COLESLAW

Sea bass is a white fish but it is unique in that it also contains omega-3 fats in the form of DHA and EPA, just like oily fish. Most white fish have very little fat in their flesh and instead store it in their liver, which is why cod-liver oil is often taken as a supplement. This makes sea bass an ideal way for people who are not keen on 'fishy' fish to still benefit from those healthy omega-3s. I like to buy good quality lemons, especially if I am eating the zest, so try to choose unwaxed or organic if you can. I often have a bottle of sharp Sicilian lemon juice in my fridge too – Sicily being, in my opinion, where the best lemons come from! You can replace the sea bass with sea bream, which has similar benefits, if preferred. The green glow coleslaw is fresh and light, making this a meal that won't weigh you down.

---

1. Preheat the oven to 200°C fan and line a ceramic baking dish with baking parchment to prevent the fish from sticking.

2. Place the fish fillets skin side down in the lined dish and gently press the herbs on to the top of each fillet. Just before you put them in the oven, drizzle with lemon juice and extra virgin olive oil, and scatter with a little lemon zest. Adding the lemon juice too early can start to 'cook' the fish, like ceviche. Cook for 8–12 minutes, or until the fish is opaque and cooked through.

3. To prepare the coleslaw, put the finely sliced cabbage, radishes cucumber and spring onions in a large bowl. Simmer the edamame beans for 3 minutes until just tender. Drain and rinse under cold water to stop the cooking process, then add them to the salad.

4. For the dressing, put the cashew nuts, garlic, spinach or rocket, herbs, nutritional yeast or Parmesan, lemon juice and zest, extra virgin olive oil and apple cider vinegar in a blender. Blend until completely smooth, adding the water slowly until you reach the desired consistency. Season with salt and pepper.

5. Toss the vegetables with the dressing just before serving. Serve the fish hot, alongside the coleslaw.

PER SERVING
PROTEIN: 40G
FIBRE: 13G
PLANT POINTS: 7.5

SERVES 4
1 rounded tablespoon smoked paprika
1 teaspoon ground cumin
1 teaspoon garlic powder
1 teaspoon sea salt
1 pork tenderloin, free range if possible (around 450g)
1 tablespoon extra virgin olive oil

Smoky beans
1 tablespoon extra virgin olive oil
1 onion, diced
1 garlic clove, crushed
2 carrots, scrubbed and diced
200g cherry tomatoes, chopped
2 x 400g tins or jars of white beans (e.g. cannellini or flageolet), rinsed and drained (480g drained weight)
1–2 teaspoons smoked paprika
a pinch of chilli powder or chilli flakes
a large handful of parsley, finely chopped
1 tablespoon apple cider vinegar or lemon juice
sea salt and freshly ground black pepper

To serve
400g Tenderstem broccoli or Savoy cabbage
2 small red apples or 1 large, julienned or grated

PORK LOIN WITH SMOKY BEANS

Pork loin is an incredibly lean cut that cooks quickly and melts in your mouth. I have used creamy beans as a base and topped it with some fresh apple. Apples are a good source of pectin, a type of soluble fibre, and of quercetin, a plant compound with anti-inflammatory properties. Keep the skin on the apples, as much of the pectin and quercetin is found there. Similarly, there's no need to peel the carrots, just give them a good scrub, as many of the nutrients are found just beneath the skin.

1. Preheat the oven to 220°C fan. In a small bowl, mix together the paprika, cumin, garlic powder and sea salt. Rub the spice mix all over the pork tenderloin (wear gloves if you prefer).

2. Heat 1 tablespoon of extra virgin olive oil in a large, heavy-based frying pan over a high heat. Sear the pork for 3 minutes on each side, then transfer to a lightly oiled ceramic oven dish. Roast in the oven for 10 minutes. Reduce the oven temperature to 200°C fan and cook for a further 5–10 minutes, until the pork is cooked through. Rest on a board for 10 minutes before slicing.

3. While the pork is cooking, make the beans. Heat 1 tablespoon of extra virgin olive oil in the same frying pan used for the pork, over a medium heat. Sauté the onion for about 5 minutes, until translucent. Stir in the garlic, carrots and cherry tomatoes, and cook for another 2 minutes. Add the beans with their liquid, the smoked paprika and a pinch of chilli. Simmer gently until thickened and creamy, usually around 10 minutes. Add the parsley and the vinegar or lemon juice and season to taste with salt and pepper.

4. Lightly steam the broccoli or Savoy cabbage, or sauté in extra virgin olive oil or butter, until just tender. Season with salt and pepper.

5. Serve the sliced pork with a generous spoonful of smoky beans, topped with freshly julienned or grated apple and alongside the warm greens.

Storage: Leftovers can be stored in the fridge in an airtight container for up to 3 days. Keep the meat and beans separate. Reheat gently until piping hot.

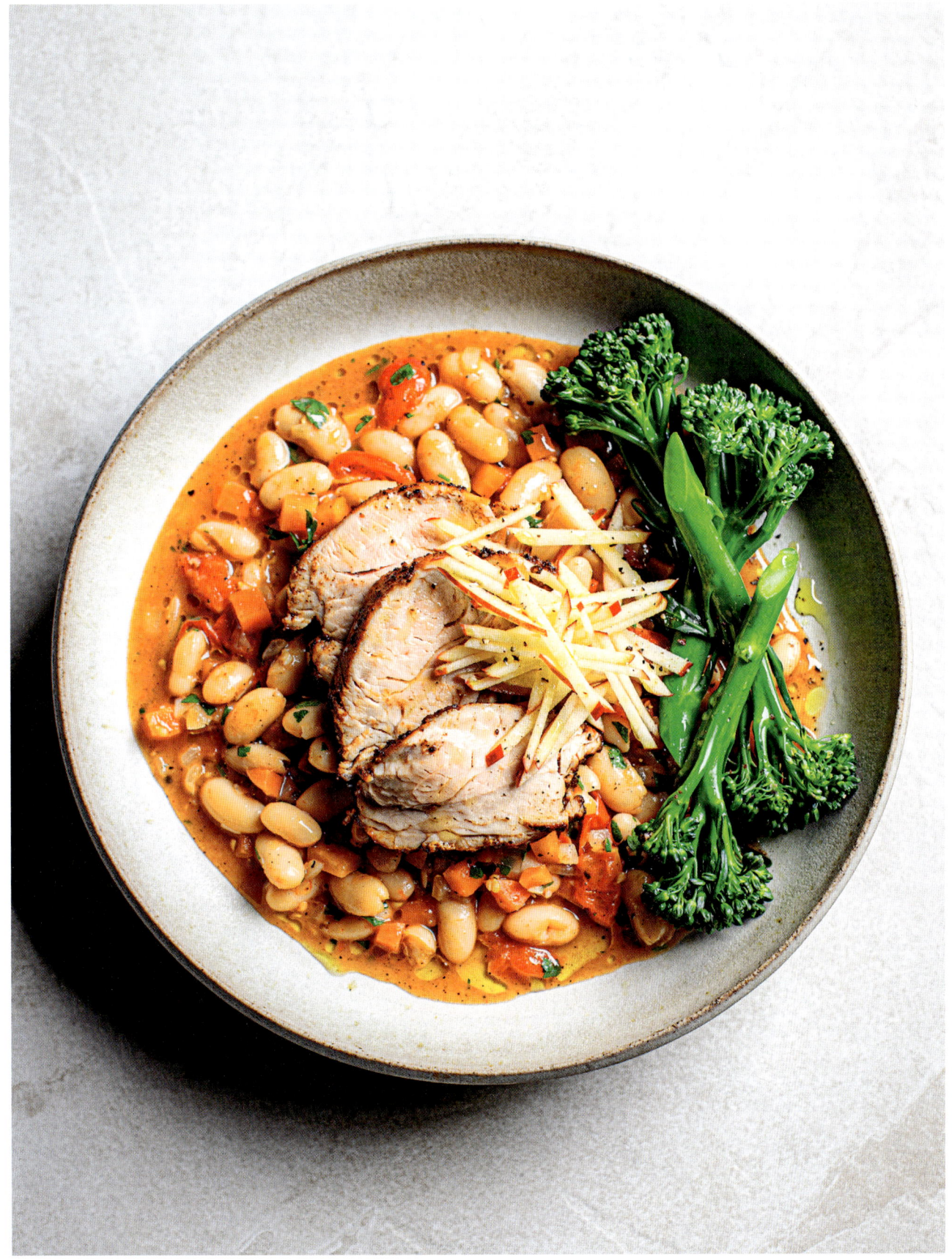

PER SERVING
PROTEIN: 40G
FIBRE: 9G
PLANT POINTS: 5.75

SERVES 4
400g chicken fillets
½ large red onion, finely diced
25g kale, destalked and roughly chopped
25g baby spinach
a pinch of chilli flakes
a small bunch of parsley, finely chopped
sea salt and freshly ground black pepper
extra virgin olive oil, for frying

Tomato salsa salad
½ large red onion, diced
400g cherry or baby plum tomatoes, diced
1 cucumber, diced
1 avocado, diced
a small handful of freshly chopped herbs (e.g. chives, parsley, coriander)
juice of ½ lemon
sea salt and freshly ground black pepper

Turmeric and coriander mayonnaise (makes 250ml)
1 whole egg, room temperature
1 tablespoon apple cider vinegar
10ml lemon juice
1 teaspoon Dijon mustard (check it is gluten-free)
1 teaspoon ground turmeric
180ml extra virgin olive oil (or 100ml extra virgin olive oil and 80ml rapeseed oil)
a small handful of coriander leaves, very finely chopped

To serve
Gluten-free flatbreads or Simple Flatbreads (page 264 or 262)
50g sauerkraut per serving

CHICKEN AND KALE BURGERS WITH TOMATO SALSA SALAD

If you are cutting down on red meat, or fancy a lighter burger, I promise you will not be disappointed! I love these burgers inside my flatbreads (page 262) with the tomato salsa, which is more like a salad, and my simple all-in-one turmeric and coriander mayo. The gorgeous colour of the turmeric with fresh coriander is a winning combination that works perfectly with so many foods. Extra virgin olive oil is so good for us but can have a strong flavour in a mayonnaise, so I like to combine it with another neutral oil, such as avocado oil or cold-pressed rapeseed oil in my mayonnaise.

---

1. Put the chicken fillets into a food processor and pulse until roughly combined but still chunky. Add the red onion, kale, spinach, chilli flakes, parsley and some salt and pepper, and pulse again to combine without over-processing. Divide the mixture into 4 large or 8 smaller portions. Roll into balls and flatten to form patties.

2. Heat a little extra virgin olive oil in a frying pan over a medium heat and cook the patties for about 4–5 minutes on each side, until golden and completely cooked through.

3. To make the salsa, combine the red onion, tomatoes, cucumber, avocado and herbs in a bowl. Squeeze over the lemon juice and season with salt and pepper.

4. To make the mayonnaise, put all the ingredients except the coriander into a narrow jar that just fits a stick blender, or a small bullet-style blender. If using a stick blender, blend starting from the bottom – once the mixture thickens and emulsifies and the oil is fully incorporated, move the blender slowly upwards to finish blending. Add the finely chopped coriander and pulse briefly to combine.

5. Warm the flatbreads and spread each one with a tablespoon of mayonnaise. Top with the cooked burgers, spoon over the tomato salsa salad and add a serving of sauerkraut to each plate.

Storage: The salsa is best fresh, but can be stored in an airtight container in the fridge for up to 24 hours. Store the mayonnaise in an airtight jar in the fridge for up to 5 days; stir before using.

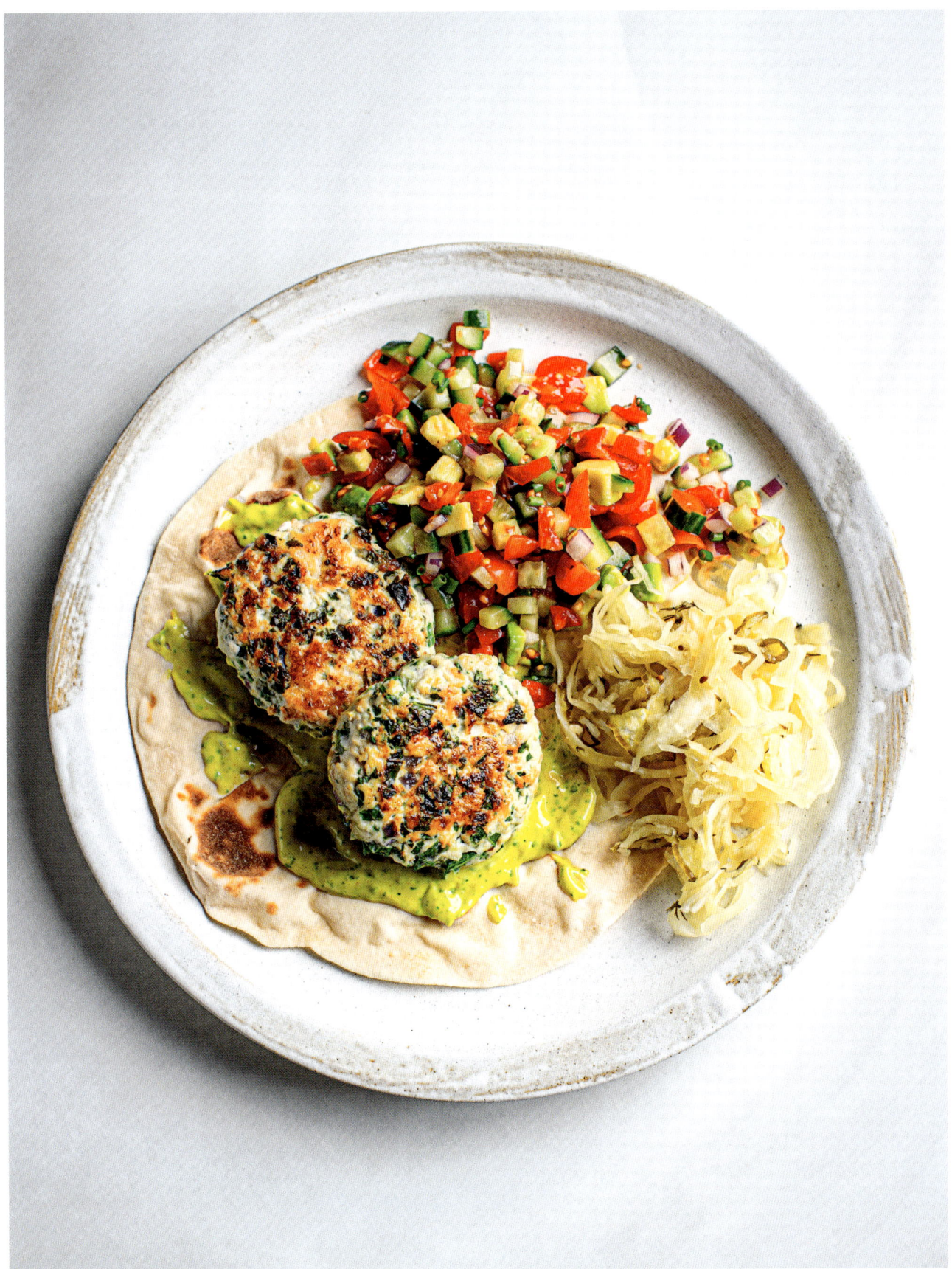

PER SERVING
PROTEIN: 29G
FIBRE: 9G
PLANT POINTS: 9.25

SERVES 4

Fishcakes
200g smoked mackerel
1 x 400g tin or jar of haricot beans (or other white beans), rinsed and drained (240g drained weight)
2 spring onions, finely sliced
10g capers, chopped
20g cornichons, finely sliced
1 tablespoon lemon juice
50g kale, destalked and finely chopped
1 egg, beaten
a small handful of finely chopped fresh parsley
½ teaspoon sea salt
freshly ground black pepper, to taste

For coating/cooking
20g chickpea (gram) flour (or other flour)
2 tablespoons extra virgin olive oil

Kale and carrot salad
200g kale, destalked and chopped
2 medium carrots, grated or julienned
1 apple, grated or julienned

Dressing
2 tablespoons apple cider vinegar
2 tablespoons extra virgin olive oil
1 teaspoon mustard e.g. Dijon (check it is gluten-free)
1 garlic clove, crushed
sea salt and freshly ground black pepper

MACKEREL FISHCAKES WITH WATERCRESS CREAM

Lots of people don't like their fish to be too 'fishy' in flavour and some people find traditional fishcakes have too much potato and not enough fish. These high-protein fishcakes get the balance just right and are packed with flavour, fibre and healthy fats. The smoked mackerel provides depth and richness, while haricot beans and kale add plant diversity and a firm texture. Served with a vibrant watercress cream and a refreshing carrot and kale salad, this dish is a delicious, colourful and nutrient-dense meal. The fishcakes can be prepared in advance and batch cooked, making them ideal for busy days. You can swap the smoked mackerel for tinned mackerel if you prefer. I like these with poached eggs, but you can serve with boiled eggs or sunny side ups if you like.

---

1. Put the smoked mackerel and drained beans into a food processor and pulse until mostly smooth. Alternatively, mash them together in a large bowl, using a fork. Transfer the mixture to a bowl and stir in the spring onions, capers, cornichons, lemon juice, kale, egg and parsley, and season with salt and pepper. Mix well until fully combined.

2. Divide the mixture into 8 and roll into balls, then flatten each into a fishcake shape. Place the chickpea flour (or other flour) on a plate and lightly coat the fishcakes. Arrange them on a plate lined with baking parchment and refrigerate for 30 minutes, or freeze for 15 minutes, to firm them up. This will help them hold together as they cook.

3. While the fishcakes are chilling, prepare the salad. Put the kale and carrot into a bowl. Combine the salad dressing ingredients in a jar or small blender and mix well. Pour over the vegetables and allow to sit for at least 30 minutes, to allow the kale and carrot to marinate. The kale will start to soften in the dressing and will become bright green and slightly wilted.

Watercress cream
100g Greek yoghurt
50g watercress
1 garlic clove, crushed
1 tablespoon lemon juice
a pinch of chilli flakes
sea salt and freshly ground black pepper

To serve
4 eggs

Tip: Poached eggs cook best when the eggs are very fresh.

4. For the watercress cream, blend all the ingredients using a food processor or stick blender until smooth and a vibrant green. Adjust the seasoning to taste.

5. Heat the extra virgin olive oil in a heavy-based frying pan over a medium heat. Cook the fishcakes in batches for 2 minutes on each side, until golden and heated through. Keep them warm in a low oven while you poach the eggs.

6. To poach the eggs, fill a wide pan with water and add a splash of vinegar. Bring to a gentle simmer. Crack each egg into an oiled ladle, gently lower into the water and release once the white starts to set. Cook for 2–3 minutes, until the whites are set but the yolks are still runny. Remove with a slotted spoon and keep warm.

7. Serve two fishcakes per person, topped with a poached egg, a spoonful of watercress cream and a generous portion of the salad.

Storage: The cooked fishcakes can be stored in an airtight container in the fridge for up to 2 days. Reheat in a frying pan or in an air fryer for 5 minutes at 180°C until piping hot.

PER SERVING
PROTEIN: 32G
FIBRE: 12G
PLANT POINTS: 6.25

SERVES 2

Tofu
200g firm, plain tofu, cut into bite-size cubes
1 garlic clove, crushed
10g chickpea (gram) flour
1½ tablespoons gochujang paste (see Tip)
1 tablespoon tamari or soy sauce (Note, soy sauce isn't gluten-free)
1 tablespoon toasted sesame oil
1 tablespoon white or black sesame seeds
freshly ground black pepper, to taste

Edamame
100g frozen edamame beans

Stir-fried vegetables
1 tablespoon toasted sesame oil
150g sprouting broccoli, cut into bite-size pieces
1 courgette, julienned, spiralised, ribboned or grated
1–2 carrots, julienned, spiralised, ribboned or grated

To serve
a sprinkling of sesame seeds
lime wedges

Tip: Gochujang paste can contain gluten, so double-check yours if you are gluten-free.

CRISPY GOCHUJANG TOFU WITH STIR-FRIED VEGETABLES

Gochujang is a fermented Korean chilli paste made from dried gochugaru chillies, and it is known for its deep, spicy and slightly sweet flavour. This is a completely balanced plant-based meal, perfect for a meat-free Monday or to add variety to your week. You can swap the tofu for chicken, prawns, salmon or beef though, if you prefer. Many people avoid tofu because of its bland taste. Instead, imagine tofu like a blank canvas that takes on all the flavours in the dish, soaking them up like a sponge. Cooked well, tofu should be crisp on the outside and soft and flavourful on the inside. Tofu can be a rich source of calcium (if calcium set) and is a great way to top up the protein in plant-based meals.

---

1. You can cook the tofu in the oven or in an air fryer, or you can pan-fry it in a little extra sesame oil. If you are using your oven, preheat it to 180°C fan; or heat your air fryer to 180°C. If you are cooking in the oven, line a baking sheet with baking parchment.

2. Press the tofu cubes gently with a clean tea towel to remove the excess water. Mix the garlic, chickpea flour, gochujang paste, tamari or soy sauce, sesame oil, sesame seeds and black pepper in a bowl. Add the tofu and toss gently to coat. Spread on the lined baking sheet and bake for 20–25 minutes, until golden and crisp outside and soft inside. Alternatively, cook in an air fryer at 180°C for 15 minutes. Or gently fry in extra sesame oil over a medium-high heat for 5–6 minutes, until crispy outside and soft in the centre.

3. Cook the edamame beans in a pan of simmering water for 3–5 minutes. Drain and set aside.

4. For the stir-fried vegetables, heat the toasted sesame oil in a heavy-based frying pan over a medium heat. Stir-fry the broccoli for 2 minutes. Add the courgette and carrot and stir-fry for another 2–3 minutes, until the vegetables are just tender but still vibrant.

5. Serve the tofu with the stir-fried vegetables and edamame beans.

Storage: Store leftovers in an airtight container in the fridge for up to 2 days. Reheat gently in a frying pan. Not suitable for freezing.

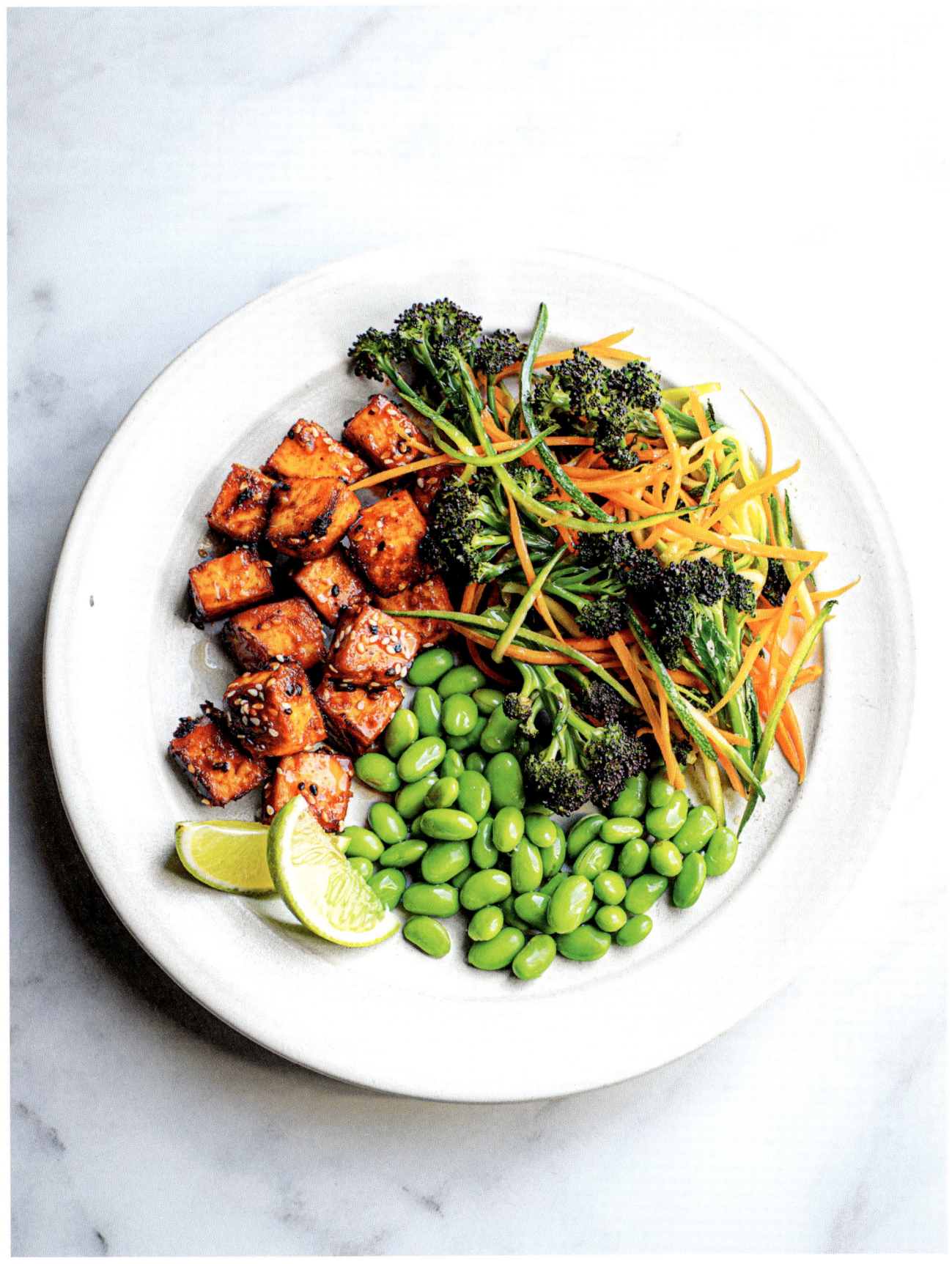

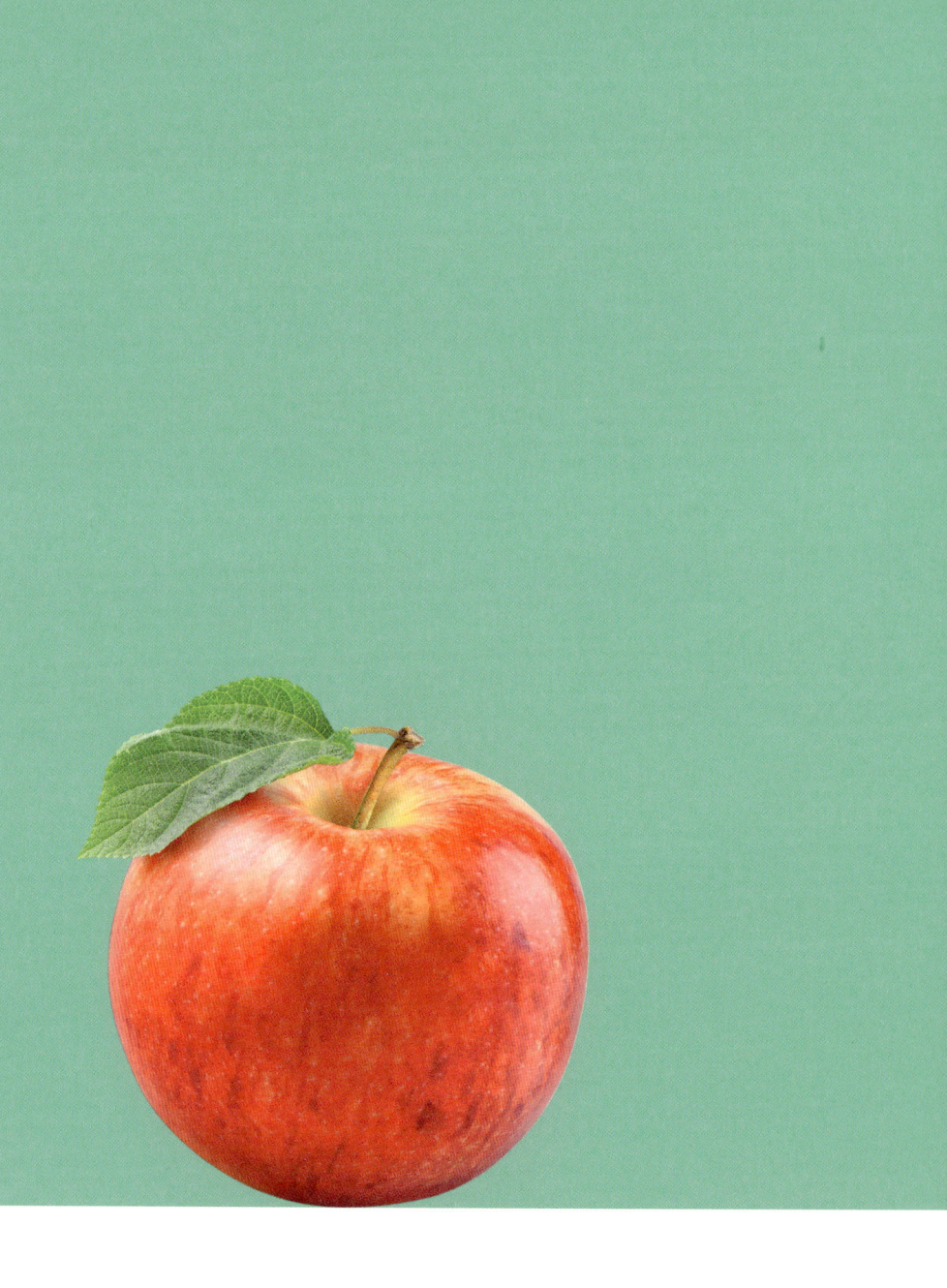

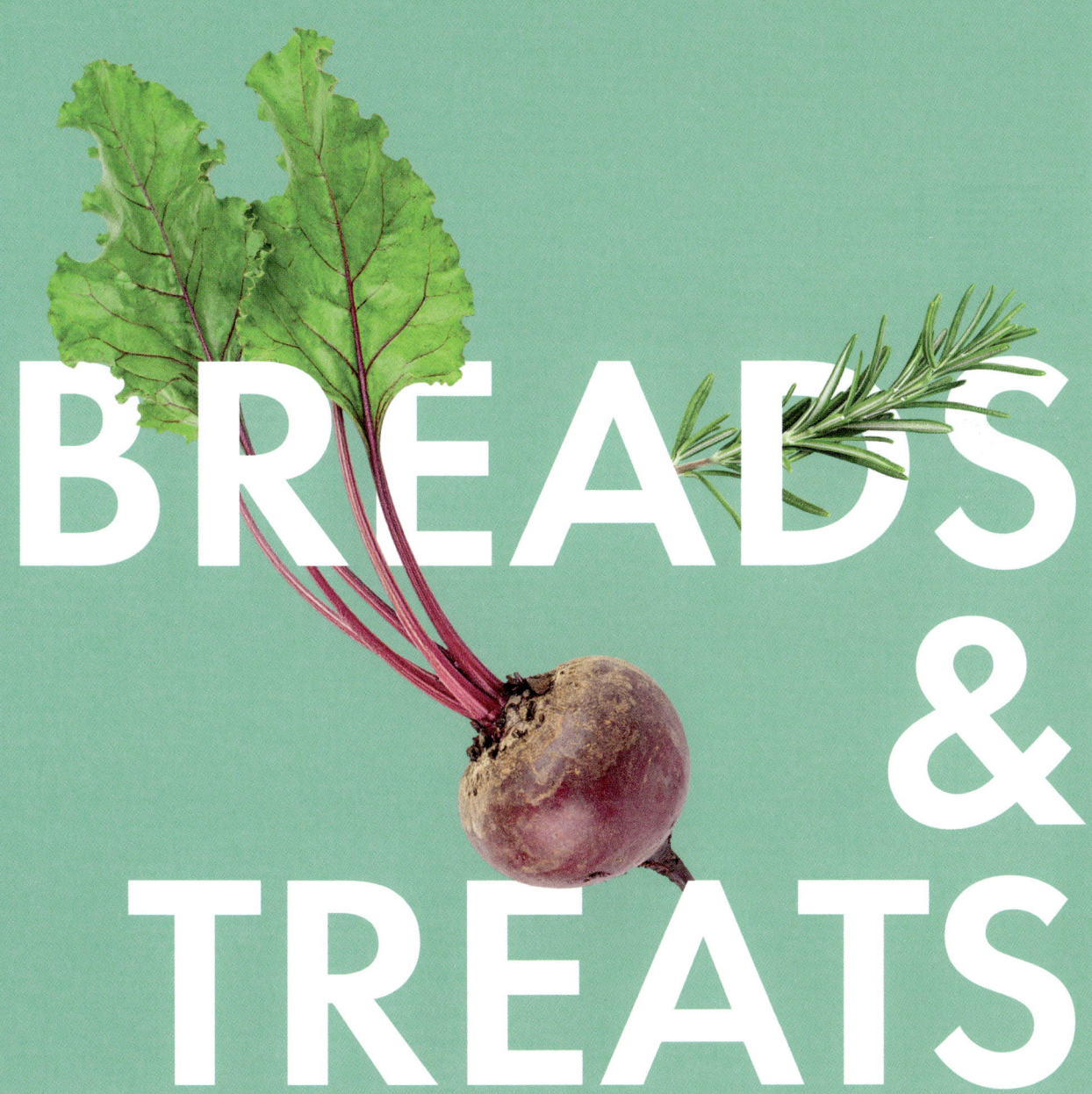

BREADS & TREATS

Aiming to reduce some of the ultra-processed foods in our diet will likely mean cutting down on some of our regular basics, such as supermarket breads and pre-prepared snacks, so this chapter has the recipes you can rely on to help you make the swap and stop you reaching for more processed alternatives. These include the staple recipes I make every week, like the Super Green Bread (page 254), Naked Loaf (page 258) and the Red Lentil Bagels (page 267) – which are the perfect brunch with smoked salmon and cream cheese (see page 128). Clocking up an impressive 10g of protein and 8g of fibre as well as two plant points in just one bagel, this is an easy way to top up any of your mealtimes.

Although my no-nonsense philosophy encourages everyone to stick to three meals a day where they can, with sufficient gaps between those meals, and to avoid snacking, I also know that life doesn't always work like that. Remember: it's about consistency, not militancy. Sometimes you need something to bridge the gap between mealtimes – or you really do just need something sweet, and I totally get that too.

When it comes to snacks and treats, I like to think of it this way: rather than grazing throughout the afternoon, why not bring any snacks up to lunchtime and eat them as part of the meal? This might look like some Rosemary and Sea Salt Seeded Crackers (page 261) with cheese on the side of your plate. It could also look like a lovely cup of matcha tea or coffee with a healthy Bliss Ball (page 290) or a date filled with homemade chocolate and hazelnut spread (page 289). Or even a Chocolate Chip Peanut Cookie (page 280)! If you are eating a snack between meals, I advise opting for something savoury, but if you're adding it as an extra to a meal, you can go for something sweeter. This can help prevent you from jumping on the blood-sugar rollercoaster where snacking becomes a necessity rather than a choice. (Also see pages 73–76 and 86–87 for more on snacking and page 88 for my snacking rules.) The secret is to plan it, add it to a meal and let your appetite guide you.

Of course, there are also times when the gaps between meals become too long. Most of us will start to get hungry again after 4–5 hours, which is completely normal. When I've had a long day and I know I'm not going to make it home in time for dinner, the Egg Muffins (page 272) have saved me numerous times, and I've included my recipes for three flavours of hummus (pages 269–271) because hummus goes with everything! I often pack a small pot of hummus along with some vegetable sticks, or to spread on top of a slice of seeded loaf (page 253).

I've also included some of my favourite desserts and treats because it really is all about balance. My No Nonsense philosophy is about eating smarter, not less, and completely cutting out foods you enjoy can easily backfire with you ending up reaching for a quick sugary fix. Once you try the Chocolate Chip Peanut Cookies or the Salted Caramel Bars (page 280 or 282), you will never look at another biscuit or chocolate bar the same way again.

Everything in this chapter is made with minimal sugars and minimally or unprocessed ingredients. But remember, this is all about trying new things and seeing how your body adapts, making small steps and not turning your life upside down in a week. Success and routines take time, so be patient and kind to yourself and make time to enjoy what you eat.

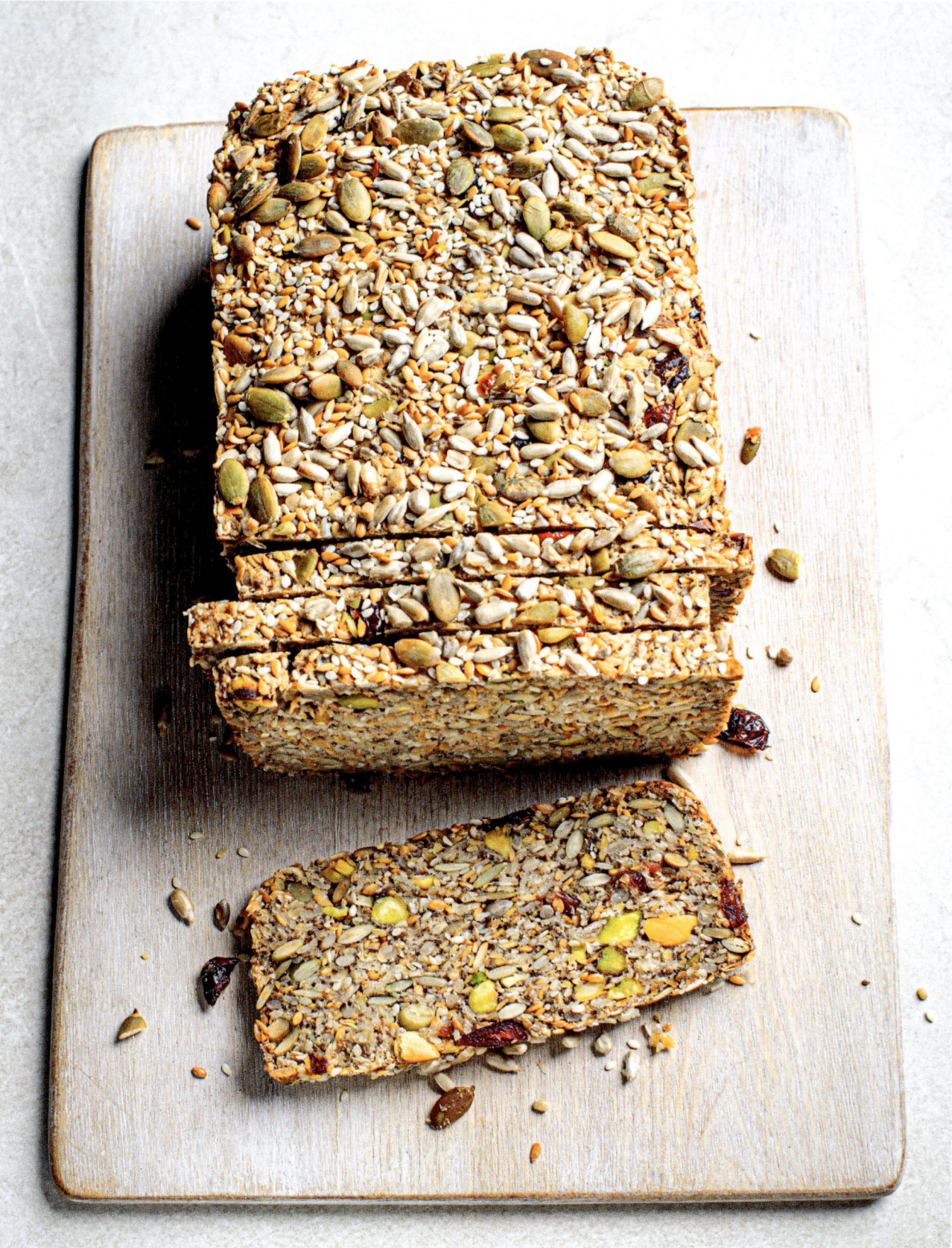

PER SLICE
PROTEIN: 8G
FIBRE: 8G
PLANT POINTS: 8.5

MAKES 18 SLICES

150g whole or milled flaxseeds
50g chia seeds
200g gluten-free (or regular) rolled oats
2 tablespoons extra virgin olive oil
100g pumpkin seeds
100g sunflower seeds
75g sesame seeds
75g pistachio nuts/hazelnuts or chopped almonds
50g dried cranberries
35g psyllium husk flakes
1 teaspoon sea salt
400–450ml filtered water
1–2 tablespoons mixed seeds, to sprinkle (optional)

SEED AND NUT LOAF

I have been making variations of this recipe for almost ten years now. It requires no kneading and is packed with healthy ingredients. Originally, I milled the oats and flaxseeds into a flour and used eggs to bind the loaf together. But with seeded breads gaining in popularity, I started swapping eggs for psyllium husk flakes and leaving the oats and flaxseeds whole to give more texture. Psyllium husk is a natural fibre derived from the outer coating of the seeds of the Plantago ovata plant. It helps bind the seeds and other ingredients together, providing structure and retaining moisture without the need for flour. I prefer to use psyllium flakes rather than the powder, as it gives a lighter texture. For a version of this loaf that is oat-free and is made entirely from nuts and seeds, see page 258.

1. Mix all the dry ingredients together in a large bowl and stir well. Add the water and mix well with a spoon or spatula. The dough should be quite thick and sticky.

2. Transfer to a 2lb/900g loaf tin, lined with baking parchment or a loaf tin parchment liner, and flatten the surface with the back of a wet spoon. Sprinkle with the extra seeds, if you like. For best results, leave to sit for around 30–60 minutes, to allow the psyllium husk and chia seeds to bind the dough together. Preheat the oven to 180°C fan.

3. Bake the loaf in the oven for 1 hour, testing it with a skewer before removing from the oven to check it is cooked through. A skewer, inserted into the middle of the loaf, should come out clean. If it isn't ready, cook for a further 10 minutes, then check again. Allow to cool a little in the tin, then turn out and cool completely on a wire rack before slicing.

Storage: Store in an airtight container for up to 5 days. Suitable for freezing for up to 2 months. Slice before freezing, separating the slices with small pieces of baking parchment.

PER SLICE
PROTEIN: 5G
FIBRE: 7G
PLANT POINTS: 9.25

MAKES 16 SLICES
100g broccoli
100g kale, stalks removed
100g baby spinach
100g gluten-free (or regular) rolled oats
100g ground almonds
3 eggs
75g pumpkin seeds
50g sunflower seeds
50g whole flaxseeds
30g chia seeds
2 tablespoons apple cider vinegar
1 teaspoon sea salt
1 teaspoon bicarbonate of soda
25g psyllium husk flakes

SUPER GREEN BREAD

The inspiration for this incredible bread came from a recipe given to me by a lovely client called Sarah. I adapted her recipe, adding more seeds, but keeping her bold levels of greens, which are the making of this loaf. Leafy greens are a great source of folate, as well as calcium for healthy bones, magnesium for its calming properties, and iron. Thought to be behind the cartoon character Popeye's strength, spinach was celebrated for its exceptionally high iron content until the 1930s, when a decimal place error was discovered in the calculation, which had originally inflated the iron by tenfold. Spinach is still a good source of iron at around 2.7mg per 100g, but just not quite as high as was once thought.

1. Preheat the oven to 180°C fan.

2. Cut the broccoli into florets and roughly chop the kale. Put them both into a food processor and pulse until very finely chopped. Add the spinach and blend again until the mixture is mostly smooth and moist but still retains some texture and moisture. Transfer to a large bowl.

3. Add all the remaining ingredients to the bowl and mix well until combined.

4. Spoon the mixture into a 2lb/900g loaf tin, lined with baking parchment or a loaf tin parchment liner, and smooth the surface with the back of a spoon. Bake for 1 hour. Check the loaf is cooked through by inserting a skewer into the middle, which should come out clean.

5. Allow the bread to cool completely in the tin before removing and slicing.

Storage: Store in an airtight container for up to 5 days. Suitable for freezing for up to 2 months; slice before freezing, separating the slices with small pieces of baking parchment.

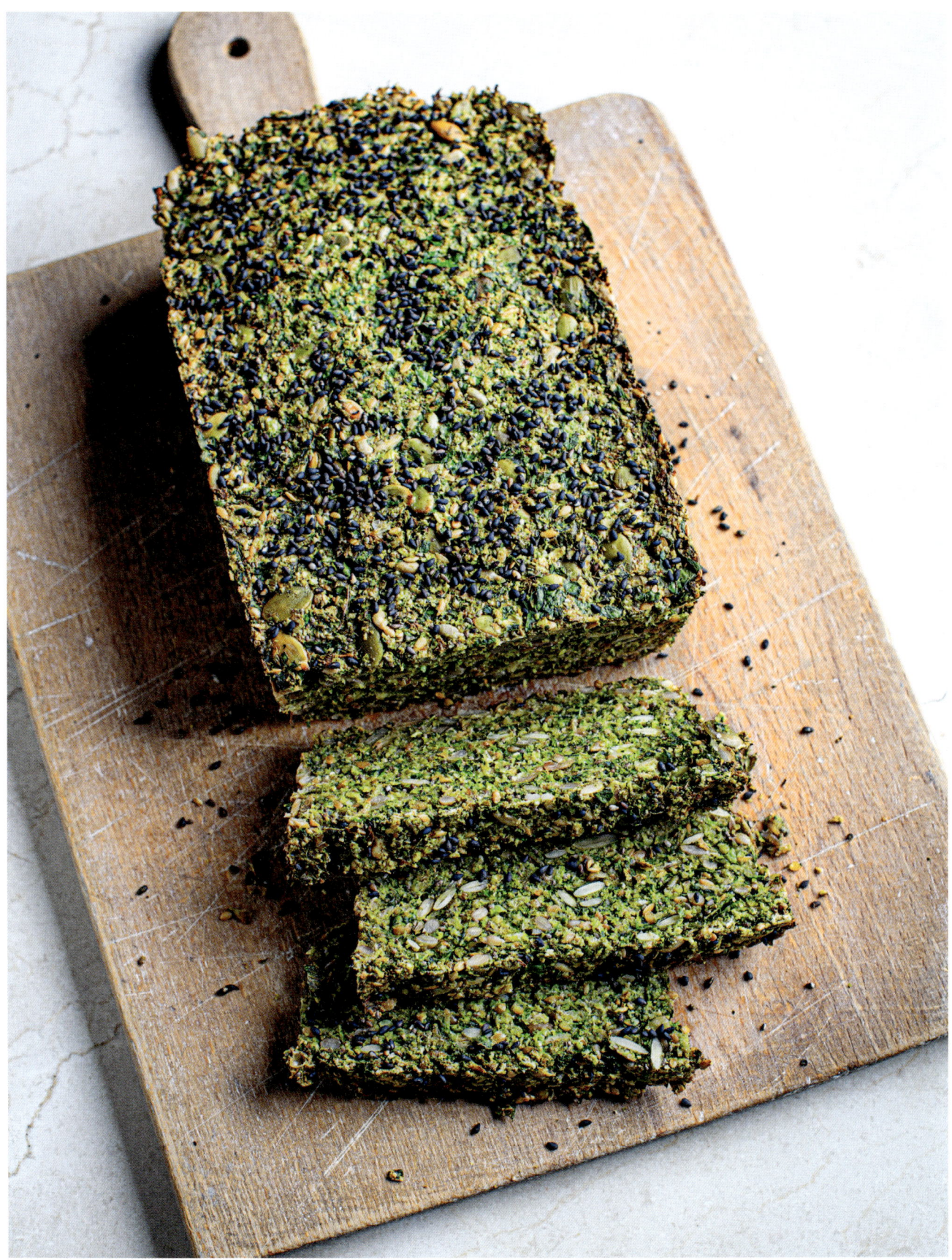

PER SLICE
PROTEIN: 9G
FIBRE: 5G
PLANT POINTS: 8.5

MAKES 16 SLICES

200g grated courgette
200g grated carrot
200g gluten-free (or regular) rolled oats
300g Greek yoghurt
50g whole or milled flaxseeds
50g chia seeds
75g sunflower seeds
75g pumpkin seeds
50g sesame seeds, plus extra to sprinkle, if desired
50g Parmesan (or vegetarian hard cheese), grated
2 eggs
1 teaspoon baking powder
1 teaspoon dried herbs (e.g. thyme and oregano)

CARROT AND COURGETTE YOGHURT LOAF

This no-knead-no-prove recipe can be ready in just over an hour! It is simple to make and does not require any specialist ingredients or kit. Packed with grated vegetables, oats and yoghurt, the loaf has a moist texture – and it is a great way to incorporate even more vegetables into your diet. Perfect freshly baked or toasted the next day, it also freezes really well. Parmesan gives it a lovely cheesy flavour and also tops up the calcium in this loaf.

---

1. Preheat the oven to 180°C fan and line a baking tray with baking parchment.

2. Use a clean tea towel or kitchen paper to squeeze out any excess liquid from the courgette. This step is important to prevent the loaf from becoming too wet and dense during baking.

3. Put all the ingredients into a large bowl and mix thoroughly until well combined. No food processor is needed, but make sure it is evenly mixed.

4. Transfer the mixture to the prepared baking tray and, using wet hands, form the mixture into a loaf shape. Try to keep the loaf an even shape and similar height, for even cooking. Press it together firmly and sprinkle the surface with extra sesame seeds, if desired.

5. Bake the loaf for 60–70 minutes, testing with a skewer before removing from the oven to check it is cooked through. Poke the skewer into the middle – it should come out clean.

Storage: Store in an airtight container (at room temperature) for up to 2–3 days. The loaf also freezes well for up to 2 months. Slice before freezing, separating the slices with small pieces of baking parchment.

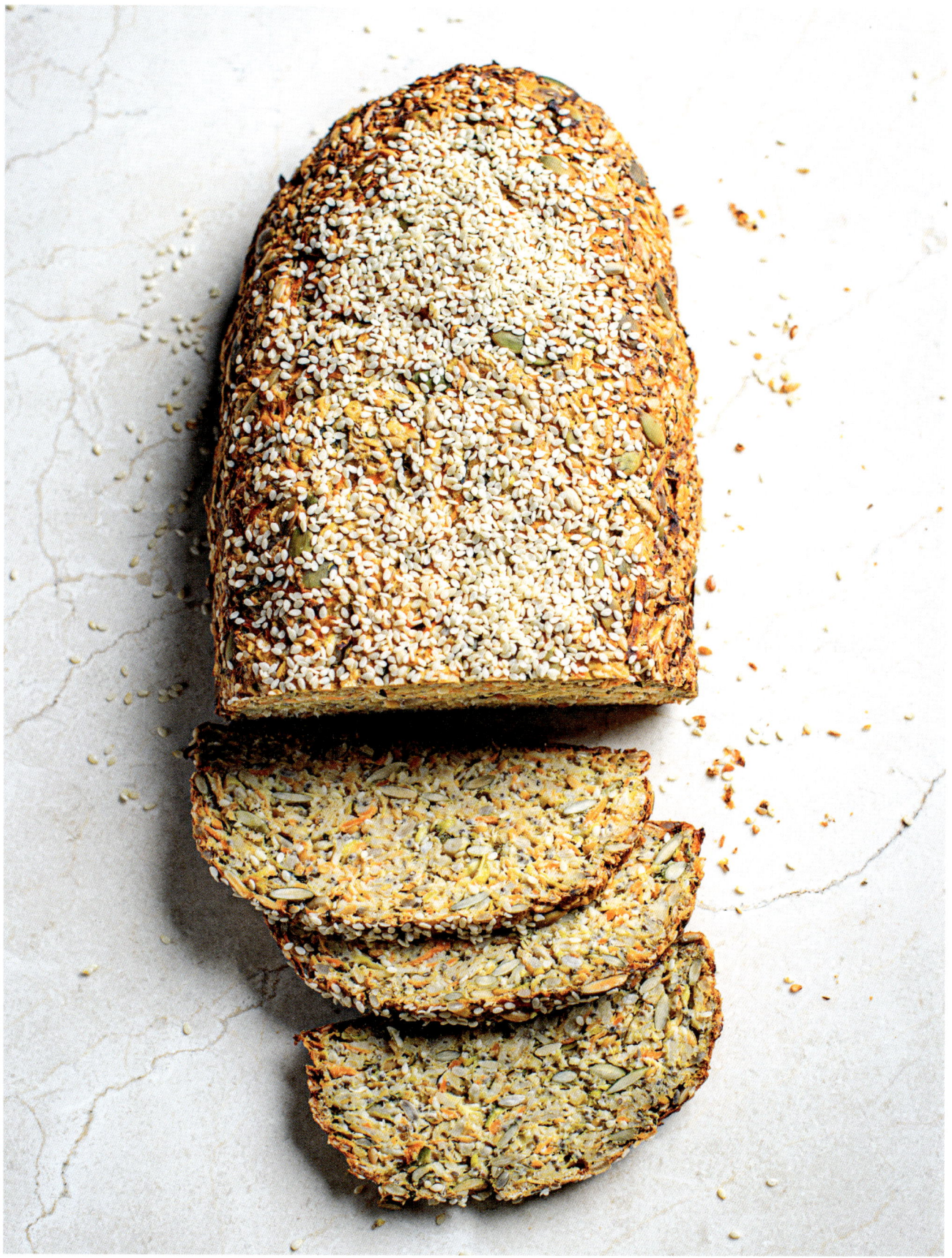

PER SLICE
PROTEIN: 7G
FIBRE: 7G
PLANT POINTS: 7.5

MAKES 18 SLICES

150g whole flaxseeds
50g chia seeds
2 tablespoons extra virgin olive oil
100g pumpkin seeds
100g sunflower seeds
75g sesame seeds
75g pistachio nuts, hazelnuts or chopped almonds
50g dried cranberries
35g psyllium husk flakes
1 teaspoon sea salt
300ml filtered water
1–2 tablespoons mixed seeds, to sprinkle (optional)

NAKED LOAF

So many people have asked me to make a loaf that is made entirely from nuts and seeds yet still tastes incredible. Always up for a challenge, this bread came about almost by accident and is the same as my Seed and Nut Loaf (page 253), but without the oats and with an adjustment to the water. Each mighty slice contains 7g of protein and 7g of fibre, which means it is a really enjoyable and simple way to top up your protein and fibre each day. I hope you enjoy it, as it tastes so delicious!

1. Put all the ingredients into a large bowl and stir thoroughly to incorporate the water. The mixture should be quite stiff.

2. Transfer the mixture to a 2lb/900g loaf tin, lined with baking parchment or a loaf tin parchment liner, and flatten the surface using the back of a wet spoon. Sprinkle over the extra seeds, if desired. Leave to sit for 30–60 minutes to allow the mixture to firm up and bind. Preheat the oven to 180°C fan.

3. Bake the loaf for 1 hour, or until golden and firm to the touch. Allow to cool completely in the tin before slicing.

Storage: Store in an airtight container for up to 5 days. Suitable for freezing for up to 2 months. Slice before freezing, separating the slices with small pieces of baking parchment.

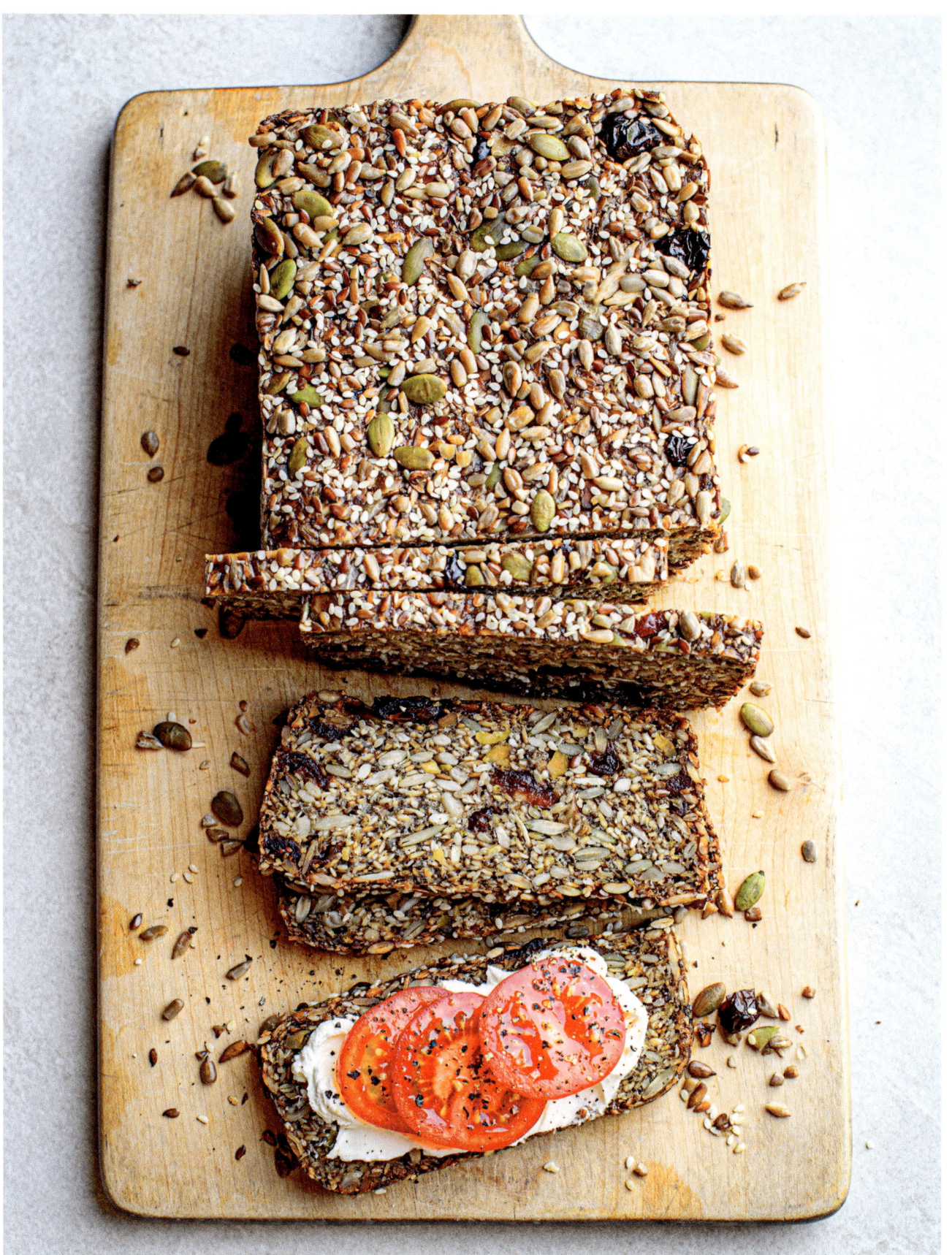

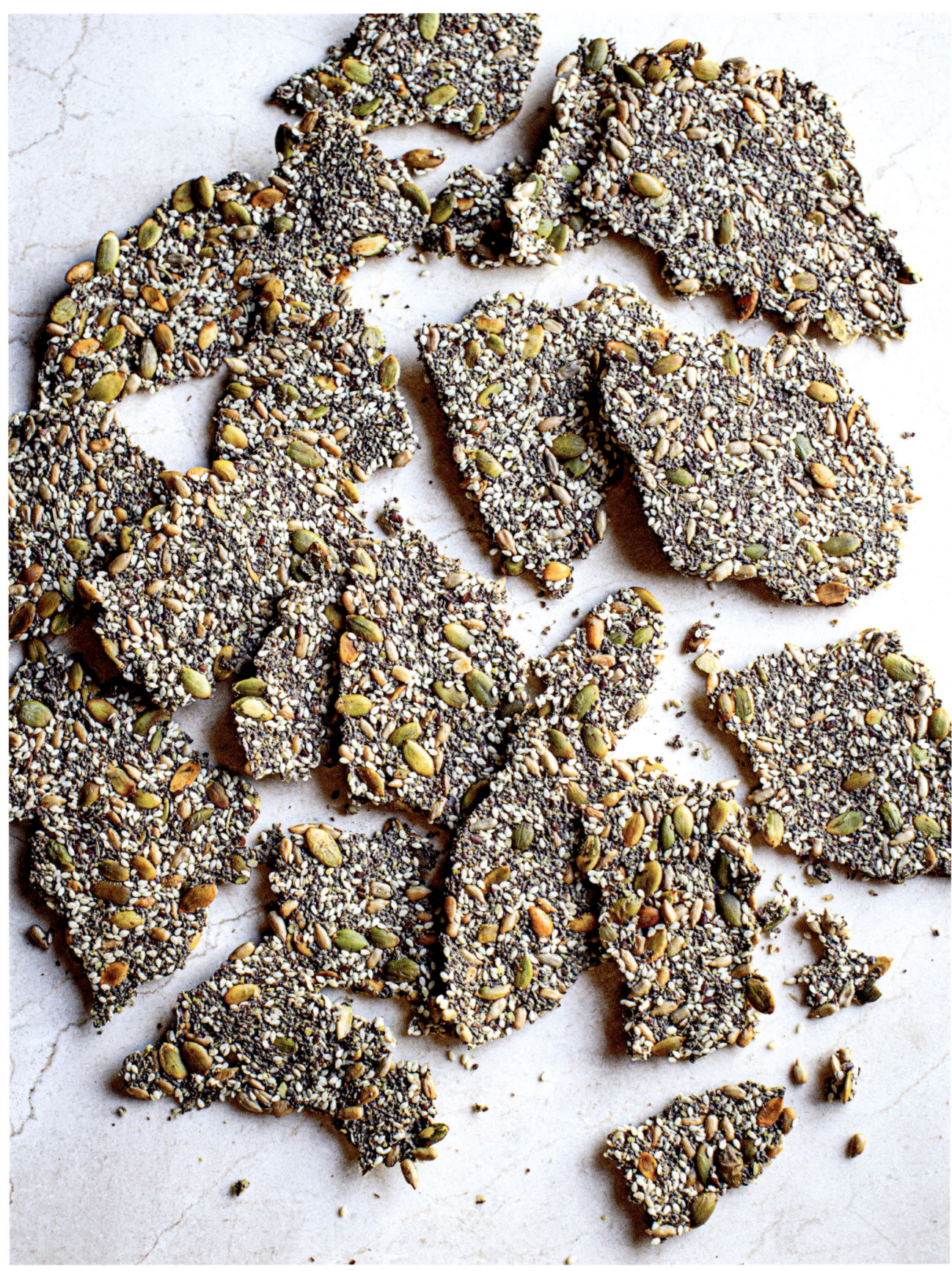

PER 30G SERVING
PROTEIN: 6G
FIBRE: 7G
PLANT POINTS: 5.25

SERVES 12
30G PER SERVING

80g milled flaxseeds
80g chia seeds
80g pumpkin seeds
80g sunflower seeds
80g sesame seeds
½ teaspoon sea salt
1 heaped teaspoon dried rosemary
250ml filtered water

ROSEMARY AND SEA SALT SEEDED CRACKERS

These crisp, seeded crackers are naturally gluten-free and packed with fibre, making them nourishing and satisfying. They are so simple to prepare at home, and bring together a variety of seeds that offer texture, flavour and plant diversity. Both the flax and chia seeds are essential to this recipe, as their high levels of soluble fibre help to bind the crackers and hold them together, but you can mix up the other seeds depending on what you have. Feel free to use different herbs to change the flavours, too.

---

1. Preheat your oven to 150°C fan. Line a large baking tray, about 45cm x 30cm, with baking parchment (or use two trays).

2. Mix all the ingredients together in a bowl and set aside for 5 minutes to allow the mixture to thicken.

3. Spoon the mixture on to the prepared tray (or trays) and either spread evenly with the back of a spoon or place another sheet of baking parchment on top and roll gently with a rolling pin, until it is around 5mm thick and 40cm x 25cm in size.

4. Bake in the preheated oven for 90 minutes. You can bake the mixture as a single sheet for a rustic finish, or alternatively, remove from the oven halfway through the cooking time and score into squares before returning to the oven.

5. Allow to cool on the tray, then either break into irregular cracker-sized pieces, or break apart along the scored lines.

Storage: Store in an airtight container for up to 4 weeks.

PER FLATBREAD
PROTEIN: 8G
FIBRE: 1G
PLANT POINTS: 0

MAKES 6

250g strong bread flour, plus extra for dusting
175g natural yoghurt (not Greek)
½ teaspoon baking powder
1 teaspoon sea salt

SIMPLE FLATBREADS

Soft and simple to prepare, these flatbreads are perfect for scooping up dips like raita and hummus (page 232 and 269–271), filling with burgers (page 242) or serving with curries (page 215). You need to use a regular yoghurt in this recipe with around 4g of protein per 100g, as Greek yoghurt makes the dough too dense and it may not rise or puff up as well when cooked. You can make these with wholemeal flour, but white flour produces a better result. I have also included a gluten-free recipe, see page 264.

1. Mix the flour, yoghurt, baking powder and salt together in a bowl until you have a rough dough. Knead on a lightly floured surface for 3–4 minutes, to develop the gluten.

2. Divide the dough into 6 equal pieces and shape each into a ball. Roll each ball out on a lightly floured surface into a circle, about 18cm in diameter.

3. Heat a heavy-based frying pan or skillet over a medium-high heat, until hot. Cook each flatbread for 1–2 minutes per side, without oil. They should puff slightly and turn light golden in colour.

Storage: Flatbreads are best eaten fresh but can be stored in an airtight container for up to 24 hours. Reheat in a dry pan or low oven. They can be frozen for up to 1 month; reheat from frozen or thaw and warm through.

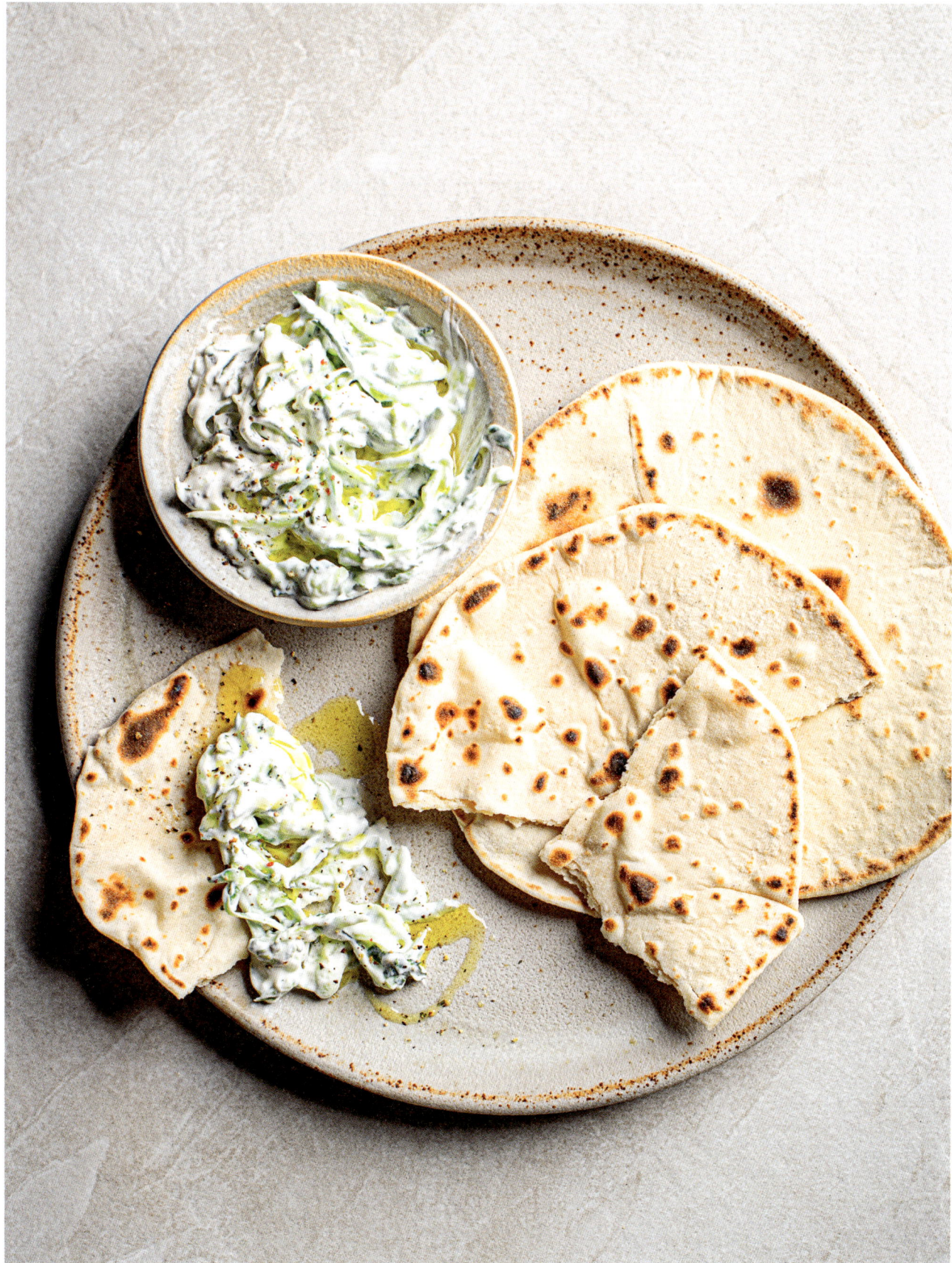

PER FLATBREAD
PROTEIN: 6G
FIBRE: 2G
PLANT POINTS: 0.25

MAKES 6

250g gluten-free self-raising flour, plus extra for dusting
225g natural yoghurt (not Greek)
15g psyllium husk flakes
1 tablespoon extra virgin olive oil
1–2 tablespoons filtered water
1 teaspoon sea salt

GLUTEN-FREE FLATBREADS

I wanted to include a gluten-free version of my flatbreads on page 262 because many people find wheat can leave them feeling bloated, or because they have a food allergy or coeliac disease. Gluten in wheat is an elastic protein that binds the wheat flour together and makes bread springy and light. It develops when the bread dough is kneaded. Psyllium husk is rich in soluble fibre, which can recreate some of this texture and helps make the flatbreads easier to roll out and cook.

---

1. Combine the gluten-free flour, yoghurt, psyllium husk flakes, extra virgin olive oil, water and salt in a bowl, or food processor, until you have a rough dough.

2. Divide the dough into 6 equal pieces and shape each into a ball. Roll each ball out on a lightly floured surface into a circle, about 18cm in diameter.

3. Heat a heavy-based frying pan or skillet over a medium-high heat, until hot. Cook each flatbread for 1–2 minutes per side without oil. They should puff up slightly and turn light golden.

Storage: Flatbreads are best eaten fresh but can be stored in an airtight container for up to 24 hours. Reheat in a dry pan or low oven. They can be frozen for up to 1 month; reheat from frozen or thaw and warm through.

PER WRAP
PROTEIN: 2G
FIBRE: 4G
PLANT POINTS: 3.25

MAKES 6

100g chickpea (gram) flour
50g baby spinach
200ml cold filtered water
1 teaspoon ground cumin
1 teaspoon ground coriander
½ teaspoon chilli powder
½ teaspoon ground turmeric
1 teaspoon sea salt
a grind of freshly ground black pepper
1 tablespoon extra virgin olive oil, plus extra for cooking

CHICKPEA PANCAKE WRAPS

Using chickpea flour to make these wraps is a nutritious alternative to regular flour. Chickpea flour contains more protein and fibre than traditional wheat flour and is gentler on our blood sugars. The wraps are deliciously simple to make and are naturally gluten-free. Chickpea flour works beautifully with a blend of different spices and these wraps really become part of the meal. Use them with the polpette (page 176) or any filling of your choice, from shredded chicken and salad to halloumi or tofu pieces.

1. Place all the ingredients in a food processor and blend at high speed until smooth. Allow the batter to rest for 15–30 minutes to thicken slightly.

2. Heat a small non-stick frying pan over a medium heat. Add a drizzle of extra virgin olive oil.

3. When the pan is hot, pour in one-sixth of the batter and swirl to coat the base. The best advice I can give is to not touch the pancake for around 2 minutes until it has completely set on top and you can see bubbles. This should allow you to easily flip the pancake over to cook the second side. Cook until lightly golden on both sides. Repeat with the rest of the batter to make 6 pancakes.

Storage: Store the cooked pancakes in an airtight container in the fridge for up to 3 days. Reheat in a dry frying pan for 1–2 minutes so they crisp up again. The batter can be kept in the fridge for up to 24 hours.

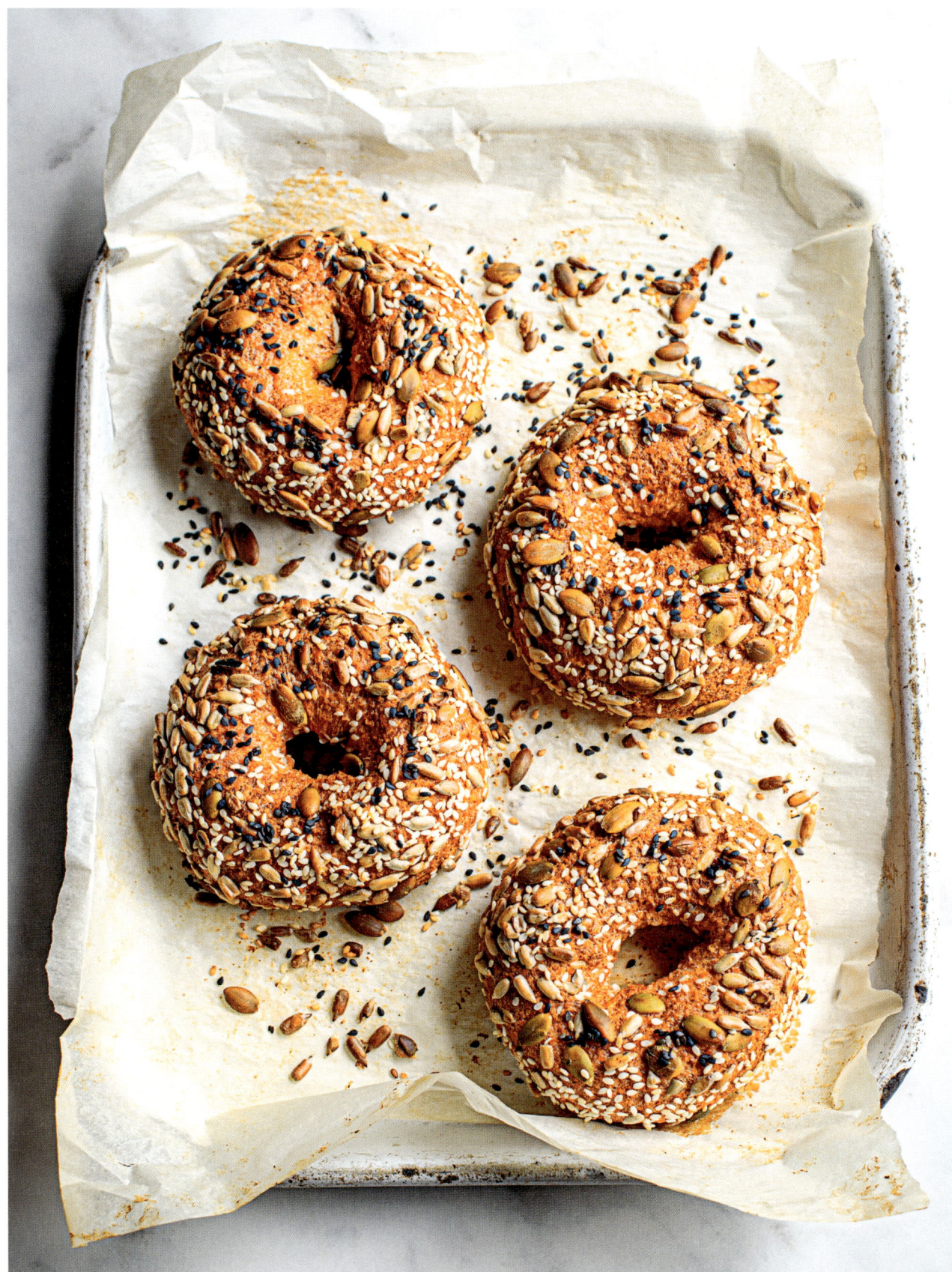

PER BAGEL
PROTEIN: 10G
FIBRE: 8G
PLANT POINTS: 3

MAKES 4

150g dried red lentils
300ml boiling water (for soaking)
100–120ml filtered water (for blending)
25g psyllium husk flakes
1 tablespoon lemon juice
1 teaspoon sea salt
1 tablespoon extra virgin olive oil
1 teaspoon baking powder
1 tablespoon mixed seeds (e.g. sunflower, pumpkin, sesame)

RED LENTIL BAGELS

I love using pulses as an alternative to flour, and this is one of my favourite recipes in the book. Red lentil bagels might sound quite adventurous, but I can assure you the results are worth it. The reason you will want to try this is because these bagels are unprocessed and are naturally high in protein and fibre. With 10g protein and 8g fibre per bagel, they are a fantastic way to help meet your daily goals. And they go with everything! I regularly serve them with salads and soups – or try them with smoked salmon and quark for my take on a classic New York-style breakfast (page 128).

Psyllium husk plays a key role here, binding the dough in a similar way to the gluten in wheat, and it is also a source of soluble fibre to feed the gut microbiome. Use whole psyllium husk flakes if possible, as these are lighter in texture and colour than psyllium powder.

---

1. Put the red lentils in a heatproof bowl and cover with the boiling water. Once cooled, leave to soak, covered, in the fridge for at least 8 hours or overnight.

2. Preheat the oven to 200°C fan and line a baking tray with non-stick baking parchment.

3. Drain and rinse the lentils in a fine-meshed sieve, then place in a food processor with half of the blending water.

4. Add the psyllium husk flakes, lemon juice, salt and extra virgin olive oil. Blend until the mixture begins to form a dough.

5. Add the remaining water slowly. I usually need the full 120ml, but yours may need less or even a dash more. The amount of water you need can vary greatly depending on how long the lentils were soaked and how much water they absorbed. The dough should be a soft Play-Doh consistency. Not too hard, or they won't rise properly, and not so soft that you cannot handle them. It should be slightly sticky to touch.

6. Lastly, add the baking powder. I add this at the end, as it will start to 'fizz' too soon if it comes into contact with the acidic lemon juice. I want the baking powder to raise the bagels in the oven and not in the processor. Pulse together again to combine.

Recipe continues overleaf

RED LENTIL BAGELS *CONTINUED*

7. Pour your mixed seeds onto a plate. Divide the dough into four portions, roll into balls, and dip one side into the mixed seeds. Flatten the balls onto the lined baking tray, seed side up. Use the end of a wooden spoon handle to create a generous hole in the centre of each one (make the hole larger than you think, as it will shrink slightly during baking).

8. Bake for 25–28 minutes, until golden on the outside, well risen, and cooked through. Keep a close eye on them! The crust should be firm to the touch. Allow to cool before serving.

Storage: Store in an airtight container for up to 3 days. Or, freeze and consume within 1 month; defrost, slice and toast.

PER SERVING
PROTEIN: 4G
FIBRE: 4G
PLANT POINTS: 3

SERVES 6

1 x 400g tin or jar of chickpeas, rinsed and drained (240g drained weight)
2 garlic cloves
2 tablespoons tahini paste
2 tablespoons extra virgin olive oil
1 tablespoon lemon juice
1 scant teaspoon sea salt
3 tablespoons cold filtered water

To serve
1 teaspoon sweet paprika
a swirl of extra virgin olive oil

NO-FRILLS HUMMUS

I deliberated whether to include this recipe, but sometimes we just want to be led back to basics so that we can put our own twist on a very classic recipe. I always like to have some hummus in the fridge to use as a side dish to my salads or even with chicken, or for dipping vegetable sticks or spreading on my Rosemary and Sea Salt Seeded Crackers (page 261) as a snack for guests to nibble on. I have included two variations: Avocado Hummus (page 270) and Roasted Beetroot Hummus with Brazil Nuts (page 271) – they are both beautifully coloured and delicious, but get creative and have a go at your own versions, too.

1. Put the chickpeas, garlic, tahini, extra virgin olive oil, lemon juice and salt into the bowl of a food processor and process at a medium speed until well combined.

2. Add the cold water slowly until the hummus reaches the perfect consistency – you may not need it all, but note that it will thicken up a little in the fridge.

3. Transfer to a bowl and sprinkle over the paprika and drizzle with extra virgin olive oil, to serve.

Option: To make the hummus into a show-stopper dip, dice 3 carrots and mix with some cumin seeds and 1 tablespoon of extra virgin olive oil. Roast in the oven at 200°C fan for 20–25 minutes, or in an air fryer at 190°C for 12–15 minutes. Top the hummus with the carrots and drizzle over some more extra virgin olive oil.

Storage: Store in an airtight container in the fridge for up to 3 days.

PER SERVING
PROTEIN: 6G
FIBRE: 6G
PLANT POINTS: 5

SERVES 6

100g frozen edamame beans
1 x 400g tin or jar of chickpeas, rinsed and drained (240g drained weight)
1 garlic clove
1 avocado
1 large tablespoon tahini paste (20g)
2 tablespoons extra virgin olive oil
1 tablespoon lemon juice
½ teaspoon sea salt

To serve
avocado slices or cooked edamame beans (optional)

AVOCADO HUMMUS

Adding avocado to hummus makes it extra creamy and also increases the fibre, while the edamame beans give it a lovely green colour and a milder flavour. This avocado hummus works well with chicken, fish, falafels, in a wrap, on a salad or with flatbreads (page 262 and 264).

---

1. Simmer the edamame beans in a pan of water for 3 minutes. Drain, then run cold water over them to cool. Drain well.

2. Put all the ingredients into a food processor and process for around 60 seconds, until smooth and combined.

3. Spoon into a serving bowl and top with a few avocado slices or freshly cooked edamame beans, if you like.

Storage: Store in an airtight container in the fridge for up to 3 days.

PER SERVING
PROTEIN: 4G
FIBRE: 4G
PLANT POINTS: 4.25

SERVES 6
500g raw beetroot
 (or 250g cooked beetroot
 if short on time)
3 tablespoons extra virgin
 olive oil, plus extra swirl
 to serve
1 teaspoon cumin seeds
 (or ground cumin if using
 pre-cooked beetroot)
a pinch of chilli flakes
1 x 400g tin or jar of chickpeas,
 rinsed and drained
 (240g drained weight)
2 garlic cloves
25g Brazil nuts
2 tablespoons lemon juice
sea salt and freshly ground
 black pepper
30ml cold filtered water

ROASTED BEETROOT HUMMUS WITH BRAZIL NUTS

Beetroots are relatively inexpensive and really are one of nature's superfoods. They are packed with antioxidants as well as fibre, folate (vitamin B9) and magnesium. But best of all, alongside their earthy flavour, they give a vibrant colour to our food. I have used Brazil nuts in this hummus as they are one of the richest natural sources of selenium, a mineral that plays a vital role in the production and metabolism of thyroid hormones. You can also cheat if you are short of time and use ready-cooked beetroot, but preferably without vinegar or sugar. Serve as a dip, a side dish, on sourdough bread or any of my breads, or with vegetable crudites.

---

1. Preheat the oven to 180°C fan. Wash, peel and dice the beetroot.

2. Combine the beetroot with 1 tablespoon of the extra virgin olive oil, the cumin seeds and chilli flakes in a baking dish. Cook for 25–30 minutes until tender. Allow to cool.

3. When cool, put the beetroot, chickpeas, garlic, Brazil nuts, remaining 2 tablespoons of olive oil and the lemon juice in a food processor (with the ground cumin, if using pre-cooked beetroot). Season with salt and pepper and process until smooth, vibrant and creamy. Add cold water to reach the correct consistency.

4. Transfer to a bowl and drizzle with a little more extra virgin olive oil, to serve.

Storage: Store in an airtight container in the fridge for up to 3 days.

PER 2 MUFFINS
PROTEIN: 15G
FIBRE: 2G
PLANT POINTS: 3

MAKES 8

1 tablespoon extra virgin olive oil
1 small bunch of red or green spring onions, finely chopped
1 red pepper, finely diced
1 yellow pepper, finely diced
4 eggs
200g cottage cheese
40g Parmesan (or vegetarian hard cheese) or Cheddar, grated
2 tablespoons freshly chopped herbs or 2 teaspoons dried herbs (e.g. parsley, chives, dill or basil), plus more to serve (optional)
sea salt and freshly ground black pepper

EGG MUFFINS

A couple of these mini egg muffins is a perfect example of a healthy, organised snack, ideal for times when meals are spaced too far apart – and they are great for packing up and taking with you. Served with crunchy crudités, they also make a balanced breakfast option the whole family can enjoy! The addition of cottage cheese boosts the protein content while adding moisture and texture. You can easily customise this recipe with other cheeses such as crumbled feta or grated Gruyère instead of the Parmesan or Cheddar. You can also vary the vegetables to suit your taste or to use up leftovers.

---

1. Preheat the oven to 180°C fan. Heat the extra virgin olive oil in a frying pan over a medium heat. Sauté the spring onions and peppers for 3–4 minutes, until softened. Remove from the heat.

2. In a bowl, whisk the eggs and stir in the cottage cheese, grated Parmesan or Cheddar and the herbs. Season with salt and pepper.

3. Line an 8-hole metal muffin tray with paper muffin cases. Alternatively, use a non-stick silicone muffin tray placed on a solid baking sheet for stability.

4. Divide the cooked vegetables evenly between the muffin moulds and pour the egg mixture over the top. Bake for 20 minutes, or until puffed up and set through.

5. Leave to cool a little before serving. Scatter over some extra fresh herbs, if you like.

Storage: Store an airtight container in the fridge for up to 2 days. Reheat in the oven at 180°C for 8–10 minutes, or in an air fryer at 160°C for 5 minutes.

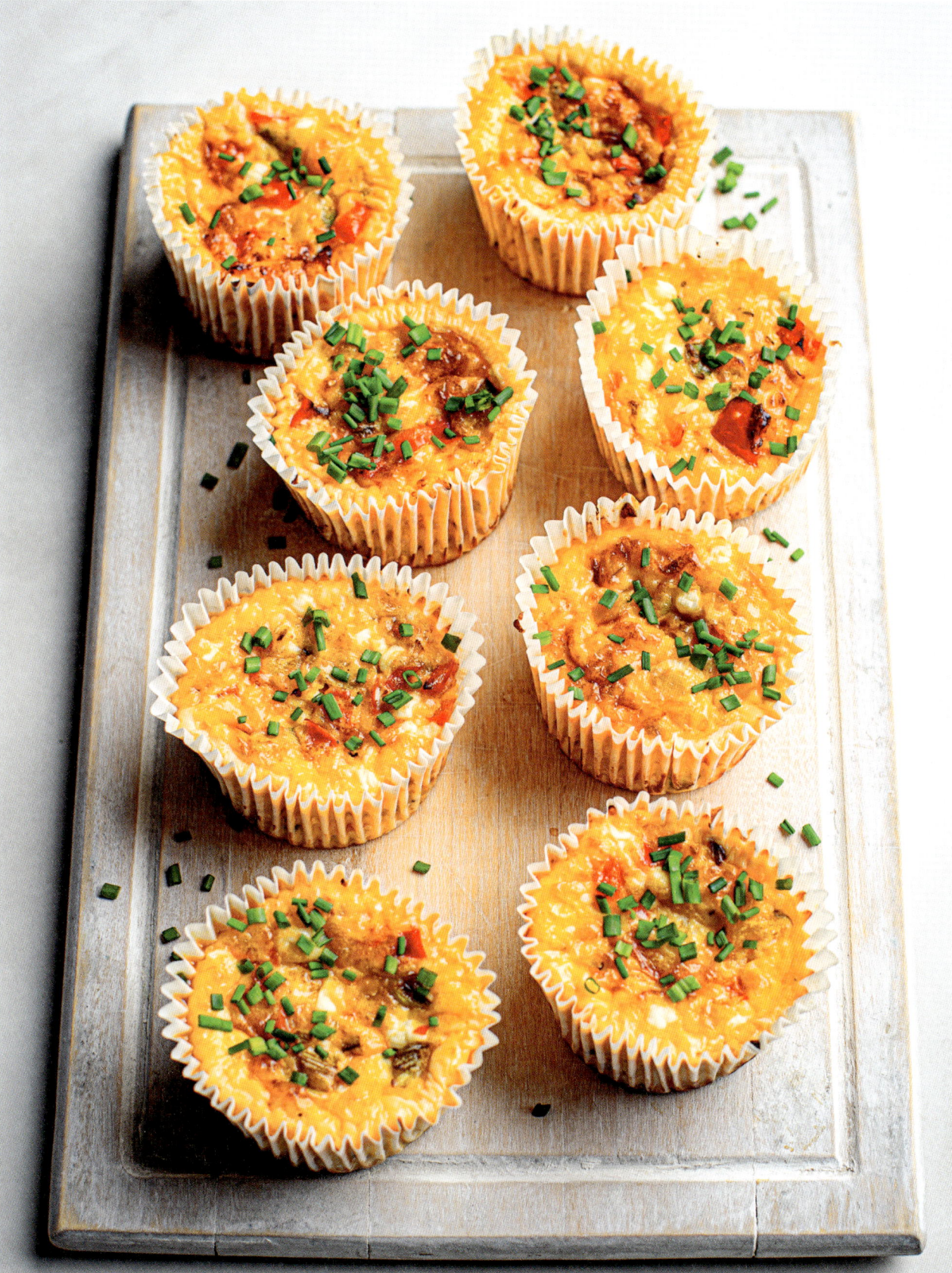

PER SQUARE
PROTEIN: 9G
FIBRE: 4G
PLANT POINTS: 9.5

MAKES 16 SQUARES

150g gluten-free (or regular) rolled oats
200g carrots, grated
1 red onion, finely diced
1 large apple, grated
3 medium eggs
175g Parmesan (or vegetarian hard cheese), finely grated
50g chia seeds
50g pumpkin seeds
50g sunflower seeds
80g walnuts, roughly chopped
50g whole or milled flaxseeds
1 level teaspoon ground turmeric

Topping (optional)
2 tablespoons mixed seeds, for sprinkling

APPLE, CARROT AND WALNUT FLAPJACKS

Savoury flapjacks are a healthier, sugar-free way to enjoy a flapjack. These flapjack squares are great on their own, served with a soup or salad, as part of a picnic, or in your lunchbox. The seeds increase the nutrients and plant points, and the apple and carrot also keep them moist. I have used Parmesan, but this recipe works well with a mix of grated halloumi (100g) and Parmesan (75g) too, if you fancy a change.

1. Preheat the oven to 180°C fan. Put all the ingredients into a bowl and mix well. The mixture should be light and slightly moist.

2. Line an ovenproof dish, around 20cm x 20cm, with baking parchment and press the mixture in firmly. Smooth over the top using the back of a spoon.

3. Sprinkle the extra seeds on top, if you like, and bake for 45 minutes, or until golden and crisp.

4. Allow to fully cool in the dish before slicing into squares.

Storage: Store in an airtight container in the fridge for up to 4 days. Suitable for freezing. Defrost and enjoy at room temperature, or reheat in a warm oven or air fryer at 180°C for 4–5 minutes.

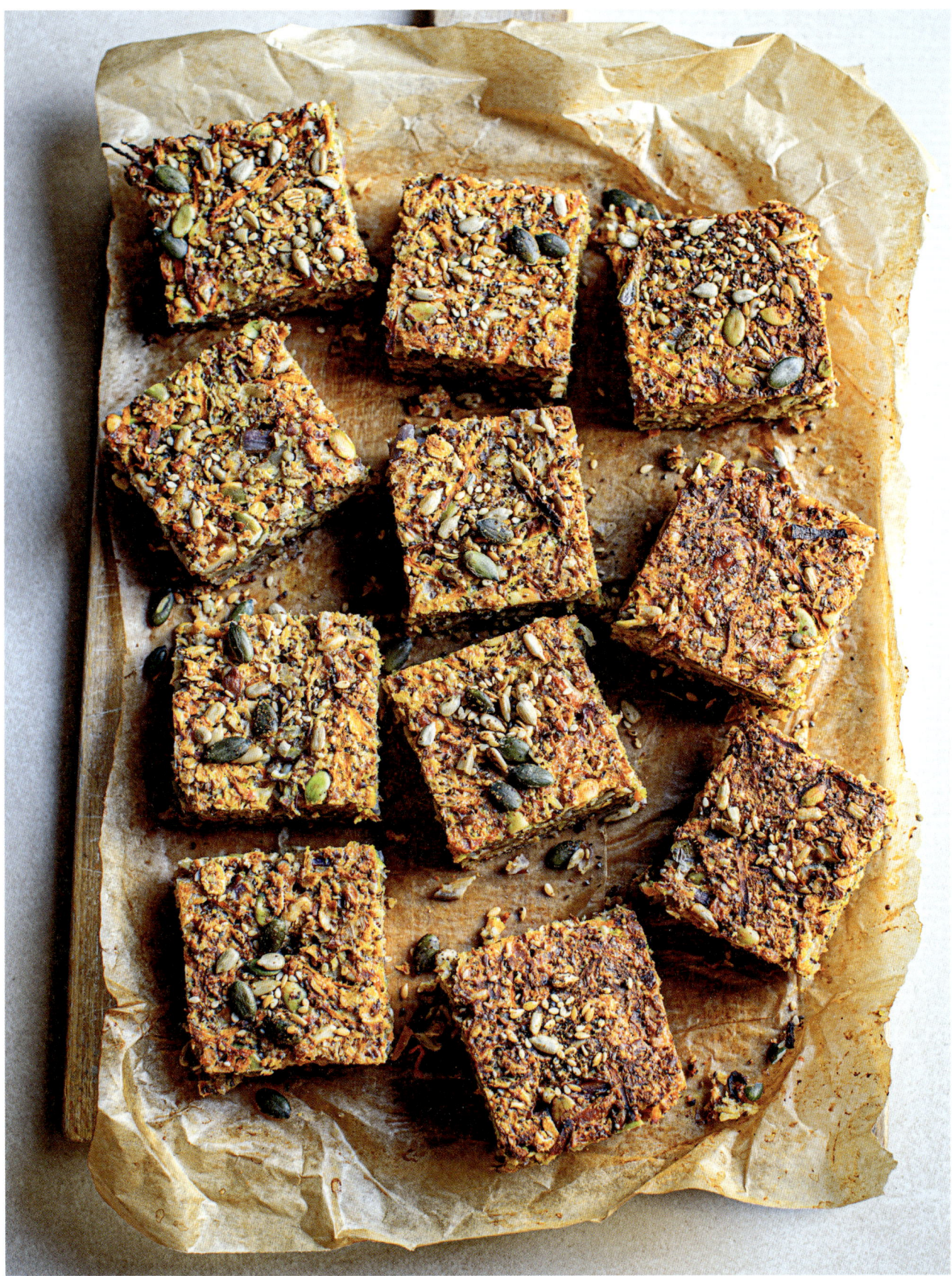

PER SERVING
PROTEIN: 7G
FIBRE: 4G
PLANT POINTS: 1.75

SERVES 4

1 tablespoon tamari or soy sauce (Note, soy sauce isn't gluten-free)
10ml toasted sesame oil
1 garlic clove, crushed
a pinch of chilli flakes
200g frozen edamame beans, defrosted

CRISPY EDAMAME BEANS

Roasted edamame beans are a high-protein, high-fibre snack and a much healthier alternative to crisps. Edamame beans are naturally low in carbohydrates and rich in plant protein (around 13g per 100g) as well as fibre (around 8g per 100g), and they also contain key nutrients such as magnesium, calcium and iron. A 100g serving of edamame contains just 124 kcals, compared to over 500 kcals for the same weight of standard crisps. Experiment with different ways of seasoning your edamame – try using other flavourings such as fajita, harissa or curry spice mix. The beans taste best eaten soon after roasting.

---

1. Preheat the oven to 180°C fan and line a baking tray with baking parchment.

2. Combine the tamari or soy sauce, toasted sesame oil, garlic and chilli flakes in a bowl. Add the edamame beans and stir well to coat.

3. Spread the mixture in an even layer on the lined baking tray and bake for 35–45 minutes, stirring halfway through the cooking time, until golden and crispy. Alternatively, put the mixture into an air-fryer basket in a single layer. Cook for 12–15 minutes at 200°C, shaking the basket halfway through, until golden and crispy.

4. Serve warm as a snack.

Serving alternative: These can also be sprinkled over salads or soups as a high-protein, high-fibre topping.

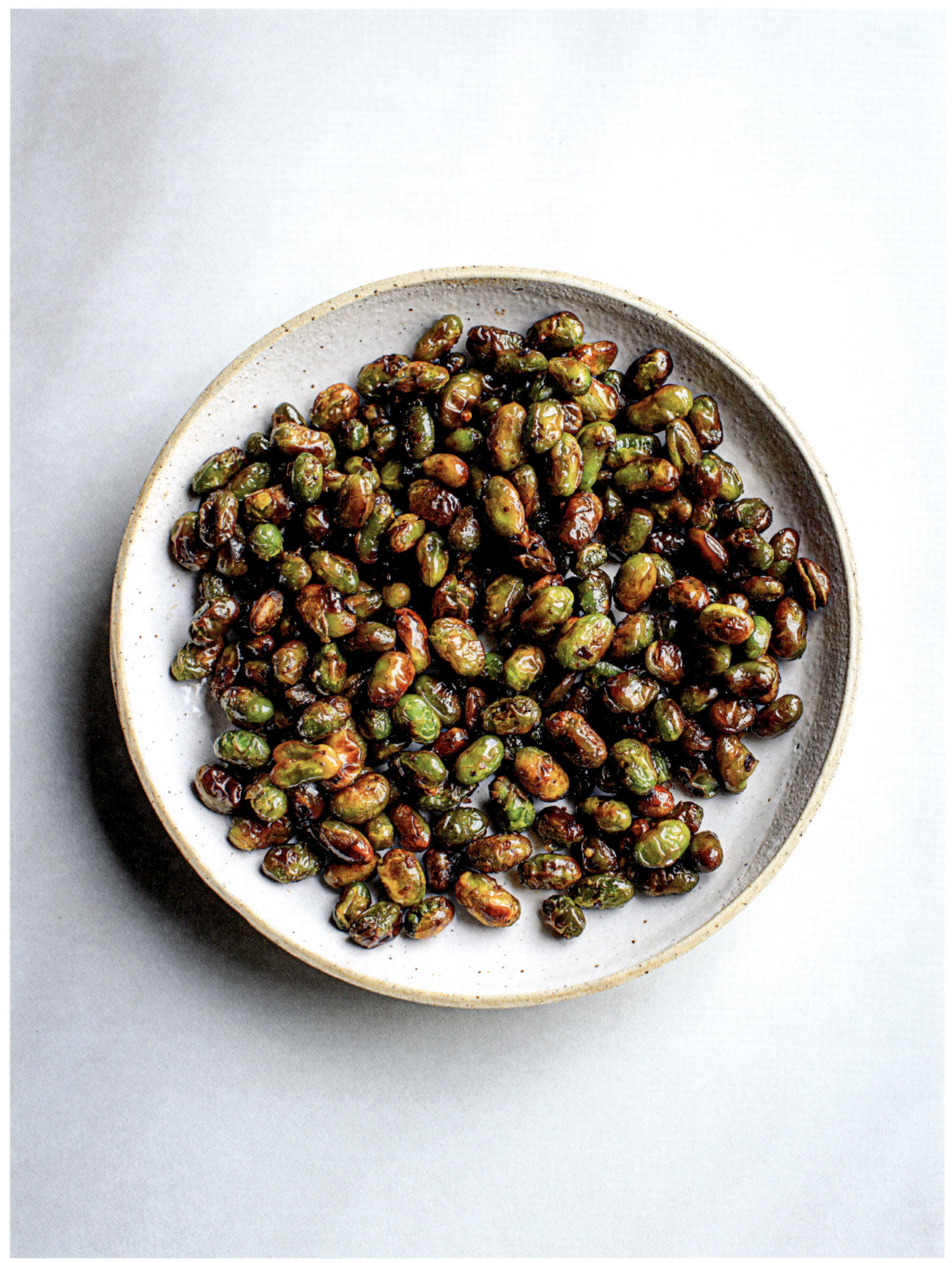

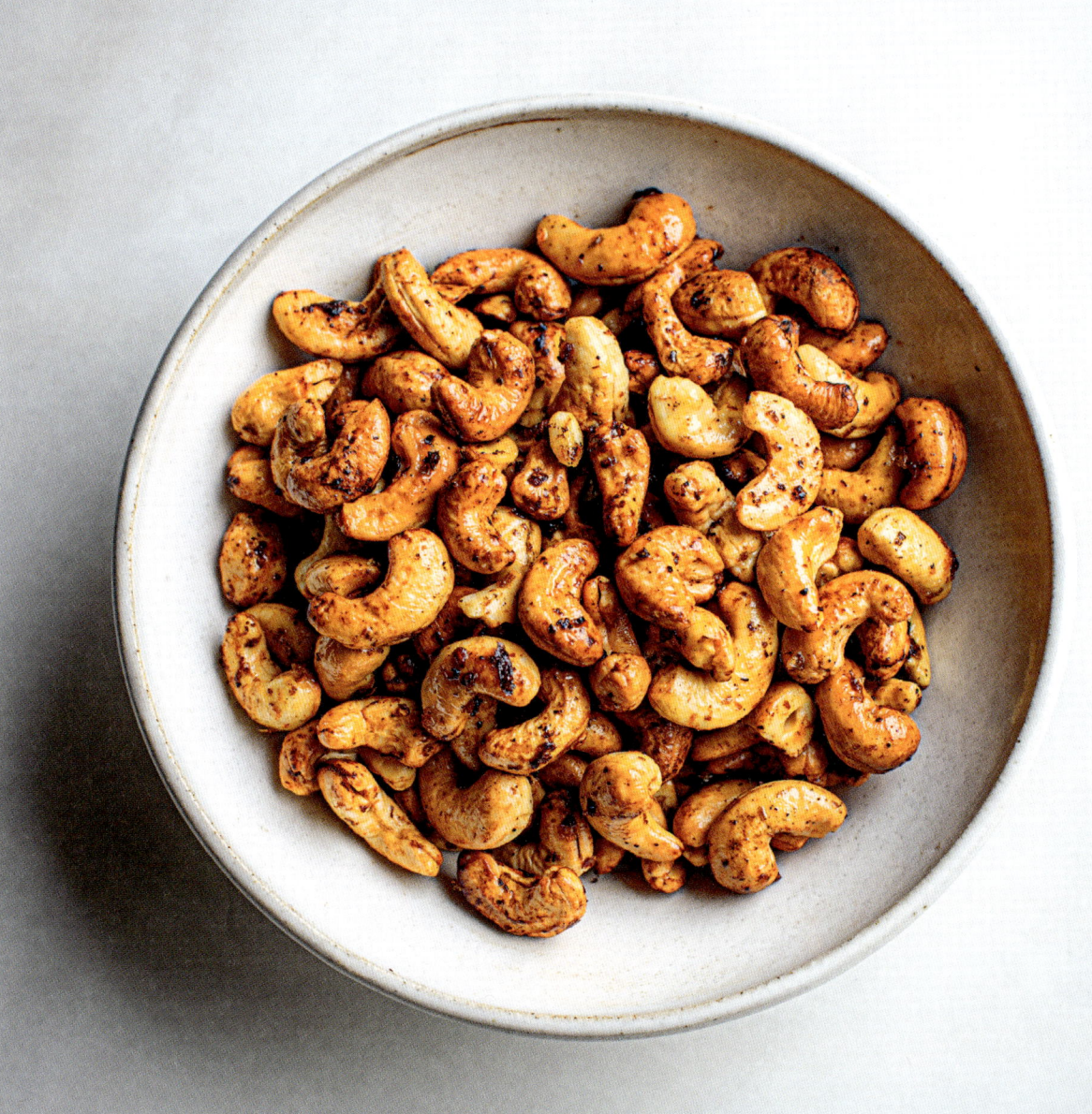

PER SERVING
PROTEIN: 4G
FIBRE: 1G
PLANT POINTS: 2.5

SERVES 8

200g raw cashew nuts
zest and juice of 1 lime
1 teaspoon extra virgin olive oil
a pinch of chilli flakes
¼ teaspoon sea salt

CHILLI AND LIME CASHEWS

This savoury treat offers a satisfying crunch, with zesty lime and warming chilli. Cashew nuts are a rich source of heart-friendly fats as well as magnesium and iron, making them a smarter snack. Using an air fryer allows for a quicker cook time while intensifying the flavour, but I have also given alternative instructions for cooking in the oven. This protein-rich snack is great for lunchboxes and for serving to guests while they are waiting for their main meal.

1. Put the cashew nuts into a bowl and add the lime juice and zest, extra virgin olive oil, chilli flakes and salt. Stir well to coat evenly.

2. Transfer the mixture to an air-fryer basket in a single layer. Cook at 180°C for 5–6 minutes until golden, crisp and fragrant, shaking the basket once halfway through to ensure even roasting. Alternatively, preheat the oven to 180°C fan and line a baking tray with baking parchment. Spread the coated cashews in a single layer on the prepared tray and bake for 10–12 minutes, stirring once, until lightly golden and crisp.

Storage: Cool completely and store in an airtight container at room temperature for up to 1 week.

PER COOKIE
PROTEIN: 6G
FIBRE: 3G
PLANT POINTS: 2

MAKES 12 COOKIES

275g good quality crunchy peanut butter
80–100g maple syrup, depending on how sweet you like them
1 teaspoon vanilla extract or paste
a pinch of sea salt
50g dark chocolate chips, above 70% cacao solids if possible (check they don't contain milk if you want the cookies to be dairy-free)

CHOCOLATE CHIP PEANUT COOKIES

These cookies are perfect if you like to keep things simple, with minimal fuss and ingredients. They are free from flour so are naturally gluten- and wheat-free, and if you choose a dairy-free dark chocolate, they can also be vegan. For me, cookies need to be soft and chewy, and this recipe delivers on both taste and texture. When using so few ingredients, quality really matters, so try to use a peanut butter that is soft and creamy rather than firm and set. I buy my peanut butter in large tubs that contain just one ingredient – peanuts. These cookies keep better in the fridge, to avoid them becoming too crumbly. You can swap the peanut butter for almond butter if you prefer.

1. Preheat the oven to 180°C fan and line a baking sheet with baking parchment.

2. Put the peanut butter, maple syrup, vanilla and salt into a food processor or a large bowl, and blend until well combined and the mixture forms a dough. Stir through the chocolate chips.

3. Divide the mixture into 12 equal pieces. Roll each piece into a ball, place them on the lined baking sheet, and flatten slightly with your hand or the back of a fork.

4. Bake for 7–8 minutes, or until just cooked and beginning to colour. You want them to stay soft, so watch the timer and don't overcook them. Allow them to cool fully, then transfer to a jar.

Storage: Store the cookies in an airtight container in the fridge for up to 1 week.

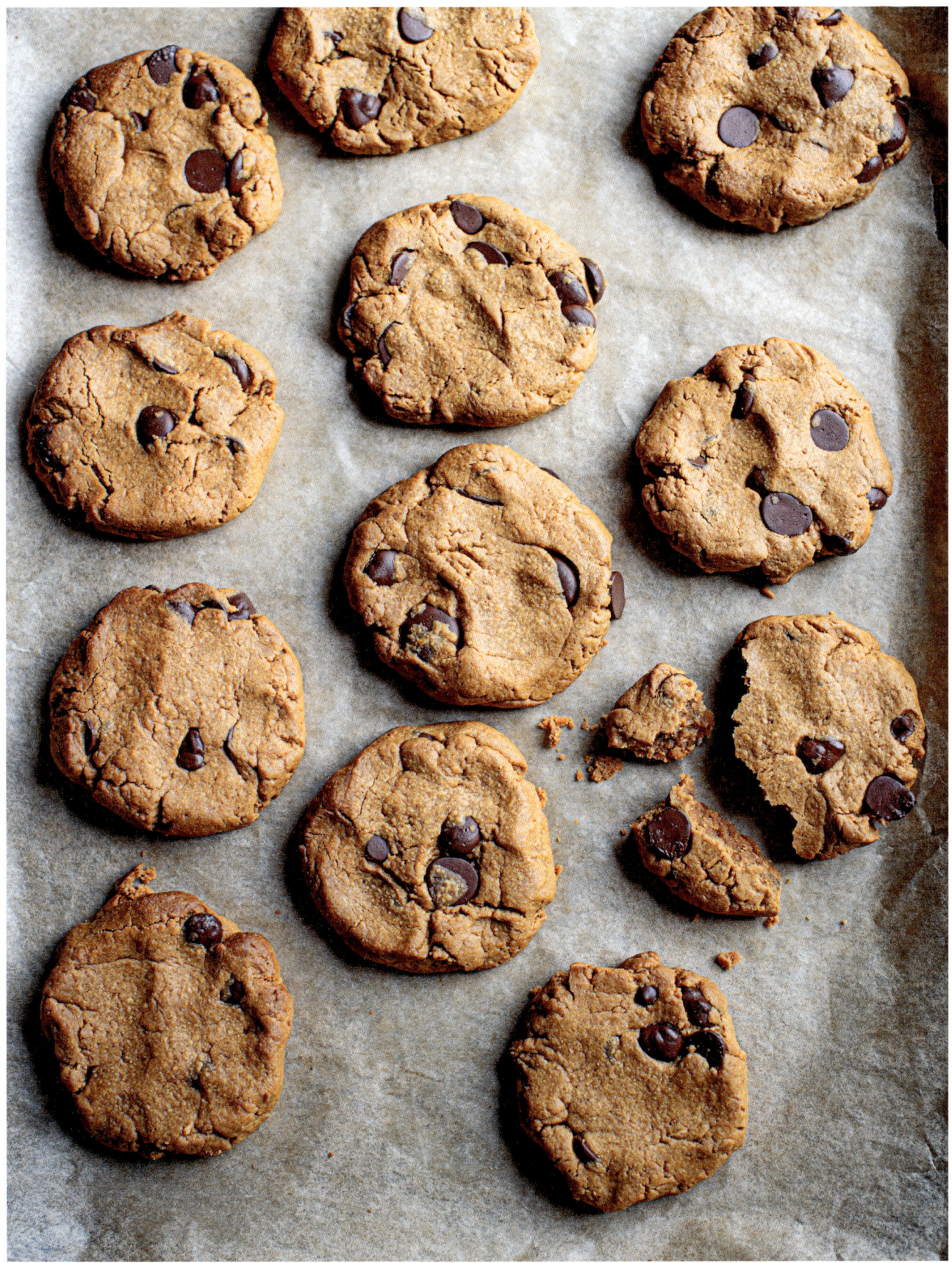

PER BAR
PROTEIN: 4G
FIBRE: 4G
PLANT POINTS: 4

MAKES 10 BARS

Base
75g gluten-free (or regular) rolled oats
75g ground almonds
a pinch of sea salt
40g butter, melted

Caramel
200g Medjool dates
120g almond butter
30–50ml almond milk
a pinch of sea salt

Topping
150g dark chocolate (check it doesn't contain milk if you want the bars to be dairy-free)
sea salt flakes

SALTED CARAMEL BARS

Delicious salted caramel bars are the perfect sweet treat. These ones contain just a handful of ingredients, and taste so much more indulgent than a shop-bought chocolate bar. I'm pretty sure they will become a firm favourite once you have tried them. I cut mine into slices and keep them in my freezer, ready for when I need something sweet after my lunch. It is best to use Medjool dates, which are naturally soft and gooey and lend themselves beautifully to the caramel layer in this recipe. To make the bars plant-based, swap the butter for a mild-flavoured oil, such as avocado oil.

1. To make the base layer, pulse the oats, ground almonds and salt in a food processor until the mixture resembles fine crumbs. Add the melted butter and pulse again. The mixture should stick together easily – if it doesn't, add a teaspoon of water and pulse again.

2. Line a 2lb/900g loaf tin with baking parchment or a loaf tin parchment liner, and press the mixture firmly into the base. Use the back of a spoon to smooth and flatten. A loaf tin works well, as it keeps the bars thick and satisfying, rather than thin and brittle. Place the tin in the freezer for 30 minutes to help the base firm up.

3. While it is chilling, put the dates, almond butter, almond milk and salt into a food processor. Blend until very smooth and caramel-like in texture. Spoon the caramel evenly over the chilled base and level with the back of a spoon. Freeze for 3–4 hours, until fully set.

4. Remove from the freezer and slice into 10 bars with a sharp knife. For easier slicing, warm the blade in hot water first and wipe dry.

5. Break the chocolate into a heatproof bowl and melt it gently over a pan of simmering water, making sure the bottom of the bowl doesn't touch the hot water. When fully melted, use a fork to dip each bar into it to completely coat on all sides. Place on a sheet of baking parchment immediately. The chocolate should set quickly if the bars are still sufficiently chilled. Drizzle over any remaining melted chocolate and decorate with sea salt flakes.

Storage: Store in an airtight container in the fridge for up to 10 days, or freeze for up to 3 months. Enjoy cold from the fridge or slightly thawed.

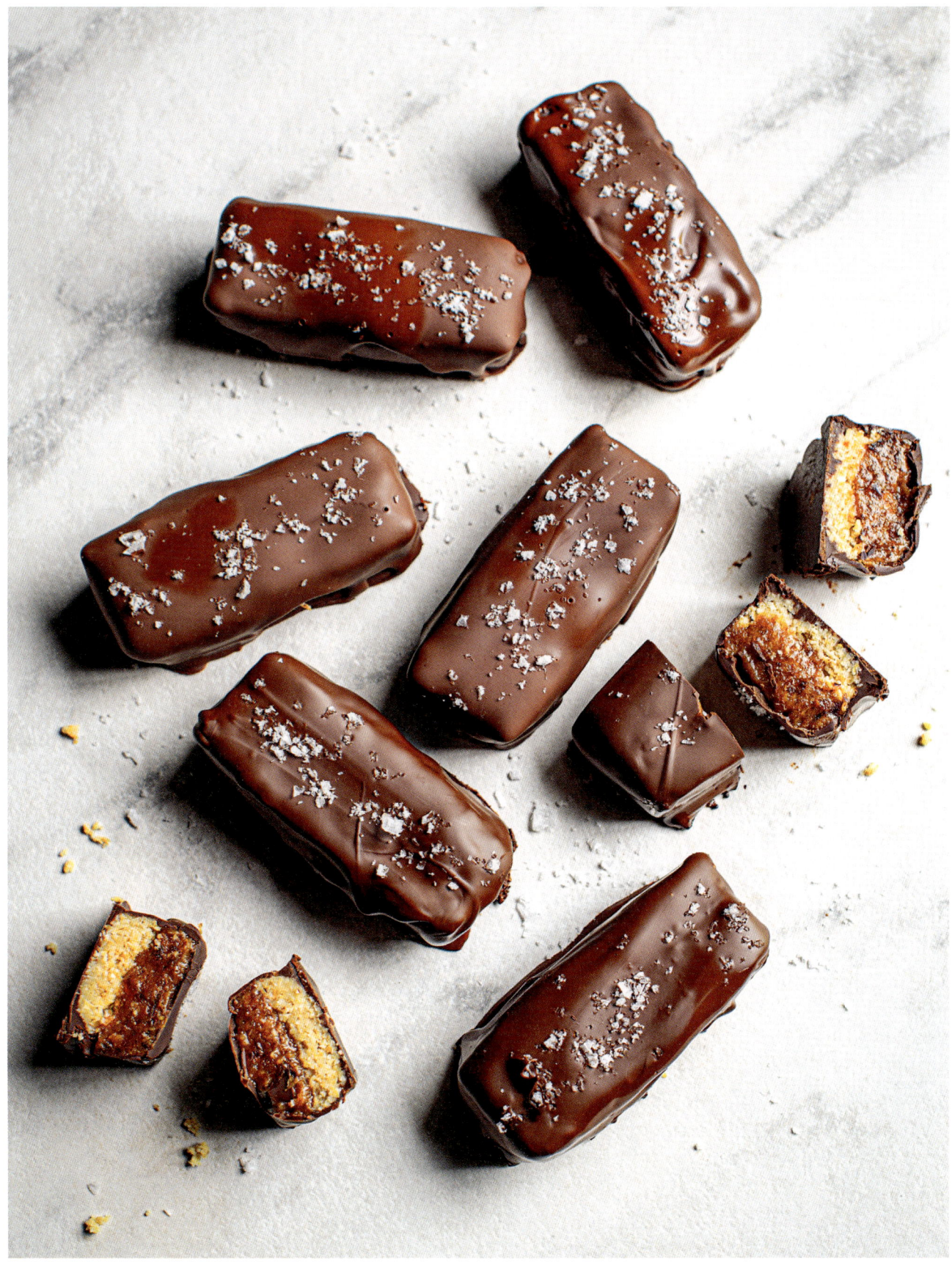

PER SQUARE
PROTEIN: 3G
FIBRE: 2G
PLANT POINTS: 2

MAKES 12 SQUARES

100g dark chocolate, at least 70% cocoa solids or, even better, 85% (check it doesn't contain milk if you want the fudge to be dairy-free)
120g tahini (or any nut butter)

Topping
a little extra tahini for swirling
sea salt flakes (optional)

TWO-INGREDIENT CHOCOLATE FUDGE

This rich and silky chocolate fudge is made with just two ingredients: dark chocolate and tahini. Tahini is made from ground sesame seeds and adds an earthy flavour. Sesame seeds are one of the richest plant sources of calcium available, making them a great addition to our diet. The tahini should not be too runny, so choose a more set one if you have a choice. You can replace the tahini with any nut butter, such as peanut or almond butter, if you prefer. The fudge comes together in minutes and sets to a satisfyingly creamy texture. I like to make it in squares, but you can also use an ice cube tray or heart-shaped silicone moulds for individual treats.

1. Line a 2lb/900g loaf tin with baking parchment or a loaf tin parchment liner. Break the chocolate into a heatproof bowl and melt it gently over a pan of simmering water, making sure the bottom of the bowl doesn't touch the hot water. Once fully melted, take off the heat and stir in the tahini, mixing well until combined. Pour the mixture into the lined tin.

2. Swirl in some extra tahini using the handle of a spoon and refrigerate for a couple of hours, until fully set.

3. Cut into 12 squares and sprinkle with sea salt flakes, if using.

Storage: Keep the fudge squares in an airtight container in the fridge, especially on warm days, as the chocolate can soften at room temperature. They will last for up to 3–5 days.

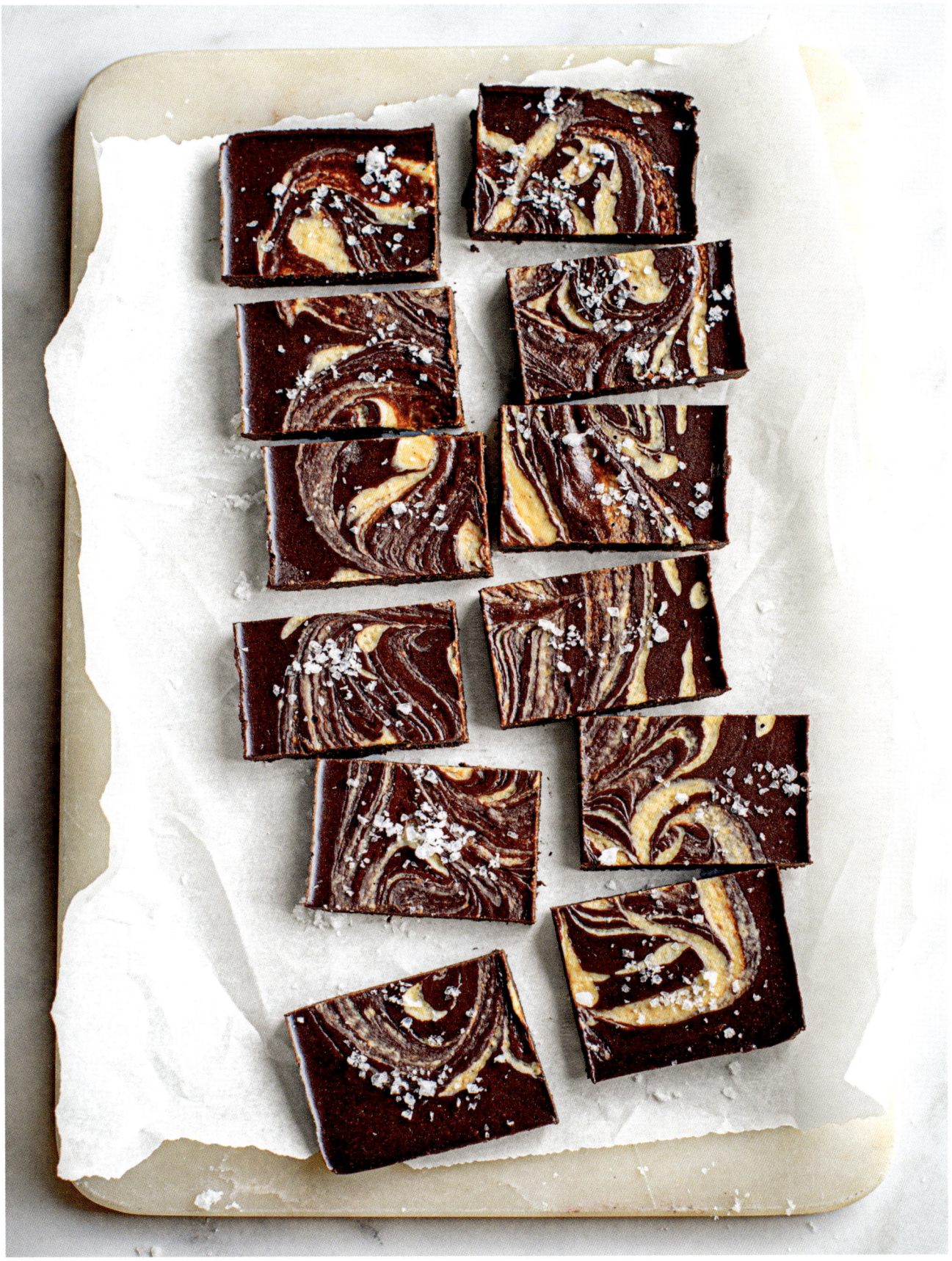

PER SERVING
PROTEIN: 1G
FIBRE: 5G
PLANT POINTS: 2.25

SERVES 2

2 pears, halved and cored
100ml filtered water
100g blueberries, frozen
4 star anise, dried

To serve
a dash of maple syrup, if required
dried blueberry, acai or pitaya powder (optional)

SPICED POACHED PEARS

This recipe came about when I was looking for a dessert for a dinner party. I wanted to create something light that would feel like a treat to end the meal, but was also a healthy option. The star anise really lifts the flavour of the pears, and the blueberries give it just a hint of blush. It even works as a breakfast with yoghurt! Frozen blueberries work particularly well in this recipe, as the freezing process breaks down the cell walls so that they release their colour (anthocyanins) more readily. The poached pears are delicious on their own, but you can also serve them with Greek yoghurt (although this will, of course, not be dairy-free).

1. Place the pears cut-side down in a frying pan. Add the water, blueberries and star anise, then cover with a lid and cook over a medium-low heat for 10 minutes. The pears will cook in the steam, so make sure the hob is on a low heat and the water is not bubbling. Use a spoon to keep covering the pears in the sauce so that they take on some of the lovely colour from the blueberries.

2. Serve warm or allow to cool. Drizzle with a little maple syrup if required, and sprinkle with a little dried berry powder or pitaya powder for an extra splash of colour, if you wish. Serve on their own or with Greek yoghurt.

Storage: Store any leftovers in an airtight container in the fridge for up to 2 days.

PER FLORENTINE
PROTEIN: 4G
FIBRE: 2G
PLANT POINTS: 6

MAKES 12
80g flaked almonds
150g mixed nuts and seeds (e.g. sunflower seeds, pumpkin seeds, sesame seeds, pistachios, hazelnuts or Brazil nuts), chop any larger nuts
20g dried cranberries
40ml maple syrup

FLORENTINES

Florentines are a light and crunchy snack that use a variety of nuts and seeds. I like to use plenty of flaked almonds, as this gives the florentines a lovely texture. I have kept the maple syrup to a minimum, with just enough to caramelise and hold the florentines together and to achieve the right level of sweetness. Florentines make great gifts for friends and are delicious with a cup of tea or coffee after a meal.

1. Preheat the oven to 180°C fan and line a baking tray with baking parchment.

2. Combine all the nuts and seeds in a large bowl. Add the cranberries and the maple syrup and stir gently until well combined.

3. Use a spoon to form 12 circular mounds of the mixture on the lined baking tray, each about 6cm in diameter.

4. Bake on the middle shelf of the oven for 7–9 minutes. Keep a close eye on them, as nuts and seeds can burn quickly. They should be turning a golden colour when cooked. Remove from the oven and allow to cool fully. The florentines will crisp up as they cool.

Storage: Store in an airtight container (at room temperature) for up to a week.

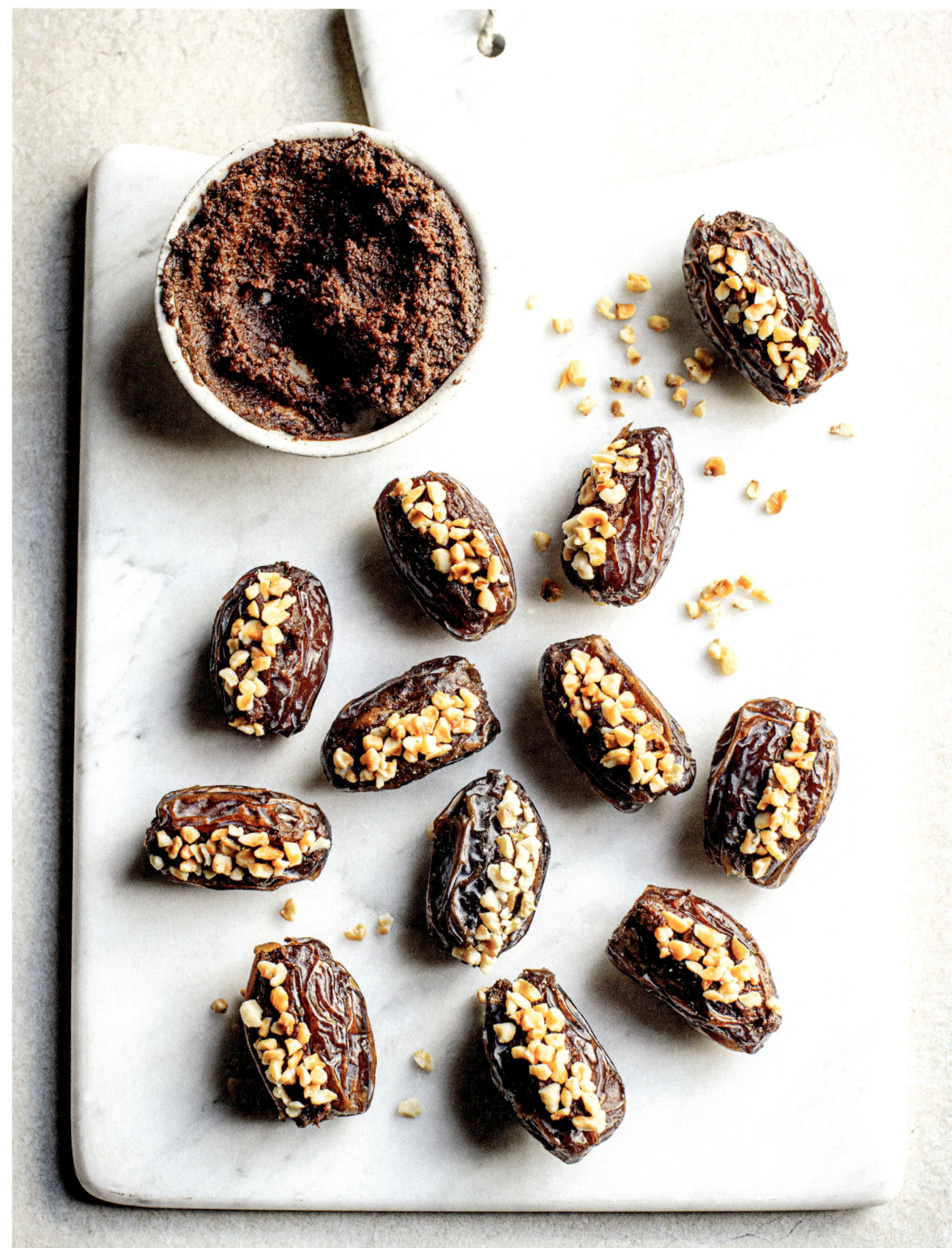

PER STUFFED DATE
PROTEIN: 2G
FIBRE: 2G
PLANT POINTS: 2

CHOCOLATE HAZELNUT SPREAD (MAKES 1 JAR)

250g shelled hazelnuts (or shelled and pre-roasted)
5 Medjool dates, pitted
30g raw cacao powder
1 teaspoon vanilla extract
75–100ml plant milk

Stuffed dates
Medjool dates
chocolate hazelnut spread
crushed hazelnuts

Tip: I recommend using dairy-free milk to extend the shelf life of the spread. Less milk results in a darker, richer consistency and flavour, whereas more milk gives a softer, more milk-chocolatey spread.

DATES STUFFED WITH CHOCOLATE HAZELNUT SPREAD

This healthier alternative to shop-bought chocolate hazelnut spread is made with less sugar and a generous amount of nuts and raw cacao. Raw cacao really is a gift from nature. Packed with 30g of fibre per 100g, it is rich in iron, magnesium and powerful antioxidants. For a special treat, I like to fill dates with the chocolate hazelnut spread! Dates are naturally rich in potassium, which helps regulate blood pressure, and they are packed with polyphenols. Gram for gram, dates are also a good source of fibre.

---

1. To roast your hazelnuts, preheat the oven to 180°C fan. Spread the hazelnuts on a baking tray and roast for 8–10 minutes, until lightly golden and fragrant. Remove from the oven and cool slightly.

2. Soak the dates in a heatproof bowl of just-boiled water to soften for around 10 minutes.

3. Process the nuts in a food processor on a medium-high speed. Initially, they will form a powder, but continue to blend and they will release their oils and become creamy. Continue blending until it has a shiny consistency and falls off a spoon easily. This can take 5–8 minutes.

4. Drain the dates and add them to the processor with the cacao powder, vanilla extract and 75ml of plant milk. Blend until completely smooth. For a creamier spread, blend again with up to 25ml more milk.

Storage: Store the spread in a sealed jar in the fridge for up to 10 days. Bring to room temperature before serving for a softer spread.

CHOCOLATE HAZELNUT FILLED DATES

Cut open a Medjool date and remove the stone and pedicel (the small part of the stem that is still attached to the fruit). Add a level teaspoon of the chocolate hazelnut spread, press gently to close, and sprinkle with some crushed hazelnuts. Store in the fridge in an airtight container for up to 5 days.

PER BLISS BALL
PROTEIN: 2G
FIBRE: 1G
PLANT POINTS: 4.5

MAKES 20 BALLS

250g raw beetroot, peeled and roughly chopped
100g pitted Medjool dates
150g desiccated coconut, plus 30g desiccated coconut for coating
50g gluten-free (or regular) rolled oats
15g raw cacao powder
1 teaspoon vanilla extract

Note: Always check when giving to someone with allergies that they are not allergic to coconut.

RED VELVET BLISS BALLS

These vibrant bliss balls combine raw cacao with all the health benefits of beetroot. Beetroots are a source of key nutrients, including folate, vitamin C, calcium and iron. Their deep red colour comes from plant compounds called anthocyanins, which have strong antioxidant properties. This recipe is tree-nut free because coconut is botanically a fruit and is not a true nut, but always check before giving to someone with an allergy.

---

1. Blend all the ingredients in a food processor on a high speed for around 30 seconds, until well combined and you can't see the oats.

2. Divide into 20 equal portions. Roll each portion into a ball, then roll in the extra desiccated coconut to coat all over.

Storage: Store in an airtight container in the fridge for up to 1 week.

PER POWER BALL
PROTEIN: 2G
FIBRE: 2G
PLANT POINTS: 5

MAKES 25 BALLS

150g ground almonds
50g desiccated coconut
250g Medjool dates, pitted
2 teaspoons matcha tea powder
a pinch of sea salt
1 teaspoon vanilla extract
1 tablespoon extra virgin olive oil
2 tablespoons cacao nibs

MATCHA POWER BALLS

The perfect quick after-lunch pick-me-up with a cup of tea or coffee, my matcha power balls are super easy to make and are a fantastic colour. Matcha, just like green tea, comes from the Camellia sinensis plant. The plants are shaded during the last month of harvest, which is thought to enhance their flavour and nutritional value. Matcha contains a calming amino acid called L-theanine, which offsets some of the effects of the caffeine, and it is also rich in catechins, plant compounds that act as antioxidants.

---

1. Blend all the ingredients, except the cacao nibs, in a food processor until fully combined. If the mixture feels too dry, add an extra date to help bind it together.

2. Stir in the cacao nibs, then use slightly wet hands to roll the mixture into 25 bite-size balls.

Storage: Store in an airtight container in the fridge for up to 5 days.

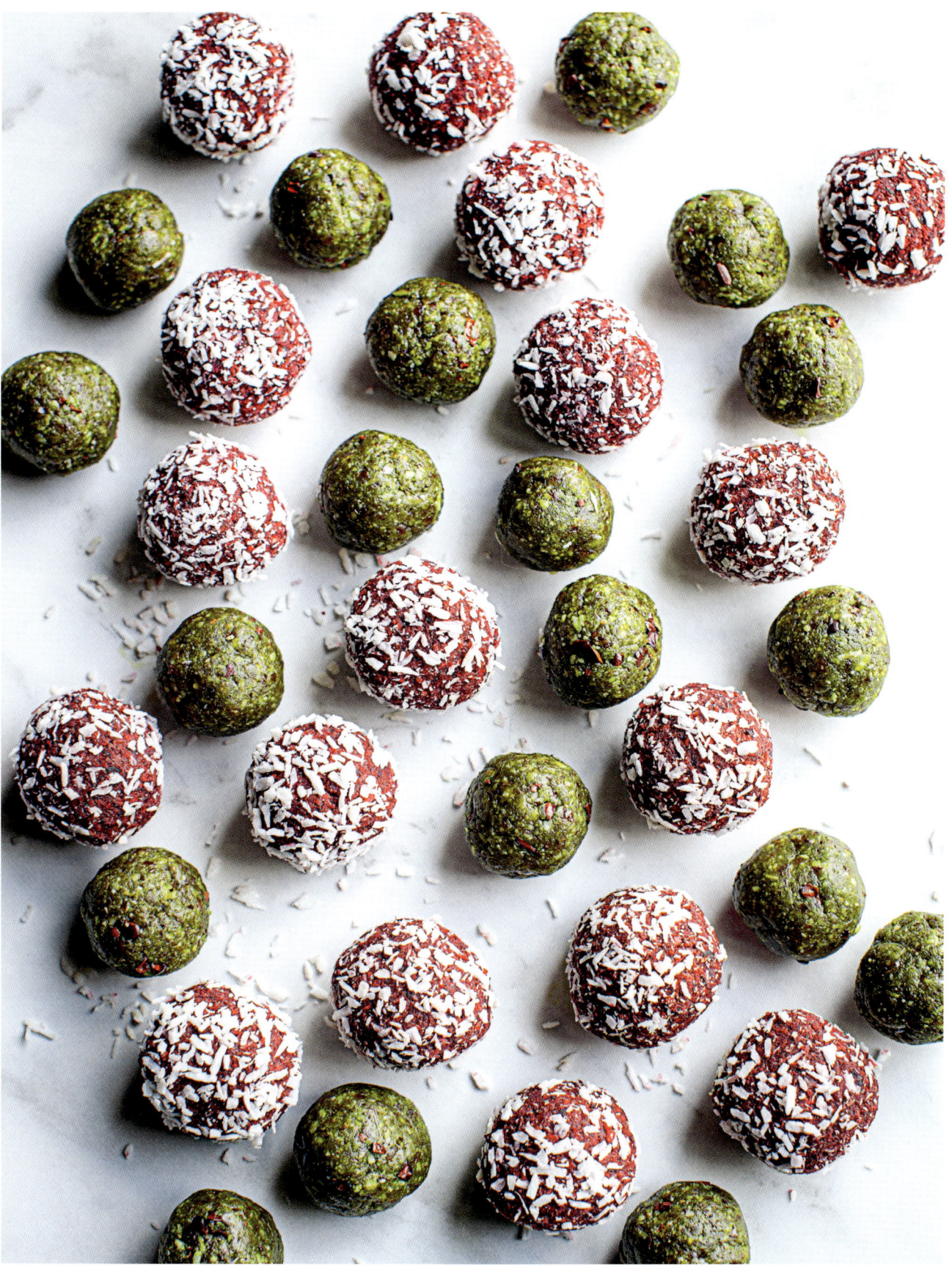

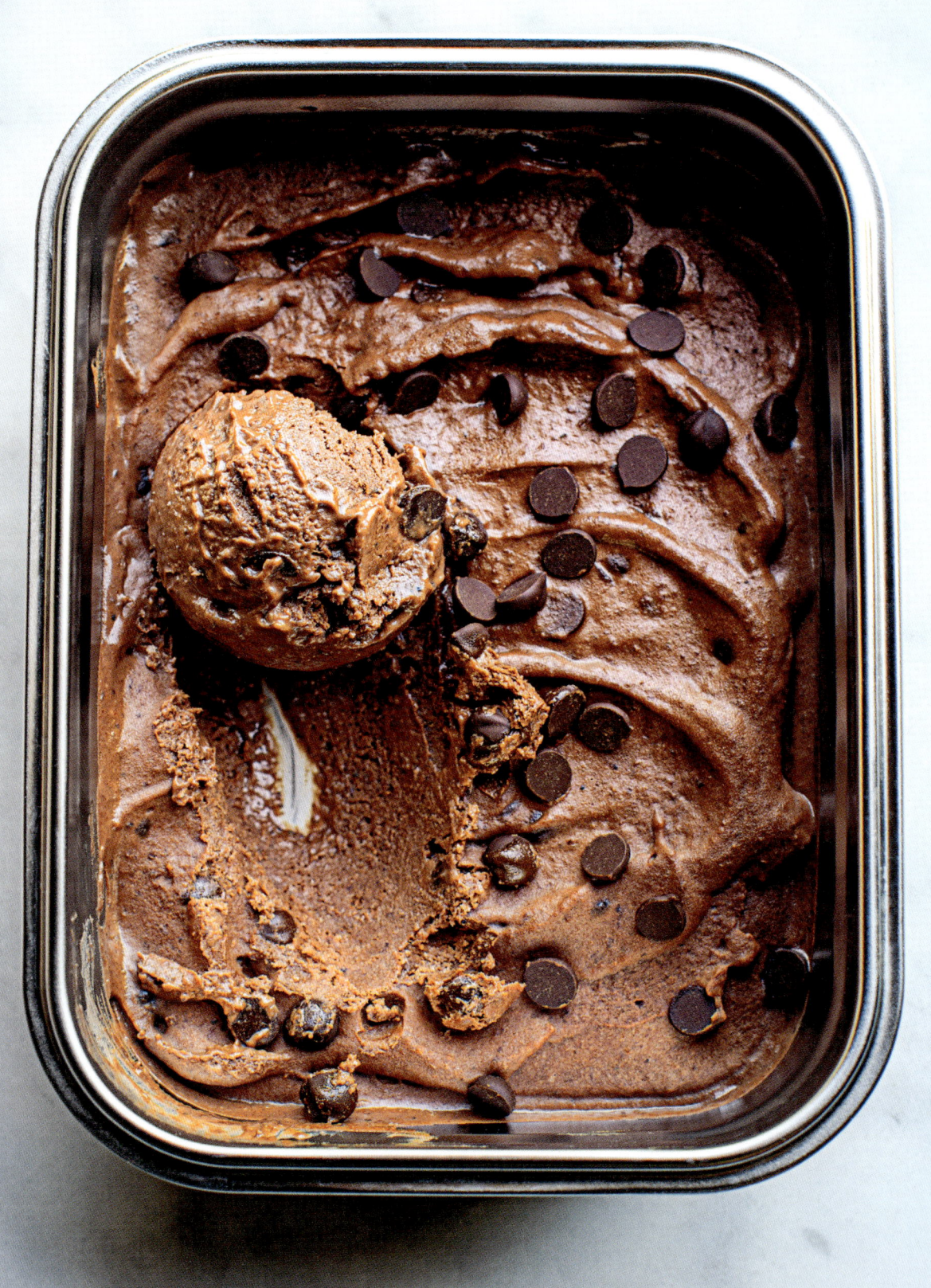

PER SERVING
PROTEIN: 8G
FIBRE: 6G
PLANT POINTS: 4

SERVES 6

1 x 400g tin or jar of black beans, rinsed and drained (240g drained weight)
100g pitted Medjool dates
50g peanut butter
150ml plant milk (e.g. almond milk)
30g cacao powder
30ml maple syrup, plus 1 extra tablespoon if desired
1 teaspoon vanilla extract

Topping
50g chocolate chips (ideally 70% cocoa solids or higher) (check they don't contain milk if you'd like the ice cream to be dairy-free)

CHOCOLATE BLACK BEAN ICE CREAM

Don't judge a recipe by its name – just as you shouldn't judge a book by its cover! This surprisingly smooth and indulgent ice cream is made with black beans. Why beans? They help create a softer texture straight from the freezer, while quietly adding fibre and an extra plant point. Homemade ice cream contains fewer additives, less sugar and less air than shop-bought options, which means they can set harder and form ice crystals. The black beans and nut butter help prevent this, resulting in a scoopable, satisfying texture with minimal ingredients.

1. Put all the ingredients into a food processor and process on high speed until completely combined and the beans are no longer visible. Add a little extra milk to loosen if the mixture is sticking to the sides. (If you prefer your ice cream sweeter, add an extra tablespoon of maple syrup.)

2. Pour into a freezer-proof bowl with a lid. Freeze for 4–5 hours for a soft-scoop texture. If the ice cream becomes too firm, leave it at room temperature for 10–15 minutes before serving, or re-blend briefly in the food processor to restore softness.

Storage: Keep in an airtight container in the freezer for up to 2 weeks. For the best texture, consume within the first few days.

PER DECORATED LOLLY
PROTEIN: 5G
FIBRE: 2G
PLANT POINTS: 4

SERVES 4

250g frozen mango cubes
100g Greek yoghurt
 (I used full-fat), chilled
100ml kefir, chilled

To serve as ice cream
50g fresh raspberries,
 per serving

To decorate the lollies
50g dark chocolate, melted
10g desiccated coconut

MANGO KEFIR INSTANT ICE CREAM AND GUT-BOOSTING LOLLIES

I wanted to incorporate the benefits of kefir and probiotic yoghurt into an ice cream that could be on the table in minutes. As an added bonus, the ice cream can be frozen into lolly moulds, to make the most delicious popsicles. I've used mango, which is bursting with flavour – and it is naturally so sweet that you don't need to add any extra sweetness. While the probiotic bacteria will go dormant in the freezer, they should come back to life again once thawed, retaining their gut-boosting benefits. Decorating the lollies is optional, but will add another two plant points as well as extra flavour and texture!

---

1. Take the mango out of the freezer and allow it to soften slightly for 5–10 minutes. Put it into a food processor and process on a high speed until it resembles mango ice.

2. Add the yoghurt and kefir and process for around 20 seconds, to make a creamy soft-scoop ice cream.

3. Serve immediately with raspberries, or pour the mixture into 4 deep lolly moulds (around 90ml each) and freeze for 4–6 hours to make delicious, healthy lollies.

4. To decorate the lollies, dip the top of each one into melted dark chocolate and then into desiccated coconut. Pop onto baking parchment to set or pop back into the freezer.

Storage: Store the ice cream in a sealed container in the freezer for up to 1 month. Allow to defrost and soften slightly before serving. The lollies will keep for up to 1 month in the freezer.

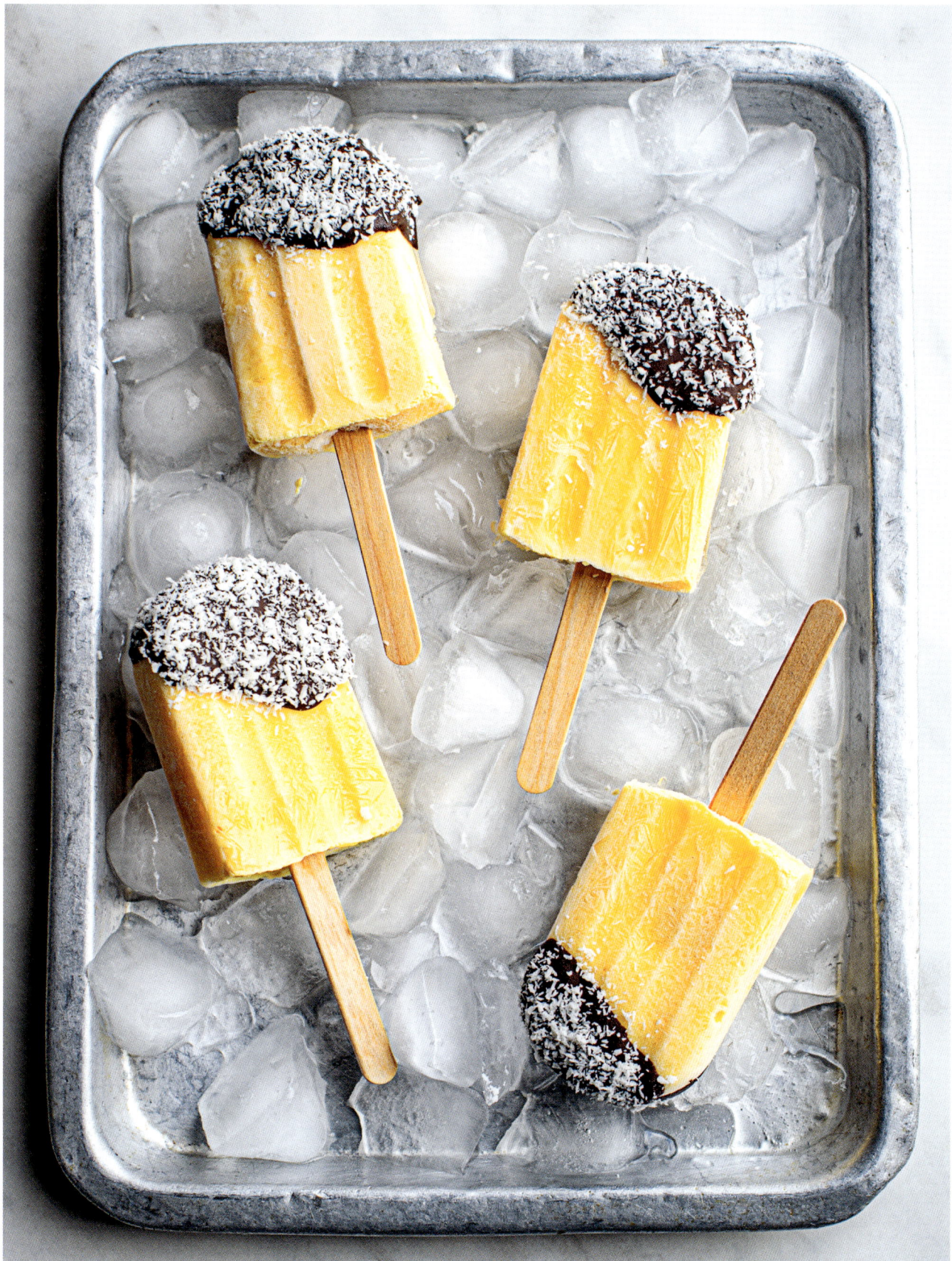

NUTRITIONAL INFORMATION

The nutritional information shown next to each recipe title is for the complete balanced recipe, as shown on the recipe page, including any 'to serve' instructions – but does not include any optional extras or variations. I have also provided nutritional information for some elements of some of the recipes, in case you wish to serve them in an alternative way. Please note that nutritional information is only ever an estimation, as values may vary depending on the ingredients you use.

BREAKFAST

	Protein	Fibre	Plants	Kcals
Jewelled Granola (40g serving) (page 107)	6g	4g	8.5	184
Jewelled Granola Breakfast Bowl (page 108)	30g	10g	11.5	462
No flaxseeds	28g	7g	10.5	411
Sunrise Sprinkles (50g serving) (page 110)	8g	8g	12	272
Sunrise Sprinkles with Yoghurt and Berries (page 112)	30g	10g	15	460
Carrot Cake Overnight Oats 1 (page 115)	30g	10g	5.5	480
With Greek soy yoghurt	23g	12g	6.5	458
Carrot Cake Overnight Oats 2 (page 116)	30g	11g	7.5	496
With Greek soy yoghurt	24g	13g	6.5	473
Large jar of Oat Mix (40g serving) (page 117)	7g	8g	4	189
Gut-Boosting Breakfast Bowl (page 118)	30g	12g	5	448
Chocolate Cherry Granola (40g serving) (page 119)	6g	5g	6.25	210
Chocolate Cherry Breakfast Bowl (page 120)	31g	7g	7.25	405
Tofu Scramble (page 122)	33g	13g	14.5	479
No bread	24g	8g	6	287
On a grilled portabello mushroom	26g	9g	7	303
Creamy Chocolate Chia Pudding (page 125)	27g	13g	5.75	342
Harissa Beans on Toast (page 126)	22g	15g	7.5	500
No bread	16	11	6.5	325
New York-Style Smoked Salmon Bagel (page 128)	25g	9g	4.5	364
Turkish Eggs Brunch (page 131)	29g	6g	6.25	416
With a slice of Super Green Bread	36g	11g	15.25	566
With a slice of seeded sourdough	36g	10g	7.25	592
Cherry Bakewell Baked Oats (page 132)	25g	10g	4	512

HEALTHY BREAD TOPPERS

	Protein	Fibre	Plants	Kcals
Sweet Potato Frittata (page 135)	28g	11g	9.5	464
No salad or seeds (serves 6)	22g	4g	3.25	338
No salad or seeds (serves 4)	33g	6g	3.25	506
Savoury Seed Mix (15g serving) (page 136)	3g	3g	6.75	81
25g serving	5g	4g	6.75	136
Hot Coconut Chia Porridge (page 137)	26g	13g	3	444
Any Bean Shakshuka (page 138)	28g	13g	6.75	531
With a slice of sourdough	34g	16g	7.75	707
Berry Pancake Stack (page 140)	27g	11g	6.25	465
With ground almonds (no flaxseeds)	27g	10g	6.25	473
Breakfast Chickpea Tortilla (page 143)	28g	15g	7.5	550
No salad	27g	15g	5.5	530
Kippers and Eggs (page 144)	33g	7g	4.25	468
Quick Hemp Milk (100ml) (page 147)	3g	0.4g	1.25	55
Hemp and Chocolate Shake (page 147)	22g	10g	4.25	441
Sardines on Toast (page 148)	25g	7g	12.25	407
No bread	16g	2g	1	157
Quark with Strawberries and Sunrise Sprinkles (page 150)	24g	11g	14.5	378
No bread	17g	4g	13	185
Avocado and Seeds (page 149)	22g	14g	11.25	561
With bread, no egg	16g	14g	11.25	486
No bread, with 1 egg	13g	9g	7.75	366
No egg or bread	7g	9g	7.75	294
Mozzarella with Tomato and Pesto (page 150)	24g	9g	11.75	512
No bread	16g	1g	3.5	277
Quick Fried Halloumi (page 151)	29g	9g	13.75	529
No bread	20g	4g	4.75	379
Smashed Eggs (page 152)	33g	7g	10.75	434
No bread	24g	2g	1.25	284
Quark and Radish (page 152)	27g	10g	15	379
No bread	18g	5g	9.75	229
Pesto Fried Eggs (page 153)	24g	11g	13.75	581
No bread	15g	4g	4.5	382
Turmeric and Coriander Folded Omelette (page 153)	21g	9g	11.25	487
No bread	13g	0g	1	252

LUNCH

	Protein	Fibre	Plants	Kcals
Grain and Lentil Healthy Carb Mix (page 159)	8g	6g	5	173
Citrus Mackerel Salad (page 160)	30g	18g	9.5	687
Roasted Vegetable, Feta and Puy Lentil Salad (page 163)	26g	14g	8.25	669
Wasabi Super Green Soup (page 164)	27g	15g	9.25	530
With Seeded Crackers	34g	21g	12.5	709
Chicken Satay Skewers (page 166)	40g	9g	12.75	407
No sauce	28g	0g	1.5	170
Sauce (per serving)	3g	1g	3	161
Asparagus and Goat's Cheese Almond Crust Flan (page 169)	35g	8g	5.75	769
No salad	34g	7g	3.75	712
Soufflé Made Simple (page 171)	32g	8g	6.5	536
No salad	22g	1g	1.25	295
Salad on its own	10g	7g	5.25	241
Sunshine Soup (page 174)	25g	15g	12.5	621
No feta dip or Seeded Crackers	5g	6g	6	216
With feta dip and ½ flatbread	22g	9g	8.5	557
Whipped Feta and Bean Dip (page 175)	26g	12g	5.5	521
No bread or crudités	13g	3g	1.5	227
Red Lentil Polpette with Chickpea Wraps (page 176)	28g	14g	12.5	590
3 x polpette (on their own)	19g	8g	5	362
Dressing (per serving)	3g	1g	1.75	112
Red lentil polpette with large salad and lemon and tahini dressing	25g	12g	9.75	518
Tomato and Carrot Soup with Red Lentil Polpette (page 179)	25g	15g	7.25	569
No polpette	6g	7g	4.75	203
Sticky Peanut Tofu Poke Bowl (page 180)	30g	14g	15.5	636

	Protein	Fibre	Plants	Kcals
Mozzarella and Vegetable Seeded Wraps with Tuna Salad (page 183)	33g	8g	9.75	427
Per wrap (no filling)	20g	5.6g	5.5	318
Spicy Lentil Soup with Halloumi and Chickpeas (page 184)	29g	14g	10.5	628
Chicken Caesar Salad with Parmesan Chickpea Croutons (page 186)				
With traditional dressing	33g	7g	5.25	464
With lighter dressing	37g	7g	5.25	358
Chicken Caesar Salad Dressings (page 188)				
Traditional dressing (40g serving)	3g	0g	0.75	174
Lighter dressing (50g serving)	7g	0g	0.5	68
Vegetable Moussaka (page 189)	30g	12g	12.5	511
Dairy-free option	25g	14g	14.5	502
Burrata and Peach Salad (page 190)	29g	8g	8.5	692
No bread	25g	5g	7.5	575
Roasted Butternut Salad with Warm Turmeric Dressing (feta) (page 193)	23g	15g	6.5	559
Made with manchego	27g	15g	6.5	642
Made with halloumi	26g	15g	6.5	579
Mackerel Pâté (page 194)	30g	11g	14	680
No bread or salad	19g	2g	2	404
Pear and Goat's Cheese Salad with Toasted Walnuts (page 196)	29g	12g	7.75	632
Tomato and Butter Bean Soup (page 197)	29g	14g	10.25	573
No bread	24g	11g	9.25	455
Dairy-free option with bread	29g	18g	16	635
Halloumi Salad with Pomegranate Salsa (page 198)	30g	8g	9	565

DINNER

	Protein	Fibre	Plants	Kcals
Pesto and Walnut Crust Salmon (page 205)	37g	10g	15	724
Pesto (15g serving)	1g	0.2g	2.5	43
Prawn Fishcakes with Soba Noodle Salad and Wasabi Dipping Sauce (page 206)	36g	8g	9.25	496
No soba noodle salad	27g	1g	3.75	216
Soba noodle salad (on its own)	9g	7g	7.5	280
Firecracker Chicken (page 208)	39g	9g	7.75	503
No rice	35g	7g	6.75	325
Sticky Tofu Noodles (page 211)	31g	13g	12	500
Lentil, Pea and Crispy Aubergine Dhal (page 212)	27g	12g	7.25	511
No flatbread	21g	12g	7.25	395
Chicken and Yellow Pea Curry with Cauliflower 'Pilau' Rice (page 215)	31g	11g	7.75	285
With cauliflower rice and flatbread	39g	12g	8.75	460
With flatbread (no cauliflower rice)	36g	10g	7.75	412
Curry (on its own)	28g	9g	6.75	237
Cauliflower rice (on its own)	3g	3g	1.5	48
Dijon Chicken with Tarragon (page 217)	40g	10g	10	486
No grain mix	34g	5g	5	356
With quinoa	39g	7g	6	502
Beef Chilli with Lentils and Chocolate (with 30g dry weight black rice, avocado and soured cream) (page 219)	25g	15g	11.75	534
Beef chilli (on its own)	22g	12g	9.75	352
With black rice	26g	14g	10.75	531
With cauliflower rice	25g	15g	11	400
With peas	27g	18g	10.75	420
With avocado and soured cream	23g	13g	10.75	418
Shepherdess Pie with Cheesy Bean and Parsnip Mash (page 221)	26g	20g	17.75	484
No greens	24g	18g	15.75	470
Rustic Butter Bean 'Gnocchi' (page 224)	29g	17g	7	494
Prawn and Tomato Pasta (page 226)	37g	8g	5	531
With red lentil pasta	42g	8g	6	539

	Protein	Fibre	Plants	Kcals
Cauliflower and Broccoli Cheese (page 227)	39g	11g	6.25	637
Made with almond milk	36g	11g	6.25	615
Creamy Lemon Pasta with Salmon Bites (page 228)	33g	7g	5.25	532
With green pea or red lentil pasta	38g	8g	5.25	530
Sticky Trout with Salad (page 231)	38g	9g	8.25	513
Tandoori Chicken Salad with Raita (page 232)	36g	10g	13.5	466
No grain mix	32g	6g	9	379
Thai Fish Curry with Sesame Zoodles (page 235)	27g	8g	7.75	495
No zoodles	24g	7g	6.75	436
Red Lentil Pizza with Yoghurt and Cucumber Salad (page 236)	31g	11g	8.25	535
No cucumber salad	28g	9g	7	498
Sea Bream with Green Glow Coleslaw (page 239)	32g	10g	9.75	498
No slaw or dressing	19g	1g	1.5	179
Green Glow Coleslaw (on its own)	13g	9g	9.75	319
Pork Loin with Smoky Beans (page 240)	40g	13g	7.5	432
Chicken and Kale Burgers (page 242)	40g	9g	5.75	565
2 burgers (on their own)	27g	1g	3.75	158
Tomato Salsa Salad (per serving)	3g	6g	4.75	155
Mayonnaise (15g serving)	0.3g	0.05	1	67
Mayonnaise (100g)	2g	0.4g	1	507
Mackerel Fishcakes with Watercress Cream (page 244)	29g	9g	9.25	526
Crispy Gochujang Tofu with Stir-Fried Vegetables (page 246)	32g	12g	6.25	526

BREADS & TREATS

	Protein	Fibre	Plants	Kcals
Seed and Nut Loaf (page 253)				
Per slice	8g	8g	8.5	235
Per loaf	143g	136g	8.5	4224
Super Green Bread (page 254)				
Per slice	5g	7g	9.25	150
Per loaf	106g	80g	9.25	2393
Carrot and Courgette Yoghurt Loaf (page 256)				
Per slice	9g	5g	8.5	192
Per loaf	149g	72g	8.5	3078
Naked Loaf (page 258)				
Per slice	7g	7g	7.5	193
Per loaf	121g	119g	7.5	3482
Rosemary and Sea Salt Seeded Crackers (page 261) (30g serving)	6g	7g	5.25	179
Simple Flatbreads (page 262)	8g	1g	0	175
Gluten-Free Flatbreads (page 264)	6g	2g	0.25	183
Chickpea Pancake Wraps (page 265)	2g	4g	3.25	83
Red Lentil Bagels (page 267)	10g	8g	3	212
No-Frills Hummus (page 269)	4g	4g	3	129
Avocado Hummus (page 270)	6g	6g	5	186
Roasted Beetroot Hummus with Brazil Nuts (page 271)	4g	4g	4.25	164
Egg Muffins (page 272)	15g	2g	3	212
Apple, Carrot and Walnut Flapjacks (page 274)	9g	4g	9.5	207
Crispy Edamame Beans (page 276)	7g	4g	1.75	102
Chilli and Lime Cashews (page 279)	4g	1g	2.5	152
Chocolate Chip Peanut Cookies (page 280)	6g	3g	2	187

	Protein	Fibre	Plants	Kcals
Salted Caramel Bars (page 282)	4g	4g	4	289
Two-Ingredient Chocolate Fudge (page 284)	3g	2g	2	116
Spiced Poached Pears (page 286)	1g	5g	2.25	156
With 75g Greek yoghurt	9g	5g	2.25	216
Florentines (page 287)	4g	2g	6	127
Dates Stuffed with Chocolate Hazelnut Spread (page 289)	2g	2g	2	98
Chocolate Hazelnut Spread				
Per 10g serving (rounded teaspoon)	1.5g	1g	1	50
Per jar	53g	28g	3.25	1999
Red Velvet Bliss Balls (page 290)	2g	1g	4.5	94
Matcha Power Balls (page 290)	2g	2g	5	97
Chocolate Black Bean Ice Cream (page 293)	8g	6g	4	230
Mango Kefir Instant Ice Cream and Gut-Boosting Lollies (page 294)	5g	2g	4	152
Ice cream with raspberries	4g	3g	2	78
Lollies, no chocolate or coconut	4g	1g	2	66

All nutritional information in this book has been calculated by referencing sources including McCance and Widdowson 7th Edition, AOAC international, USDA's FoodData Central (FDC) and averages across a number of supermarkets.

HOW TO ADAPT PROTEIN GOALS FOR YOUR BODY?

As discussed on page 44, protein requirements can vary between individuals depending on factors such as activity levels and training goals, as well as general health. There is no one-size-fits-all approach when it comes to protein. You know your body best, so adjust portions to what feels right for you.

1.2g/kg/day is a good aim for most people, but some people might benefit from eating slightly more protein, potentially up to 1.4g/kg/day, if they are more active and as they get older. Around the menopause, oestrogen levels decline, which can increase muscle loss (sarcopenia) as well as bone loss (which can gradually lead to osteopenia or osteoporosis). Muscles can become less responsive to the usual signals that stimulate growth and repair, meaning that adequate protein, as well as exercise, are important during this stage of life. Men may also require slightly more protein as they age.

It's also important to note that optimum protein requirements are based on lean body mass (healthy muscle mass). You'll see I've stopped the chart at 95kg, as there is likely to be no extra benefit to increasing protein further than this. Above this weight, more of our body weight is likely to comprised of body fat. Additionally it would also be quite difficult – and probably not very enjoyable – to consume higher levels of protein than this.

Chart to calculate your daily protein requirements in grams.

Weight (kg)	Weight (stones)	Weight (lbs)	0.75	0.8	1.0	1.2	1.4	1.6	1.8	2
45	7 stone 1lb	99	34	36	45	54	63	72	81	90
50	7 stone 12lb	110	38	40	50	60	70	80	90	100
55	8 stone 10lb	122	41	44	55	66	77	88	99	110
60	9 stone 7lb	133	45	48	60	72	84	96	108	120
65	10 stone 3lb	143	49	52	65	78	91	104	117	130
70	11 stone 1lb	155	53	56	70	84	98	112	126	140
75	11 stone 12lb	166	56	60	75	90	105	120	135	150
80	12 stone 9lb	177	60	64	80	96	112	128	144	160
85	13 stone 6lb	188	64	68	85	102	119	136	153	170
90	14 stone 3lb	199	68	72	90	108	126	144	162	180
95	15 stone	210	71	76	95	114	133	152	171	190

NOTE: This table is for adults over the age of 18 and is for information only and not a direct recommendation.

REFERENCES

For sources and references relating to the opening sections of the book, please scan:

INDEX

A
adenosine triphosphate (ATP) 13
alcohol 17
alliums 35
almond butter & milk
 salted caramel bars 282
almonds
 asparagus and goat's cheese almond crust flan 169–70
 cherry Bakewell baked oats 132
 florentines 287
 matcha power balls 290
 salted caramel bars 282
 sunrise sprinkles 110
 super green bread 254
amino acids 42
anchovies
 lighter Caesar dressing 188
 traditional Caesar dressing 188
antioxidants 43, 64, 68
any bean shakshuka 138
appetite 15, 33, 43, 52
apples
 apple, carrot and walnut flapjacks 274
 soufflé made simple, with broccoli, hazelnut and cranberry salad 171–2
 spicy lentil soup with halloumi and chickpeas 184
asparagus
 asparagus and goat's cheese almond crust flan 169–70
 kippers and eggs 144
 Turkish eggs brunch 131
aubergines
 lentil, pea and crispy aubergine dhal 212
 vegetable moussaka 189
avocado
 avocado and seeds 150
 avocado hummus 270

B
bacteria 20–1. see also microbiome
 bifidobacterium 21, 90
 lactobacillus 21, 68, 90, 118
bagels
 New York-style smoked salmon bagel 128
 red lentil bagels 267–8
bananas
 berry pancake stack 140
 cherry Bakewell baked oats 132
 hemp and chocolate shake 147
batch cooking 80–2
beans 38. see also individual types
beef chilli with lentils and chocolate 219–20
beetroot
 red velvet bliss balls 290
 roasted beetroot hummus with brazil nuts 271
berries, mixed
 berry pancake stack 140
 gut-boosting breakfast bowl 118
 sunrise sprinkles with yoghurt and berries 112
berry pancake stack 140
bifidobacterium 21, 90
black beans
 any bean shakshuka 138
 beef chilli with lentils and chocolate 219–20
 chocolate black bean ice cream 293
blood sugar 15, 16, 18–19, 32
 and diet 22, 36, 37, 42–3, 52, 75
 glycaemic index 39

blueberries
 spiced poached pears 286
the brain 64
 and dopamine 22, 33
 gut-brain axis 55
brazil nuts
 roasted beetroot hummus with brazil nuts 271
 sunrise sprinkles 110
bread 49, 302
 carrot and courgette yoghurt loaf 256
 chickpea pancake wraps 265
 gluten-free flatbreads 264
 naked loaf 258
 red lentil bagels 267–8
 seed and nut loaf 253
 simple flatbreads 262
 super green bread 254
bread/toast toppings
 avocado and seeds 150
 harissa beans on toast 126
 kippers and eggs 144
 mackerel pâté 194
 mozzarella with tomato and pesto 151
 pesto fried eggs 153
 quark and radish 152
 quark with strawberries and sunrise sprinkles 150
 quick fried halloumi 151
 sardines on toast 148
 shopping for 90–1
 smashed eggs 152
 tofu scramble 122
 turmeric and coriander folded omelette 153
breakfast 32, 92, 102–4, 296–7
breakfast chickpea tortilla 143

broccoli
　cauliflower and broccoli cheese 227
　crispy gochujang tofu with stir-fried vegetables 246
　soufflé made simple, with broccoli, hazelnut and cranberry salad 171–2
　super green bread 254
　wasabi super green soup 164
buckwheat
　grain and lentil healthy carb mix 159
burgers
　chicken and kale burgers with tomato salsa salad 242
burrata and peach salad 190
butter beans
　rustic butter bean 'gnocchi' 224
　tomato and butter bean soup 197
butternut squash
　roasted butternut salad with warm turmeric dressing 193
　sunshine soup 174

C

cabbage
　chicken satay skewers 166
　sea bream with green glow coleslaw 239
　sticky peanut tofu poke bowl 180
cacao
　chocolate black bean ice cream 293
　chocolate cherry breakfast bowl 120
　chocolate cherry granola 119
　creamy chocolate chia pudding 125
　dates stuffed with chocolate hazelnut spread 289
　hemp and chocolate shake 147
　matcha power balls 290
　red velvet bliss balls 290
calcium 13, 83
calories 16, 32
cannellini beans
　whipped feta and bean dip 175
carbohydrates 12, 17, 31, 37–8, 40
　and blood sugars 18, 37
　fast acting 18–19
　natural 18
　refined 38, 40
　simple swaps 41
carrot cake overnight oats 1: 115
carrot cake overnight oats 2: 116
carrots
　apple, carrot and walnut flapjacks 274
　carrot and courgette yoghurt loaf 256
　carrot cake overnight oats 1: 115
　carrot cake overnight oats 2: 116
　crispy gochujang tofu with stir-fried vegetables 246
　harissa beans on toast 126
　mozzarella and vegetable seeded wraps with tuna salad 183
　pork loin with smoky beans 240
　roasted vegetable, feta & puy lentil salad 163
　spicy lentil soup with halloumi and chickpeas 184
　sticky peanut tofu poke bowl 180
　sunshine soup 174
　tomato and butter bean soup 197
　tomato and carrot soup with red lentil polpette 179
　vegetable moussaka 189

cashew nuts
　chilli and lime cashews 279
　sea bream with green glow coleslaw 239
　sunshine soup 174
cauliflower
　cauliflower and broccoli cheese 227
　chicken and yellow pea curry with cauliflower 'pilau' rice 215–16
celery
　mozzarella and vegetable seeded wraps with tuna salad 183
　tomato and butter bean soup 197
Cheddar
　cauliflower and broccoli cheese 227
　shepherdess pie with cheesy bean and parsnip mash 221–2
cherries
　cherry Bakewell baked oats 132
　chocolate cherry granola 119
chia seeds
　apple, carrot and walnut flapjacks 274
　carrot and courgette yoghurt loaf 256
　carrot cake overnight oats 1: 115
　carrot cake overnight oats 2: 116
　chocolate cherry granola 119
　creamy chocolate chia pudding 125
　gut-boosting breakfast bowl 118
　hemp and chocolate shake 147
　hot coconut chia porridge 137
　jewelled granola 107
　large jar of oat mix 117
　mozzarella and vegetable seeded wraps with tuna salad 183
　naked loaf 258

rosemary and sea salt seeded crackers 261
savoury seed mix 136
seed and nut loaf 253
sunrise sprinkles 110
super green bread 254
chicken
chicken and kale burgers with tomato salsa salad 242
chicken and yellow pea curry with cauliflower 'pilau' rice 215–16
chicken Caesar salad with Parmesan chickpea croutons 186
chicken satay skewers 166
Dijon chicken with tarragon 217
firecracker chicken 208
tandoori chicken salad with raita 232
chickpea (gram) flour
breakfast chickpea tortilla 143
chickpea pancake wraps 265
red lentil polpette with chickpea wraps 176
chickpeas
avocado hummus 270
chicken Caesar salad with Parmesan chickpea croutons 186
citrus mackerel salad 160
no-frills hummus 269
roasted beetroot hummus with brazil nuts 271
roasted butternut salad with warm turmeric dressing 193
spicy lentil soup with halloumi and chickpeas 184
chilli
beef chilli with lentils and chocolate 219–20
chilli and lime cashews 279

chocolate
beef chilli with lentils and chocolate 219–20
chocolate black bean ice cream 293
chocolate cherry breakfast bowl 120
chocolate cherry granola 119
chocolate chip peanut cookies 280
dates stuffed with chocolate hazelnut spread 289
florentines 287
hemp and chocolate shake 147
salted caramel bars 282
two-ingredient chocolate fudge 284
cholesterol 52, 63
citrus mackerel salad 160
coconut
hot coconut chia porridge 137
mango kefir instant ice cream and gut-boosting lollies 294
matcha power balls 290
red velvet bliss balls 290
coconut milk
chicken satay skewers 166
Thai fish curry with sesame zoodles 235
coleslaw
green glow coleslaw 239
convenience foods 29
cookies
chocolate chip peanut cookies 280
cooking 80–2
coriander
turmeric and coriander folded omelette 153
turmeric and coriander mayonnaise 242

cottage cheese
egg muffins 272
smashed eggs 152
courgettes
breakfast chickpea tortilla 143
carrot and courgette yoghurt loaf 256
crispy gochujang tofu with stir-fried vegetables 246
mozzarella and vegetable seeded wraps with tuna salad 183
Thai fish curry with sesame zoodles 235
vegetable moussaka 189
crackers
rosemary and sea salt seeded crackers 261
cranberries, dried
florentines 287
jewelled granola 107
naked loaf 258
seed and nut loaf 253
soufflé made simple, with broccoli, hazelnut and cranberry salad 171–2
sunrise sprinkles 110
cravings 29, 33, 43, 52. see also blood sugar
cream cheese
creamy lemon pasta with salmon bites 228
mackerel pâté 194
sardines on toast 148
creamy chocolate chia pudding 125
creamy lemon pasta with salmon bites 228
crispy gochujang tofu with stir-fried vegetables 246
croutons: chicken Caesar salad with Parmesan chickpea croutons 186

cruciferous vegetables 35
cucumber
    asparagus and goat's cheese almond crust flan 169–70
    chicken Caesar salad with Parmesan chickpea croutons 186
    halloumi salad with pomegranate salsa 198
    red lentil pizza with yoghurt and cucumber salad 236
    sticky peanut tofu poke bowl 180
    tandoori chicken salad with raita 232
cumin seeds
    roasted beetroot hummus with brazil nuts 271

D
dairy-free diets 82–5
dates
    chocolate black bean ice cream 293
    dates stuffed with chocolate hazelnut spread 289
    matcha power balls 290
    red velvet bliss balls 290
    salted caramel bars 282
dhal
    lentil, pea and crispy aubergine dhal 212
diabetes 19
diet, balanced 28, 29–38
    benefits of 14, 15, 16, 25
    changing to 24, 25
    healthy food plate 30
digestive system 20–1. see also microbiome
    and appetite 32–3
    and fasting 74

Dijon chicken with tarragon 217
dinners 92, 202–3, 300–1
dips
    whipped feta and bean dip 175
dopamine 22, 33
dressings
    lemon tahini dressing 176
    lighter Caesar dressing 188
    salad dressing 231
    sea bream with green glow coleslaw 239
    sticky peanut tofu poke bowl 180
    traditional Caesar dressing 188
    turmeric and coriander mayonnaise 242
    warm turmeric dressing 193
    watercress cream 244–5
dysbiosis 20

E
edamame beans
    avocado hummus 270
    chicken satay skewers 166
    crispy edamame beans 276
    crispy gochujang tofu with stir-fried vegetables 246
    sea bream with green glow coleslaw 239
    sticky peanut tofu poke bowl 180
    sticky tofu noodles 211
    sticky trout with salad 231
    Thai fish curry with sesame zoodles 235
eggs 89
    any bean shakshuka 138
    asparagus and goat's cheese almond crust flan 169–70
    berry pancake stack 140
    egg muffins 272
    kippers and eggs 144

pesto fried eggs 153
smashed eggs 152
soufflé made simple, with broccoli, hazelnut and cranberry salad 171–2
sweet potato and feta frittata 135
traditional Caesar dressing 188
Turkish eggs brunch 131
turmeric and coriander folded omelette 153
emulsifiers 22
equipment 91
exercise 17

F
Fajita spice mix 184
fasting 17, 72, 73, 74
fat, visceral 19
fats 12, 41, 60–7
    importance of 64
    sources of 65
    types of 60–2
fermented foods 21, 23, 61
feta
    roasted butternut salad with warm turmeric dressing 193
    roasted vegetable, feta & puy lentil salad 163
    soufflé made simple, with broccoli, hazelnut and cranberry salad 171–2
    sweet potato and feta frittata 135
    wasabi super green soup 164
    whipped feta and bean dip 175
fibre 7–8, 31, 51–9
    importance of 18, 21, 51, 52, 54–5
    increasing intake 53, 55–7
    and protein 31, 32
    sources of 35, 58–9, 68
    types of 51–2

firecracker sauce 208
fish 89
fishcakes
   mackerel fishcakes with watercress cream 244–5
   prawn fishcakes with soba noodle salad and wasabi dipping sauce 206
flapjacks
   apple, carrot and walnut flapjacks 274
flatbreads
   gluten-free flatbreads 264
   simple flatbreads 262
flaxseeds
   apple, carrot and walnut flapjacks 274
   carrot and courgette yoghurt loaf 256
   carrot cake overnight oats 2: 116
   gut-boosting breakfast bowl 118
   jewelled granola breakfast bowl 108
   large jar of oat mix 117
   mozzarella and vegetable seeded wraps with tuna salad 183
   naked loaf 258
   rosemary and sea salt seeded crackers 261
   savoury seed mix 136
   seed and nut loaf 253
   sunrise sprinkles 110
   super green bread 254
florentines 287
food 28, 89
   craving 22, 29, 33, 43, 52
   relationship with 8, 14, 15, 24
   ultra-processed 16, 22–3, 33
'food noise' 14, 29

freekeh
   grain and lentil healthy carb mix 159
   halloumi salad with pomegranate salsa 198
fruit 35, 36, 53, 89. *see also* plants
fudge
   two-ingredient chocolate fudge 284

G
ghrelin 15
GLP-1 (glucagon-like peptide) 8, 15, 52
glucose 13, 18–19
gluten-free diets 86
gluten-free flatbreads 264
glycaemic index 39
glycogen 12, 18, 19, 73
goat's cheese
   asparagus and goat's cheese almond crust flan 169–70
   pear and goat's cheese salad with toasted walnuts 196
grain and lentil healthy carb mix 159
   Dijon chicken with tarragon 217
   tandoori chicken salad with raita 232
gram flour. *see* chickpea flour
granola
   chocolate cherry breakfast bowl 120
   chocolate cherry granola 119
   jewelled granola 107
   jewelled granola breakfast bowl 108
gut-boosting breakfast bowl 118
gut-brain axis 55
gut health 15, 20–1, 73, 90. *see also* microbiome

polyphenols 54, 64, 66, 68–9
prebiotics 68
probiotics 61, 90, 94, 118, 294

H
habits, forming 24, 25
halloumi
   halloumi salad with pomegranate salsa 198
   quick fried halloumi 151
   spicy lentil soup with halloumi and chickpeas 184
ham: burrata and peach salad 190
harissa beans on toast 126
hazelnuts
   carrot cake overnight oats 1: 115
   carrot cake overnight oats 2: 116
   dates stuffed with chocolate hazelnut spread 289
   florentines 287
   soufflé made simple, with broccoli, hazelnut and cranberry salad 171–2
hemp and chocolate shake 147
hemp seeds
   hemp and chocolate shake 147
   quick hemp milk 147
   savoury seed mix 136
   sunrise sprinkles 110
herbs
   egg muffins 272
   sea bream with green glow coleslaw 239
hot coconut chia porridge 137
hummus
   avocado hummus 270
   no-frills hummus 269
   roasted beetroot hummus with brazil nuts 271
hydration 53

I

ice cream
  chocolate black bean ice cream 293
  mango kefir instant ice cream and gut-boosting lollies 294
inflammation 21, 54, 73
insulin 19
iodine 13, 83
iron 13, 83

J

jewelled granola 107
jewelled granola breakfast bowl 108

K

kale
  chicken and kale burgers with tomato salsa salad 242
  super green bread 254
  tofu scramble 122
  wasabi super green soup 164
kefir 90
  gut-boosting breakfast bowl 118
  mango kefir instant ice cream and gut-boosting lollies 294
kidney beans
  beef chilli with lentils and chocolate 219–20
kimchi
  sweet potato and feta frittata 135
  Turkish eggs brunch 131
kippers and eggs 144

L

lactobacillus 21, 68, 90, 118
large intestine 20, 21
large jar of oat mix 117
legumes 38, 53
lemons
  avocado hummus 270
  creamy lemon pasta with salmon bites 228
  lemon tahini dressing 176
  no-frills hummus 269
  red lentil polpette with chickpea wraps 176
  roasted beetroot hummus with brazil nuts 271
  sea bream with green glow coleslaw 239
  traditional Caesar dressing 188
lentils (green or black) 38
  grain and lentil healthy carb mix 159
  shepherdess pie with cheesy bean and parsnip mash 221–2
  sticky trout with salad 231
lentils (puy) 38
  beef chilli with lentils and chocolate 219–20
  grain and lentil healthy carb mix 159
  pear and goat's cheese salad with toasted walnuts 196
  roasted vegetable, feta & puy lentil salad 163
lentils (red) 38
  lentil, pea and crispy aubergine dhal 212
  red lentil bagels 267–8
  red lentil pizza with yoghurt and cucumber salad 236
  red lentil polpette with chickpea wraps 176
  spicy lentil soup with halloumi and chickpeas 184
  tomato and butter bean soup 197
  tomato and carrot soup with red lentil polpette 179
  vegetable moussaka 189
lighter Caesar dressing 188
limes
  chilli and lime cashews 279
the liver 19
lollies
  mango kefir instant ice cream and gut-boosting lollies 294
lunch 92, 156–7, 298–9

M

mackerel
  citrus mackerel salad 160
  mackerel fishcakes with watercress cream 244–5
  mackerel pâté 194
macronutrients 12, 29–38. see also carbohydrates; fats; protein
magnesium 13, 94
mango kefir instant ice cream and gut-boosting lollies 294
maple syrup
  chocolate black bean ice cream 293
  chocolate chip peanut cookies 280
  florentines 287
matcha power balls 290
meals 96–9
  cooking 80–2
  macronutrients 29–38
  planning 30, 31, 32, 92, 93–5
  timing 72–6
meat 60–1, 89
mental health 43
microbiome 20–1, 54–5
  and diet 51, 68
  and fasting 73

micronutrients 13
migrating motor complex (MCC) 74
milk
   cherry Bakewell baked oats 132
   chocolate black bean ice cream 293
   creamy chocolate chia pudding 125
   hot coconut chia porridge 137
   quick hemp milk 147
minerals 13
monkfish
   Thai fish curry with sesame zoodles 235
monounsaturated fats (MUFAs) 61
moussaka
   vegetable moussaka 189
mozzarella
   mozzarella and vegetable seeded wraps with tuna salad 183
   mozzarella with tomato and pesto 151
   red lentil pizza with yoghurt and cucumber salad 236

N

naked loaf 258
New York-style smoked salmon bagel 128
no-frills hummus 269
noodles
   prawn fishcakes with soba noodle salad and wasabi dipping sauce 206
   sticky tofu noodles 211
nutrition principles 7–8, 31, 77
   balanced meals 29–38
   fats 60–7
   fibre 51–9
   plants 68–71

protein 42–9
   timing meals 72–6
nutritional information 296–303
nuts 53. *see also* individual types

O

oats 105
   apple, carrot and walnut flapjacks 274
   berry pancake stack 140
   carrot and courgette yoghurt loaf 256
   carrot cake overnight oats 1: 115
   carrot cake overnight oats 2: 116
   cherry Bakewell baked oats 132
   chocolate cherry granola 119
   jewelled granola 107
   large jar of oat mix 117
   red lentil polpette with chickpea wraps 176
   red velvet bliss balls 290
   salted caramel bars 282
   super green bread 254
obesity 19
oestrogen balance 52
oils 66–7
olive oil 61, 64, 66–7
omega-3 fatty acids 61, 62, 83
omega-6 fatty acids 61
omelette
   turmeric and coriander folded omelette 153
oranges
   citrus mackerel salad 160
   firecracker chicken 208
   halloumi salad with pomegranate salsa 198
   mackerel pâté 194
   sunshine soup 174

P

pancakes
   berry pancake stack 140
Parmesan
   apple, carrot and walnut flapjacks 274
   chicken Caesar salad with Parmesan chickpea croutons 186
   egg muffins 272
   lighter Caesar dressing 188
   traditional Caesar dressing 188
   vegetable moussaka 189
parsnips
   shepherdess pie with cheesy bean and parsnip mash 221–2
pasta
   cauliflower and broccoli cheese 227
   creamy lemon pasta with salmon bites 228
   prawn and tomato pasta 226
pastry, flans etc.
   asparagus and goat's cheese almond crust flan 169–70
pâté
   mackerel pâté 194
peaches
   burrata and peach salad 190
peanut butter
   chicken satay skewers 166
   chocolate black bean ice cream 293
   chocolate chip peanut cookies 280
   sticky peanut tofu poke bowl 180
peanuts
   sticky tofu noodles 211
pears
   pear and goat's cheese salad with toasted walnuts 196

spiced poached pears 286
peas
   lentil, pea and crispy aubergine dhal 212
   sweet potato and feta frittata 135
   wasabi super green soup 164
pecans
   burrata and peach salad 190
peppers
   egg muffins 272
   firecracker chicken 208
   harissa beans on toast 126
   mozzarella and vegetable seeded wraps with tuna salad 183
   soufflé made simple, with broccoli, hazelnut and cranberry salad 171–2
   spicy lentil soup with halloumi and chickpeas 184
   sticky peanut tofu poke bowl 180
   Thai fish curry with sesame zoodles 235
   tofu scramble 122
   vegetable moussaka 189
peptide YY (PYY) 15
pesto
   green walnut and basil pesto 205
   mozzarella with tomato and pesto 151
   pesto fried eggs 153
   quick fried halloumi 151
   red lentil pizza with yoghurt and cucumber salad 236
phytonutrients 35, 43, 68–9
pistachio nuts
   florentines 287
   gut-boosting breakfast bowl 118
   jewelled granola 107
   naked loaf 258
   seed and nut loaf 253
   sunrise sprinkles 110

pizza
   red lentil pizza with yoghurt and cucumber salad 236
plant milks 49, 84
plant protein 43, 49, 85
plants
   importance of 68–9
   increasing intake 69–71
polpette
   red lentil polpette with chickpea wraps 176
   tomato and carrot soup with red lentil polpette 179
polyphenols 54, 64, 66, 68–9
polyunsaturated fats (PUFAs) 61
pomegranate seeds
   burrata and peach salad 190
   halloumi salad with pomegranate salsa 198
   jewelled granola breakfast bowl 108
   roasted butternut salad with warm turmeric dressing 193
   sticky tofu noodles 211
pork loin with smoky beans 240
porridge
   hot coconut chia porridge 137
potatoes
   breakfast chickpea tortilla 143
prawns
   prawn and tomato pasta 226
   prawn fishcakes with soba noodle salad and wasabi dipping sauce 206
prebiotics 68
probiotics 61, 90, 94, 118, 294
processed food 23
protein 7–8, 12, 31, 42–9, 89
   combining sources 31, 32, 33
   importance of 42–3
   increasing 45–7

plant protein 43, 49, 85
   requirements 44–5, 304
   sources of 48–9, 84
psyllium husk
   gluten-free flatbreads 264
   naked loaf 258
   red lentil bagels 267–8
   red lentil pizza with yoghurt and cucumber salad 236
   seed and nut loaf 253
   super green bread 254
pulses. see legumes
pumpkin seeds
   apple, carrot and walnut flapjacks 274
   carrot and courgette yoghurt loaf 256
   cauliflower and broccoli cheese 227
   chocolate cherry granola 119
   florentines 287
   jewelled granola 107
   naked loaf 258
   red lentil bagels 267–8
   roasted butternut salad with warm turmeric dressing 193
   rosemary and sea salt seeded crackers 261
   savoury seed mix 136
   seed and nut loaf 253
   sunrise sprinkles 110
   super green bread 254
   wasabi super green soup 164

Q

quark
   chocolate cherry breakfast bowl 120
   New York-style smoked salmon bagel 128

quark and radish 152
quark with strawberries and sunrise sprinkles 150
quick fried halloumi 151
quick hemp milk 147
quinoa
   grain and lentil healthy carb mix 159
   sticky peanut tofu poke bowl 180

R

radishes
   asparagus and goat's cheese almond crust flan 169–70
   quark and radish 152
   sea bream with green glow coleslaw 239
   sticky peanut tofu poke bowl 180
raita 232
red lentil bagels 267–8
red lentil polpette with chickpea wraps 176
red velvet bliss balls 290
resistant starch 36, 51–2
rice
   beef chilli with lentils and chocolate 219–20
   firecracker chicken 208
roasted beetroot hummus with brazil nuts 271
roasted butternut salad with warm turmeric dressing 193
roasted vegetable, feta & puy lentil salad 163
rocket
   halloumi salad with pomegranate salsa 198
   roasted butternut salad with warm turmeric dressing 193
roasted vegetable, feta & puy lentil salad 163
rosemary and sea salt seeded crackers 261
rustic butter bean 'gnocchi' 224

S

salads
   burrata and peach salad 190
   chicken and kale burgers with tomato salsa salad 242
   chicken Caesar salad with Parmesan chickpea croutons 186
   chicken satay skewers 166
   citrus mackerel salad 160
   halloumi salad with pomegranate salsa 198
   mozzarella and vegetable seeded wraps with tuna salad 183
   pear and goat's cheese salad with toasted walnuts 196
   prawn fishcakes with soba noodle salad and wasabi dipping sauce 206
   red lentil pizza with yoghurt and cucumber salad 236
   roasted butternut salad with warm turmeric dressing 193
   roasted vegetable, feta & puy lentil salad 163
   soufflé made simple, with broccoli, hazelnut and cranberry salad 171–2
   sticky peanut tofu poke bowl 180
   sticky trout with salad 231
   tandoori chicken salad with raita 232
salmon
   creamy lemon pasta with salmon bites 228
   New York-style smoked salmon bagel 128
   pesto and walnut crust salmon 205
salsa
   pomegranate salsa 198
   tomato salsa salad 242
salted caramel bars 282
sardines on toast 148
satay sauce
   chicken satay skewers 166
satiety 15, 33, 43, 52
saturated fats 60–1
sauces
   cheese sauce 189, 227
   dairy-free cheese sauce 189
   firecracker sauce 208
   satay sauce 166
   wasabi dipping sauce 206
sauerkraut
   citrus mackerel salad 160
   Turkish eggs brunch 131
savoury seed mix 136
   avocado and seeds 150
   pesto and walnut crust salmon 205
   shepherdess pie with cheesy bean and parsnip mash 221–2
   sweet potato and feta frittata 135
SCFAs (short-chain fatty acids) 54
sea bream with green glow coleslaw 239
seeds 53. see also individual types
selenium 13, 83
serotonin 55
sesame seeds
   carrot and courgette yoghurt loaf 256
   cauliflower and broccoli cheese 227
   crispy gochujang tofu with stir-fried vegetables 246

firecracker chicken 208
florentines 287
jewelled granola 107
mozzarella and vegetable seeded wraps with tuna salad 183
naked loaf 258
prawn fishcakes with soba noodle salad and wasabi dipping sauce 206
red lentil bagels 267–8
rosemary and sea salt seeded crackers 261
savoury seed mix 136
sticky trout with salad 231
wasabi super green soup 164
shakes
   hemp and chocolate shake 147
shepherdess pie with cheesy bean and parsnip mash 221–2
shopping 89–91
simple flatbreads 262
small intestine 20, 74
smashed eggs 152
snacks 14–15, 17, 29, 43, 53, 250–1
   healthy 76, 88
   and inflammation 73
   reducing 72, 75, 86–8
soluble fibre 36, 51, 52, 105
soufflé made simple, with broccoli, hazelnut and cranberry salad 171–2
soup 157
   spicy lentil soup with halloumi and chickpeas 184
   sunshine soup 174
   tomato and butter bean soup 197
   tomato and carrot soup with red lentil polpette 179
   wasabi super green soup 164
spice mixes
   Fajita spice mix 184

Tandoori spice mix 232
spiced poached pears 286
spicy lentil soup with halloumi and chickpeas 184
spinach
   chickpea pancake wraps 265
   pear and goat's cheese salad with toasted walnuts 196
   red lentil polpette with chickpea wraps 176
   sea bream with green glow coleslaw 239
   soufflé made simple, with broccoli, hazelnut and cranberry salad 171–2
   super green bread 254
   wasabi super green soup 164
split peas
   chicken and yellow pea curry with cauliflower 'pilau' rice 215–16
spring onions
   egg muffins 272
   pear and goat's cheese salad with toasted walnuts 196
star anise
   spiced poached pears 286
sticky peanut tofu poke bowl 180
sticky tofu noodles 211
sticky trout with salad 231
strawberries
   quark with strawberries and sunrise sprinkles 150
sugar 15, 17, 18, 36. see also blood sugar
sugar snap peas
   chicken satay skewers 166
sunflower seeds
   apple, carrot and walnut flapjacks 274
   carrot and courgette yoghurt loaf 256

carrot cake overnight oats 2: 116
cauliflower and broccoli cheese 227
chocolate cherry granola 119
florentines 287
jewelled granola 107
large jar of oat mix 117
naked loaf 258
red lentil bagels 267–8
rosemary and sea salt seeded crackers 261
savoury seed mix 136
seed and nut loaf 253
spicy lentil soup with halloumi and chickpeas 184
sunrise sprinkles 110
super green bread 254
wasabi super green soup 164
sunrise sprinkles 110
   quark with strawberries and sunrise sprinkles 150
   sunrise sprinkles with yoghurt and berries 112
sunshine soup 174
super green bread 254
supplements 13
sweet potatoes
   shepherdess pie with cheesy bean and parsnip mash 221–2
   spicy lentil soup with halloumi and chickpeas 184
   sweet potato and feta frittata 135

T
tahini
   avocado hummus 270
   lemon tahini dressing 176
   no-frills hummus 269
   two-ingredient chocolate fudge 284

tamari
　sticky peanut tofu poke bowl 180
tandoori chicken salad with raita 232
tarragon
　Dijon chicken with tarragon 217
Thai fish curry with sesame zoodles 235
thyroid gland 13
Time-Restricted Eating (TRE) 72–6
tofu 85
　crispy gochujang tofu with
　　stir-fried vegetables 246
　sticky peanut tofu poke bowl 180
　sticky tofu noodles 211
　tofu scramble 122
tomatoes
　any bean shakshuka 138
　burrata and peach salad 190
　chicken and kale burgers with
　　tomato salsa salad 242
　chicken and yellow pea curry with
　　cauliflower 'pilau' rice 215–16
　chicken Caesar salad with
　　Parmesan chickpea croutons 186
　chicken satay skewers 166
　lentil, pea and crispy aubergine
　　dhal 212
　mozzarella with tomato and pesto 151
　pork loin with smoky beans 240
　prawn and tomato pasta 226
　red lentil pizza with yoghurt and
　　cucumber salad 236
　roasted butternut salad with warm
　　turmeric dressing 193
　rustic butter bean 'gnocchi' 224
　tofu scramble 122
　tomato and butter bean soup 197
　tomato and carrot soup with red
　　lentil polpette 179

vegetable moussaka 189
tortillas
　breakfast chickpea tortilla 143
traditional Caesar dressing 188
treats
　nutritional information 302–3
triglycerides 62, 63
Triple 30 nutrition principles
　7–8, 31, 77
　balanced meals 29–38
　fats 60–7
　fibre 51–9
　plants 68–71
　protein 42–9
　timing meals 72–6
trout
　sticky trout with salad 231
tuna
　mozzarella and vegetable seeded
　　wraps with tuna salad 183
Turkish eggs brunch 131
turmeric
　roasted butternut salad with
　　warm turmeric dressing 193
　turmeric and coriander folded
　　omelette 153
　turmeric and coriander
　　mayonnaise 242
two-ingredient chocolate
　fudge 284
tyrosine 13

U
ultra-processed food 16, 22–3, 33

V
vegan products 49, 84–5
vegetables 35, 53, 89. see also
　individual types; plants

vegetables, mixed
　crispy gochujang tofu with
　　stir-fried vegetables 246
　mozzarella and vegetable seeded
　　wraps with tuna salad 183
　roasted vegetable, feta & puy
　　lentil salad 163
　super green bread 254
vegetarian & vegan diets 82–5
visceral fat 19
vitamins 13, 54, 82–3

W
walnuts
　apple, carrot and walnut
　　flapjacks 274
　pear and goat's cheese salad
　　with toasted walnuts 196
　pesto and walnut crust salmon 205
　roasted vegetable, feta & puy
　　lentil salad 163
　sunrise sprinkles 110
wasabi
　prawn fishcakes with soba noodle
　　salad and wasabi dipping
　　sauce 206
　wasabi super green soup 164
watercress
　citrus mackerel salad 160
　mackerel fishcakes with watercress
　　cream 244–5
　smashed eggs 152
weight gain 12
weight management 16, 17, 43, 52,
　73, 75
whipped feta and bean dip 175
white beans
　harissa beans on toast 126
　mackerel fishcakes with watercress
　　cream 244–5

pork loin with smoky beans 240
shepherdess pie with cheesy bean and parsnip mash 221–2
whipped feta and bean dip 175
whole foods 16, 18, 28, 53, 58
wraps
    chickpea pancake wraps 265
    mozzarella and vegetable seeded wraps with tuna salad 183
    red lentil polpette with chickpea wraps 176

Y
yoghurt 84, 90
    asparagus and goat's cheese almond crust flan 169–70
    berry pancake stack 140
    carrot and courgette yoghurt loaf 256
    carrot cake overnight oats 1: 115
    carrot cake overnight oats 2: 116
    creamy chocolate chia pudding 125
    gluten-free flatbreads 264
    hot coconut chia porridge 137
    jewelled granola breakfast bowl 108
    lighter Caesar dressing 188
    mango kefir instant ice cream and gut-boosting lollies 294
    mozzarella and vegetable seeded wraps with tuna salad 183
    prawn fishcakes with soba noodle salad and wasabi dipping sauce 206
    red lentil pizza with yoghurt and cucumber salad 236
    simple flatbreads 262
    sunrise sprinkles with yoghurt and berries 112
    tandoori chicken salad with raita 232
    Turkish eggs brunch 131

Z
zinc 13, 83

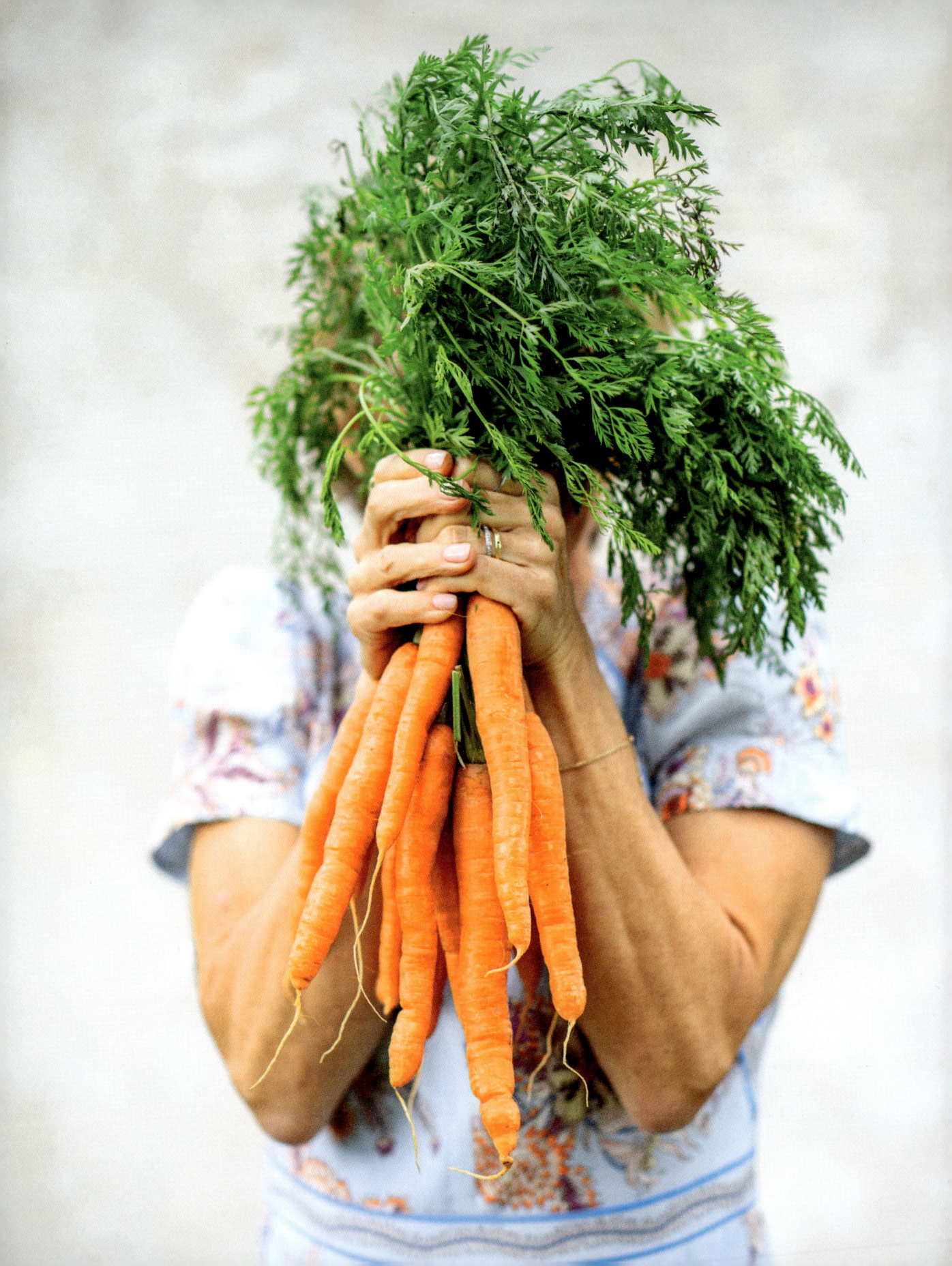

ACKNOWLEDGEMENTS

I have always wanted to write a book, but I was particular about what it should be. I dreamed of a book with enough science to inspire and motivate, but also full of colour and recipes that would show how to apply that science in everyday life. From a proposal scribbled in a notepad on a plane to Ibiza, this idea has grown into the book you are holding today. I am pretty proud of how it turned out!

I would like to thank you for choosing this book and I very much hope it becomes a well-thumbed addition to your kitchen, and that it helps to simplify food in a way that feels intuitive and natural.

My acknowledgements go back a long way, as so many things had to align to bring me to this point in my career. The privilege of studying nutrition at King's College London at the age of twenty-one and to the team at King's College who sparked a passion for nutrition that is still with me today.

I owe my thanks to every client I have worked with over the past twenty years, each of whom has helped shape me into the practitioner I am today by continually challenging me to deepen my knowledge and refine my skills. Through my clinics, you have also taught me how to communicate nutrition in a way that is clear, practical and accessible to all. You are all the reason why I do what I do. Your questions make sure that I never stop learning, but it is your emails, testimonials and live feedback that remind me how important it is to share this knowledge. And of course, to everyone who has followed me on social media and been part of this journey too, without you this would not have been possible. It is your support and following that created the wave that turned into this book.

I would like to thank everyone on my publishing team. To Alice Russell at Mirador for taking me on board after an astonishingly brief phone call and to Melissa Hemsley for guiding me towards her. To Alice King for her weekly catch-ups and keeping us all in the loop. To all the team at Pan Macmillan, my editor Lizzy Gray for your clarity and above all your vision, as well as Dawn Burnett and Sian Gardiner and everyone at Pan Macmillan who have made this project come to life, and for taking a chance on me and believing in me. To Alex and Emma Smith for the photography and design, Annie Rigg for her food styling and Laura Bayliss for her patience and taking on board all my changes, right up until the last moment, sorry. To Sarah Bennie, you have also been pivotal in the success of this book.

To all my friends who tested my recipes, with some of you still making them regularly! I believe that Rebecca is yet to get bored of her weekly Firecracker Chicken. To Fee, for always being a friend to lean on and for never getting tired of me talking about nutrition, and for just being there, a true friend. To Rachael, my PA, for being my second brain and making sure I know what I am up to each day!

A big thank you to my family, especially Frank for giving me support and honest feedback on all my recipes, and my children Alex and Issi for their even more brutal feedback, and for always spending time with me in the kitchen as they grew up and who have gone on to become great cooks too.

To all those at the British Association for Nutritional Therapy and Lifestyle Medicine. Studying Nutritional Therapy was also fundamental in shaping the way I work today, combined with the thousands of hours I have spent in practice talking to clients. This has given me the privilege of working with thousands of people globally, some with complex health conditions, which has been incredibly rewarding.

I hope that this book cuts through some of the noise around nutrition, puts you firmly back in the driving seat of your health and shows you how food really can transform our health and change the way we feel every single day. I want you to feel confident, inspired and to have sufficient knowledge to give you ultimate food freedom. Thank you.

First published 2026 by Bluebird
an imprint of Pan Macmillan
The Smithson, 6 Briset Street, London EC1M 5NR
EU representative: Macmillan Publishers Ireland Ltd, 1st Floor,
The Liffey Trust Centre, 117–126 Sheriff Street Upper, Dublin 1 D01 YC43
Associated companies throughout the world

ISBN 978-1-0350-7631-4

Copyright © Dominique Ludwig, 2026
Photography Copyright © Smith & Gilmour, 2026

The right of Dominique Ludwig to be identified as the author of this work has been asserted in accordance with the Copyright, Designs and Patents Act 1988.

All rights reserved. No part of this publication may be reproduced, stored in a retrieval system, or transmitted, in any form, or by any means (including, without limitation, electronic, mechanical, photocopying, recording or otherwise) without the prior written permission of the publisher.

Pan Macmillan does not have any control over, or any responsibility for, any author or third-party websites (including, without limitation, URLs, emails, barcodes and QR codes) referred to in or on this book.

9 8 7 6

A CIP catalogue record for this book is available from the British Library.

Photography, Design and Art Direction: Smith & Gilmour
Food Stylist: Annie Rigg
Prop Stylist: Hannah Wilkinson

Printed and bound in Italy

This book is sold subject to the condition that it shall not, by way of trade or otherwise, be lent, hired out, or otherwise circulated without the publisher's prior consent in any form of binding or cover other than that in which it is published and without a similar condition including this condition being imposed on the subsequent purchaser. The publisher does not authorize the use or reproduction of any part of this book in any manner for the purpose of training artificial intelligence technologies or systems. The publisher expressly reserves this book from the Text and Data Mining exception in accordance with Article 4(3) of the European Union Digital Single Market Directive 2019/790.

Visit www.panmacmillan.com to read more about all our books and to buy them.

Disclaimer: Nutritional guidance in this book has been provided by the author, an accredited Nutritionist, but it should not be considered individual professional medical or dietary advice.